Advanced OPERATIVE DENTISTRY

Commissioning Editor: Alison Taylor
Development Editor: Carole McMurray
Project Manager: Kiruthiga Kasthuriswamy
Designer: Kirsteen Wright
Illustration Manager: Bruce Hogarth

Advanced OPERATIVE DENTISTRY
A PRACTICAL APPROACH

Edited by

Professor David Ricketts

Professor of Cariology and Conservative Dentistry/Honorary Consultant in Restorative Dentistry
Leader of the Section of Operative Dentistry, Fixed Prosthodontics and Endodontology,
Dundee Dental School, University of Dundee, UK

Professor David Bartlett

Professor of Prosthodontics/Honorary Consultant in Restorative Dentistry
Head of Prosthodontics, Kings College London Dental Institute, Guy's Hospital, London, UK

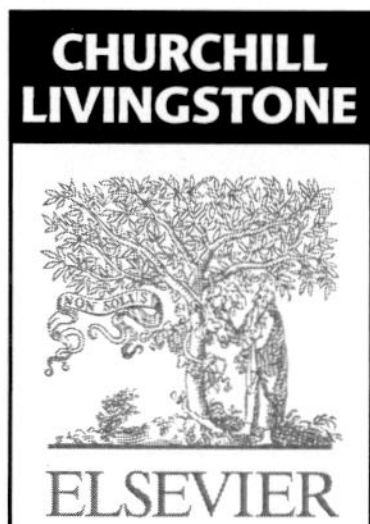

Edinburgh London New York Oxford Philadelphia St Louis Sydney Toronto 2011

CHURCHILL
LIVINGSTONE
ELSEVIER

ISBN 978 0 7020 3126 7

British Library Cataloguing in Publication Data
A catalogue record for this book is available from the British Library

Library of Congress Cataloging in Publication Data
A catalog record for this book is available from the Library of Congress

Notices

Knowledge and best practice in this field are constantly changing. As new research and experience broaden our understanding, changes in research methods, professional practices, or medical treatment may become necessary.

Practitioners and researchers must always rely on their own experience and knowledge in evaluating and using any information, methods, compounds, or experiments described herein. In using such information or methods they should be mindful of their own safety and the safety of others, including parties for whom they have a professional responsibility.

With respect to any drug or pharmaceutical products identified, readers are advised to check the most current information provided (i) on procedures featured or (ii) by the manufacturer of each product to be administered, to verify the recommended dose or formula, the method and duration of administration, and contraindications. It is the responsibility of practitioners, relying on their own experience and knowledge of their patients, to make diagnoses, to determine dosages and the best treatment for each individual patient, and to take all appropriate safety precautions.

To the fullest extent of the law, neither the Publisher nor the authors, contributors, or editors, assume any liability for any injury and/or damage to persons or property as a matter of products liability, negligence or otherwise, or from any use or operation of any methods, products, instructions, or ideas contained in the material herein.

Printed in China

Contents

Contributors

Professor David Bartlett
Professor of Prosthodontics/Honorary Consultant in Restorative Dentistry,
Head of Prosthodontics, Kings College London Dental Institute,
Guy's Hospital, London, UK

Professor David Ricketts
Professor of Cariology and Conservative Dentistry/Honorary Consultant in Restorative Dentistry,
Section Leader,
Section of Operative Dentistry, Fixed Prosthodontics and Endodontology,
Dundee Dental School,
Dundee, UK

Dr Graham Chadwick
Senior Lecturer/Honorary Consultant in Restorative Dentistry,
Dundee Dental School,
Dundee, UK

Dr Angela Gilbert
Senior Lecturer in Restorative Dentistry,
Dundee Dental School,
Dundee, UK

Dr Andrew Hall
Senior Lecturer/Honorary Consultant in Restorative Dentistry,
Dundee Dental School,
Dundee, UK

Dr John Radford
Senior Lecturer/Honorary Consultant in Restorative Dentistry,
Dundee Dental School,
Dundee, UK

Professor William Saunders
Professor of Endodontology/Honorary Consultant in Restorative Dentistry,
Dundee Dental School,
Dundee, UK

Dr Brian Stevenson
Lecturer/Honorary Specialist Registrar in Restorative Dentistry,
Dundee Dental School,
Dundee, UK

Dr Carol Tait
Senior Clinical Teaching Fellow,
Dundee Dental School,
Dundee, UK

Preface

Advanced operative procedures in dentistry encompass all dental subjects and disciplines such as oral surgery, the placement and restoration of dental implants and endodontics to name a few; however, these subjects are comprehensively addressed in other texts. This book therefore concentrates on fixed prosthodontics which involves the preparation of teeth for laboratory-made indirect restorations such as crowns, bridges, veneers, inlays and onlays. Where alternative, more conservative treatments are possible – for example the placement of direct composite to alter the shape of teeth – these are also described.

The necessity for advanced indirect restorations is the result of disease or conditions which have compromised the dentition. It is important to appreciate that using restorations does not treat the diseases or conditions, and their identification and prevention underpin successful treatment. The first five chapters of this book therefore focus on the main diseases and conditions (dental caries, periodontal disease, endodontic problems, tooth wear and aesthetic problems) which can lead to the need for advanced operative techniques and addresses how these techniques can impact on the remaining dentition and oral health. In the ensuing chapters details of materials, techniques and tooth preparation are described which aim to empower the reader to achieve a high standard of care for their patients.

Indirect restorations are made in a dental laboratory and clear communication between dentist and laboratory technician is essential. This takes the form of accurate impressions, occlusal registration and aspects of appearance such as the shade and contour required, all of which are devoted an individual chapter. Clear prescription of restoration design and material choice is also required and these are discussed in relation to the individual restorations. In many dental schools little or no laboratory work is carried out by undergraduate dental students; however, an understanding of how indirect restorations are made is important as certain aspects of tooth preparation have to be followed to facilitate laboratory construction. Laboratory procedures can also impact upon how materials and restorations are handled at the chairside. As such, these aspects of laboratory work are described throughout the book.

The provision of advanced indirect restorations is costly and can often have an impact on the remaining dentition and dental health. The advantages and disadvantages associated with their provision have to be balanced for each individual patient for them to be able to give informed consent. These principles underlie successful treatment planning, execution and hence patient care, and are the principles behind this text.

Chapter 1

Management of dental caries

David Ricketts, Graham Chadwick, Andrew Hall

CHAPTER CONTENTS

DENTAL CARIES THE DISEASE

Dental caries is a disease that is common to all dentate individuals. At the hydroxyapatite crystal level it could be considered a ubiquitous phenomenon. For dental caries to occur a bacterial biofilm has to accumulate on a tooth surface. The bacteria within the biofilm metabolize dietary sugar substrates producing acids which, over time, lead to demineralization of the tooth tissue. Thus the requirements for the carious process may be depicted by the Venn diagram seen in Figure 1.1. However, this diagram is overly simplistic and implies that the disease process and its progression are inevitable. Clinically, this is not the case. Some tooth surfaces that are frequently covered in plaque do not develop clinically detectable caries whereas other tooth surfaces covered with plaque in the same mouth do. Many other factors, such as dietary habits, fluoride and saliva impact upon the disease process which is complex and dynamic in nature. From the earliest stage, continued demineralization is not inevitable and lesion arrest is possible by simply disrupting the plaque biofilm on the surface of the tooth at regular intervals. Very early lesions which are not detected clinically may therefore not progress to clinically detectable white spot lesions and the carious process is better represented by Figure 1.2.

It is often said that if an early white spot lesion develops, remineralization can take place. While complete remineralization and resolution of the lesion is unlikely, the clinically apparent remineralization of a white spot lesion may also be due to its surface abrasion following improved oral hygiene procedures. Remineralization or regrowth of partially demineralized apatite crystals in the surface zone of an enamel lesion (Figure 1.3) has been reported. However, the relatively well-mineralized surface zone acts also as a diffusion barrier to ions, making it less likely that, in the underlying body of the lesion, supersaturation with respect to apatite will occur with subsequent mineral deposition. Prevention of the disease is therefore our primary aim. However, for many patients, this primary prevention fails and lesions develop. Caries risk assessment and early caries detection are important so that further prevention can be targeted to those patients and lesions that are in need. In this situation a method of monitoring the lesion is also important to determine the outcome of our preventive approach; that is, has the lesion arrested or progressed.

Primary prevention can fail for a number of reasons. It may be due to the fact that the patient has not visited

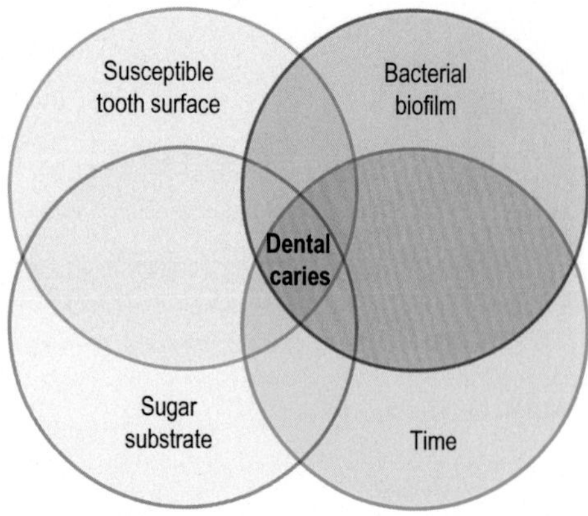

Figure 1.1 Venn diagram depicting the requirements for caries to occur.

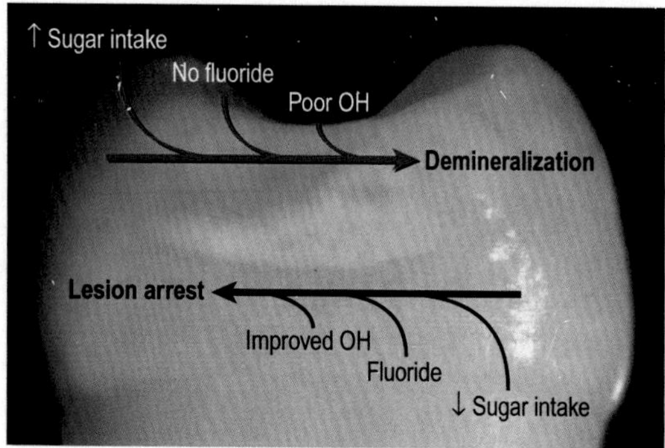

Figure 1.2 Diagram depicting the dynamic nature of the carious process and how it can be influenced by some external factors.

a dentist to receive such advice or, worse still, they may have attended a dentist or dental care professional and not been given preventive advice and treatment. However, for some patients, regardless of their attendance pattern, the preventive advice is ignored or they are unable to follow it through no fault of their own. For example, an elderly patient may know that oral hygiene procedures are important in caries prevention, but they may not have the manual dexterity, due to a physical disability, to carry them out efficiently.

When primary prevention fails, demineralization within the carious lesion can progress to a stage that it becomes heavily infected with bacteria and no longer manageable with preventive procedures alone. Indeed, the surface of the lesion can break down and a microcavity or frank cavity can result which can no longer be kept clean of plaque. In these situations caries removal and restoration with an appropriate dental material is required. The patient has now entered the restorative cycle.

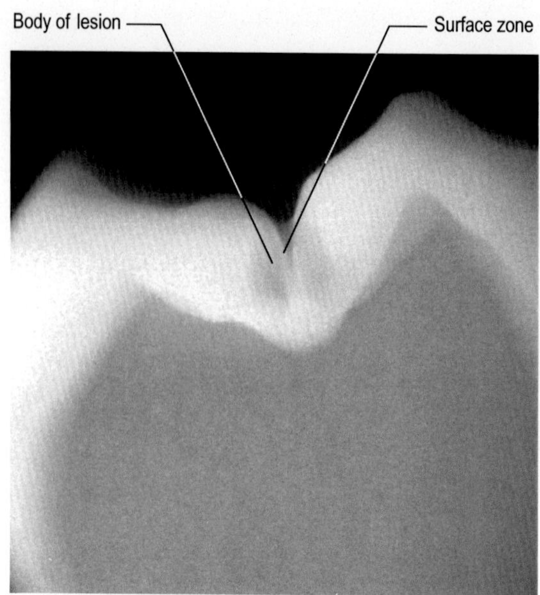

Figure 1.3 High definition macroradiograph of a section of a tooth showing two enamel lesions on the bilateral walls of a fissure. The relatively well-mineralized surface zone and body of the lesion can clearly be seen.

THE RESTORATIVE CYCLE

A significant proportion of a dentist's work time is spent replacing restorations and the most common reason given to justify this clinical decision is the presence of secondary caries. This is caries that develops under or adjacent to a restoration placed to repair a carious lesion. The term secondary caries is, however, misleading as it implies that the restoration is somehow the cause. In certain situations this is true when the restorative procedures have been carried out incorrectly. For example, ledges create plaque stagnation areas, poor contact points allow food packing and poor adaptation with an inadequate bond of materials to tooth tissue leads to microleakage (Figure 1.4). Most 'secondary caries' is actually new caries that has just formed adjacent to the restoration and is better termed as such: caries adjacent to a restoration (CAR). The appearance of caries, following restoration of a tooth, illustrates the continued high caries risk of the patient and also shows that restoration alone does not change this. In order to prevent recurrence it is fundamental that the caries risk be managed. If successful, this might avoid the need for more advanced restorative work, and ensure its predictability when carried out.

Unlike directly placed restorations, which are packed and adapted to cavity walls and margins, indirect restorations are made on models from impressions taken of

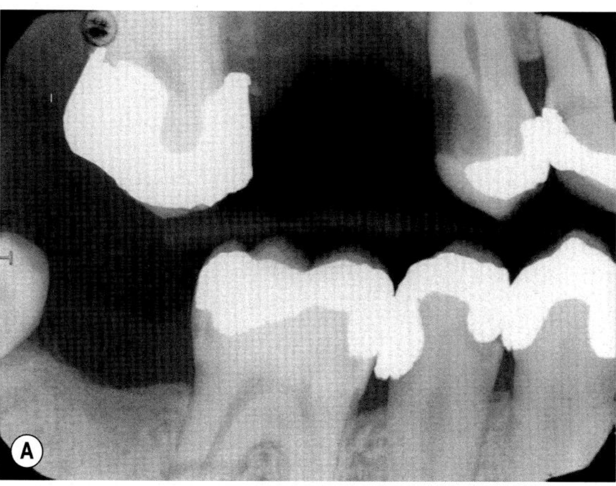

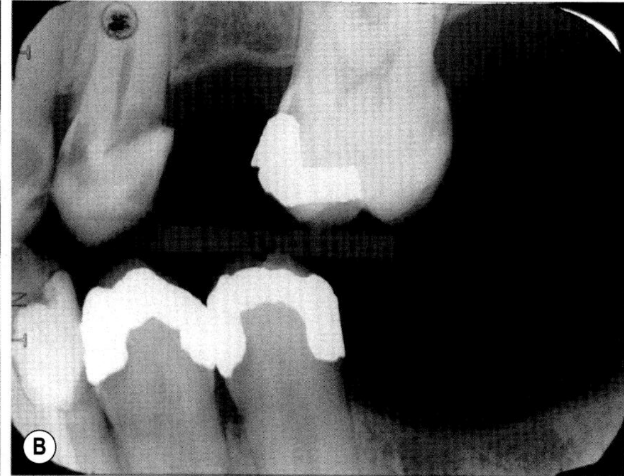

Figure 1.4 Bitewing radiographs of a high caries risk patient. The amalgam restorations placed in the lower right second premolar tooth distally, the upper right second molar mesially and the composite restoration upper left first premolar distally have ledges and are poorly contoured, encouraging food packing and caries adjacent to the restorations.

tooth preparations. As such, discrepancies in the marginal fit, seating and hence the width of cement lute exposed to the oral cavity can occur. Marginal discrepancies in the order of 70 µm have been reported in well-fitting restorations. When fitting an indirect restoration it is important to assess its fit to ensure the marginal discrepancies are kept to a minimum. A dental probe is useful for checking this and for ledges. Poor plaque control in relation to ill-fitting and contoured restorations not only increases the patient's risk to new caries, but also to periodontal disease if the margins are close to the gingival tissues.

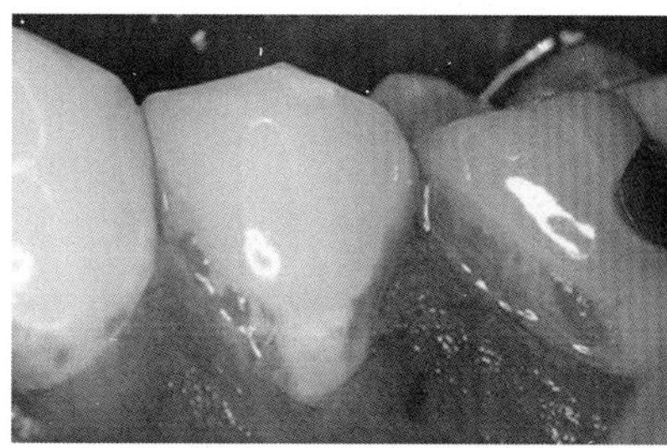

Figure 1.5 Disclosed biofilm on the buccal surface of the lower left second premolar tooth has partially been removed exposing the white spot lesion beneath. The biofilm on the mesial surface of the first molar tooth completely obscures the detection of the white spot lesion beneath.

CARIES DETECTION AND DIAGNOSIS

It is important when examining a patient for primary caries or caries adjacent to restorations that the teeth are examined clean. The carious process initially takes place in the biofilm on the surface of the tooth and the product of that process is the initial lesion in the tooth. To see the lesion and make a diagnosis the biofilm needs to be removed (Figure 1.5). It is also essential that the teeth are examined both wet and dry. The importance of drying is illustrated in Figure 1.6. When light illuminates a sound tooth, the light can either be transmitted, or it can undergo refraction or reflection. Refraction is the ability of a tooth to bend (scatter) light and will vary according to the refractive index of the material the light passes through. The porosities created in enamel during the carious process are normally filled with water (refractive index = 1.33) which has a refractive index close to enamel (1.66). In this situation little light scattering occurs. If the lesion is dried and the water is replaced with air which has a lower refractive index (1.0), the larger difference in refractive indices between enamel and air results in greater light scattering, enabling easier recognition of the white spot lesion. The occlusal lesion in Figure 1.7 clearly illustrates this and it stands to reason that a lesion that needs to be dried to enable its diagnosis is less severe than one that is seen even on a wet surface. The examination of clean teeth under both wet and dry conditions forms the basis for a clinical visual classification system known as the International Caries Detection and Assessment System (ICDAS II). This system characterizes lesions of increasing severity by correlating the visual appearance of the lesions with their histological depth (Table 1.1). The ICDAS II criteria can also be applied to caries adjacent to restorations. For further information on the ICDAS, visit the website http://www.icdas.org/index.htm.

A number of caries detection devices have been invented to aid detection and monitoring of early carious lesions; however, their use has mainly focussed on primary caries.

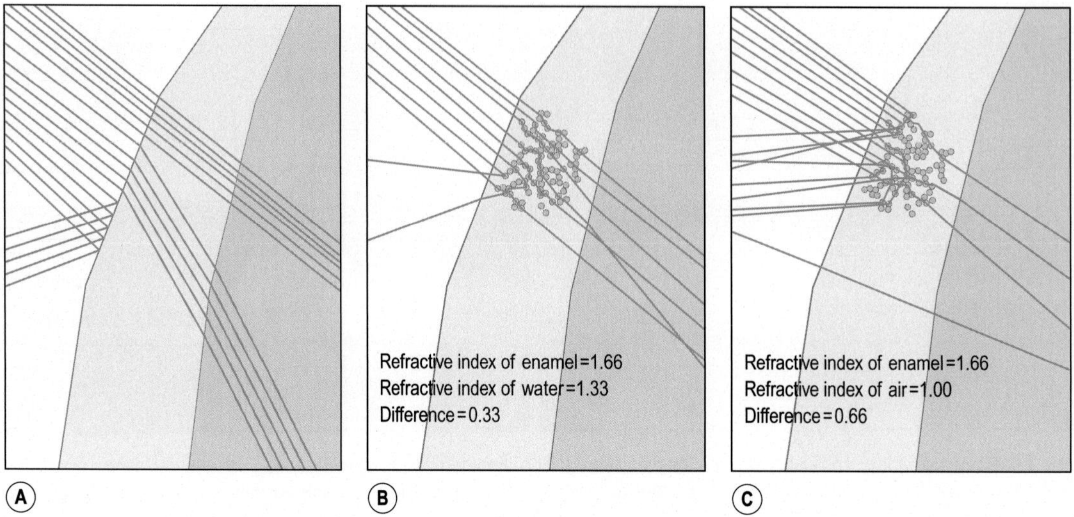

Figure 1.6 When light illuminates sound enamel (A) it undergoes transmission, refraction and reflection, porosities created during the carious process are normally filled with water (B) with a refractive index close to that of enamel. As a consequence, there is little light scattering. When the lesion is dried and air fills the porosities (C) the difference in refractive index with enamel is greater and greater light scattering occurs, making the white spot lesion easier to detect.

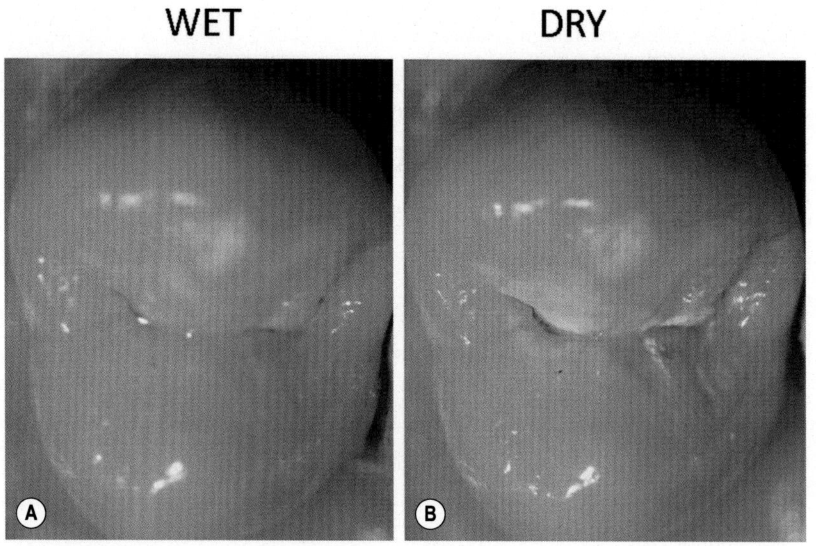

Figure 1.7 White spot lesion at entrance to the fissure (A) is seen more clearly when dry (B).

When a restoration is placed their use is often complicated; for example, the laser fluorescence devices, the DIAGNOdent and the newer DIAGNOdent pen (Figure 1.8), which detect fluorescence from bacterial porphyrins, cannot differentiate between staining around a restoration margin and caries as they both fluoresce. Similarly, false-positive readings could occur if electrical conductance methods were used around metallic restorations. The clinical visual examination, supplemented with an intraoral radiograph, remains the examination of choice for the evaluation of restoration margins and adjacent caries. A dental probe can be used to remove plaque, assess the fit of a restoration and assess for any loss in tooth surface integrity (cavitation), but it must not be used with pressure to detect stickiness as this can lead to errors in diagnosis and more importantly damage to early lesions.

Table 1.1 International Caries Detection and Assessment System (ICDAS II)[a]

ICDAS CRITERIA	COLLAPSED CRITERIA FOR CLINICAL USE	CORRESPONDING HISTOLOGY
0 No or slight change in enamel translucency after prolonged air drying (>5 s).	**0** No or slight change in enamel translucency after prolonged air drying (>5 s).	**0** No enamel demineralization or a narrow surface zone of opacity (edge phenomenon).
1 Opacity or discoloration hardly visible on a wet surface, but distinctly visible after air drying.	**1** Opacity or discoloration hardly visible on a wet surface, but distinctly visible after air drying.	**1** Enamel demineralization limited to the outer 50% of the enamel layer.
2 Opacity or discoloration distinctly visible without air drying.	**2** Opacity or discoloration distinctly visible without air drying.	**2** Demineralization involving between 50% of the enamel and the outer third of dentine.
3 Localized enamel breakdown in opaque or discoloured enamel. **4** Greyish discoloration from the underlying dentine.	**3** Localized enamel breakdown in opaque or discoloured enamel and/or greyish discoloration from the underlying dentine.	**3** Demineralization involving the middle third of dentine.
5 Cavity in opaque or discoloured enamel exposing the dentine – involving less than half of the tooth surface **6** Cavity in opaque or discoloured enamel exposing the dentine – involving > half tooth surface.	**4** Cavity in opaque or discoloured enamel exposing the dentine.	**4** Demineralization involving the inner third of the dentine.

[a]The original codes and description of lesions are seen in the left column, a collapsed version more appropriate for clinical practice in the middle and the corresponding lesion depth as would be seen histologically on the right.

The identification or detection of a carious lesion as outlined here is only one part of the diagnostic process. Lesion characteristics, including severity (depth and mineral loss) and activity, as well as caries risk factors (see later), are all taken into consideration. It is only when all this information is processed that a true diagnosis, prognosis and treatment plan can be made.

CARIES RISK ASSESSMENT

The patient seen in Figures 1.4 and 1.9 is a young patient who has received multiple restorations, a number of endodontic treatments and several extractions as a result of caries. There is new primary caries and caries adjacent to existing restorations which has led to loss of restorations and tooth fracture. This patient has a high risk of developing caries unless a treatment plan dominated by a preventive approach is adopted. Simply re-restoring the teeth is not addressing the caries problem.

What is caries risk?

Caries risk is a prediction as to whether a patient is likely to develop new caries in the future. This is a complex process, which a dentist does on a day-to-day basis, by either consciously or subconsciously assessing the impact of factors which affect caries. It is important to note that caries risk can change throughout a patient's life and a dentist can have a positive impact on reducing this risk. Events in a patient's life can also have a negative effect on caries risk; for example, an elderly patient may be placed on medication which causes a dry mouth. In addition, this patient may require a removable partial prosthesis which will complicate oral hygiene procedures.

For the patient in Figures 1.4 and 1.9, extensive and advanced restorative procedures are likely to be necessary. But before they can be considered his caries risk has to be modified. Even though it is obvious that he is currently at a high caries risk, an assessment should be made to establish the main risk factors and a treatment plan formulated to address them. Once this preventive approach has been instituted, stabilization of active caries is required and

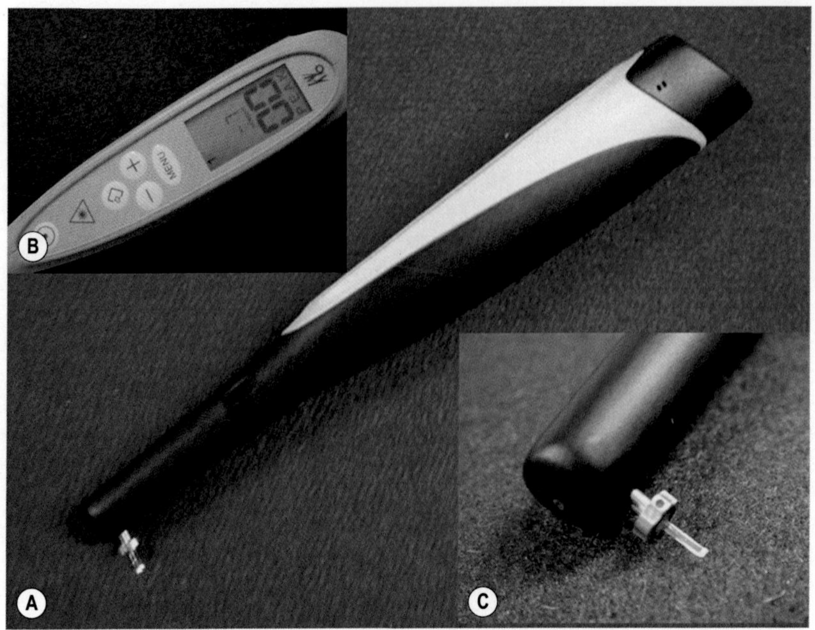

Figure 1.8 The DIAGNOdent pen laser fluorescence device (A) with display on the back of the handle (B) and the approximal sapphire tip (C).

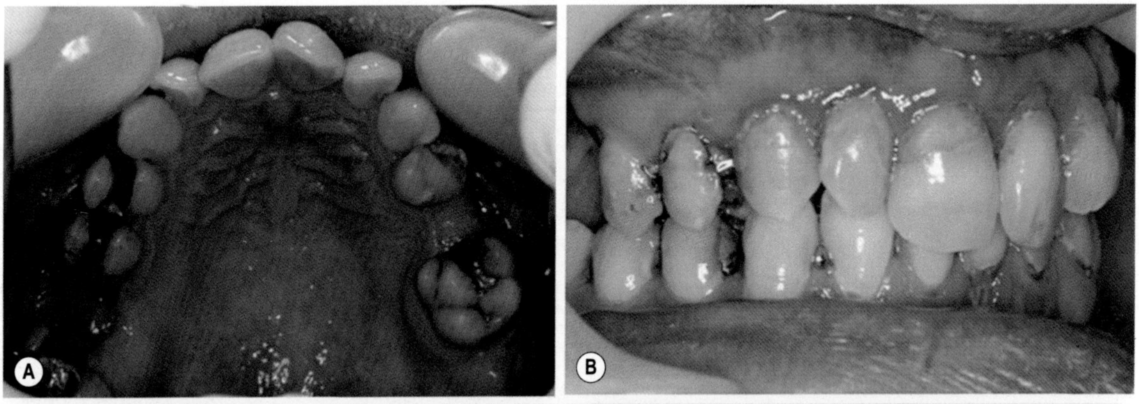

Figure 1.9 Clinical images of a high caries risk patient with multiple restorations and new carious lesions. The patient's bitewing radiographs are seen in Figure 1.4.

elimination of plaque-retentive factors such as poorly contoured restorations should take place. Reassessment of caries risk is then required over a period of time before advanced operative techniques are considered.

Caries risk factors

Social deprivation

Caries prevalence, and hence risk, has been shown to be closely associated with social deprivation in many countries. For example, in Scotland, DEPprivation CATegories (DEPCAT) have been derived from censuses in small post code areas. Variables taken into consideration in deriving DEPCAT scores are:

- Overcrowding
- Male unemployment
- Low social class
- No car.

DEPCAT score 1 is the most affluent and DEPCAT score 7 the least affluent. Figures 1.10 and 1.11 clearly demonstrate the relationship between caries prevalence and social deprivation, with the least affluent areas having fewer caries-free individuals and the highest average decayed (at the dentine level), missing and filled teeth ($d_3$mft). Whilst these figures are derived on a population basis, dentists need to be aware of this association, and careful assessment of caries risk on an individual patient basis needs to be carried out prior to advanced operative procedures.

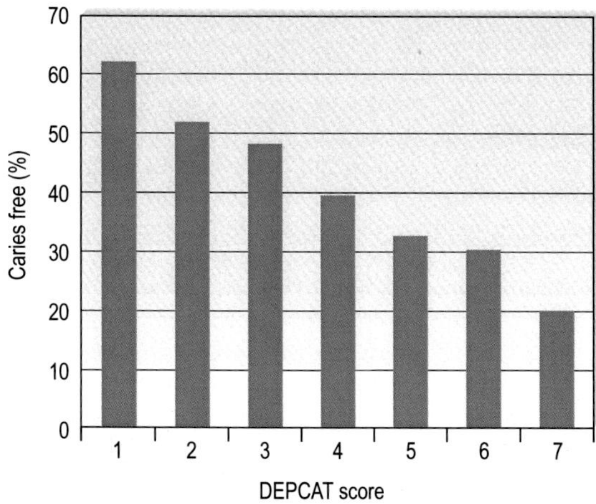

Figure 1.10 The relationship between social deprivation categories (DEPCAT score) and the percentage of the population who are caries free, the least affluent (score 7) having the fewest caries-free teeth for 5-year-old children.
(From Sweeney PC, Nugent Z, Pitts NB. Deprivation and dental caries status of 5-year-old children in Scotland. Community Dent Oral Epidemiol 1999;27:152–159.)

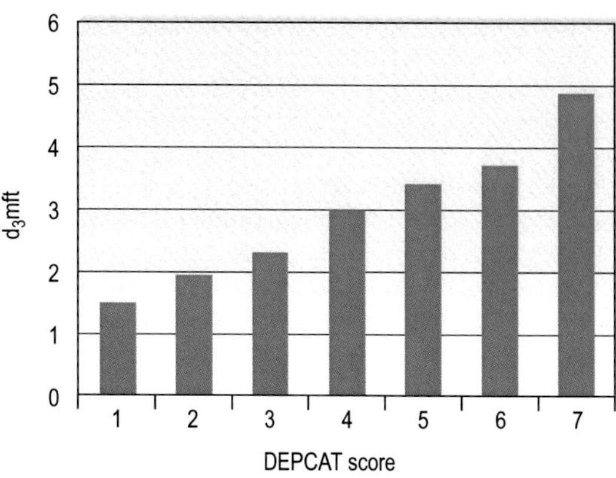

Figure 1.11 The relationship between social deprivation categories (DEPCAT score) and the percentage of the population who have dentine caries, missing or filled teeth ($d_3$mft), the least affluent (score 7) having the highest $d_3$mft for 5-year-old children.
(From Sweeney PC, Nugent Z, Pitts NB. Deprivation and dental caries status of 5-year-old children in Scotland. Community Dent Oral Epidemiol 1999;27:152–159.)

Past caries experience

A strong predictor of future caries is previous caries experience. A dental history and chart are important to assess dental attendance, how often restorations and re-restoration have been required, and whether teeth have been lost due to caries. The clinical and radiographic examination will reveal any new carious lesions. Following preventive advice, preventive treatment and stabilization of caries, assessment of the patient's compliance with attendance and treatment will be required. This will be followed by reassessment of caries risk over a period of 6–12 months before embarking on a more advanced phase of the treatment plan.

Oral hygiene

The level of oral hygiene can be assessed in a number of ways. At its simplest, the Silness and Löe index can be used to measure the amount and distribution of plaque accumulation around teeth. Commonly this is done on buccal and labial surfaces of undisclosed key teeth such as first molar, incisor and premolar teeth (e.g. UR6, UR1, UL4, LL6, LR1, LR6).

Silness and Löe plaque index:

- 0 = No plaque visible
- 1 = Plaque visible on a probe
- 2 = Plaque visible with the naked eye
- 3 = Plaque visible all around tooth.

This is useful as a screening tool, but to assess the level of oral hygiene throughout the mouth of a patient and to establish whether there has been a change in oral hygiene with time, full mouth plaque scores should be recorded. For this, the tooth is divided into four surfaces: mesial, buccal, distal and lingual. The teeth are disclosed and the presence of plaque is recorded on a chart. The proportion of surfaces covered in plaque can then be calculated to give an objective figure at baseline with which comparison is made when reassessing caries risk. Figure 1.12 shows a typical plaque chart.

Many patients with poor oral hygiene may not have received any guidance on oral hygiene instruction and its implementation. Such guidance and implementation is a core feature in an effective preventive program. Disclosing plaque is an important first step for patients to see where the plaque builds up, where they are missing with their current oral hygiene procedures and to note the relationship between plaque accumulation and dental caries. The choice of toothbrush and appropriate tooth brushing technique must be discussed and demonstrated to the patient. Use of interdental aids, such as dental floss and interdental brushes, needs to be gradually introduced, so as not to overwhelm the patient.

It also is important when providing patients with fixed and removable prostheses that they are designed in such a way as to facilitate these oral hygiene procedures. Special additional hygiene procedures may need to be advised and then demonstrated; for example, the use of super floss, also known as three-in-one floss, beneath bridge pontics and connectors.

Diet

An association between dietary sugars and caries has long been established. Once sugar is consumed, the bacteria within the biofilm are able to produce acid, resulting in a rapid fall in plaque pH. When this falls below a critical pH, often considered to be in the region of pH 5.5, the plaque fluid becomes undersaturated with respect to tooth mineral, and demineralization of the tooth occurs. It may take some time for the pH and plaque fluid mineral saturation to return to resting levels. In terms of plaque and salivary pH this is characterized by the Stephan curve. A subsequent sugar snack may cause another dip in pH. Frequent sugar intakes may keep the biofilm undersaturated with respect to tooth mineral and below the critical pH for several hours each day. Sticky, sugary foods may also remain around the teeth for prolonged periods of time and have a similar effect.

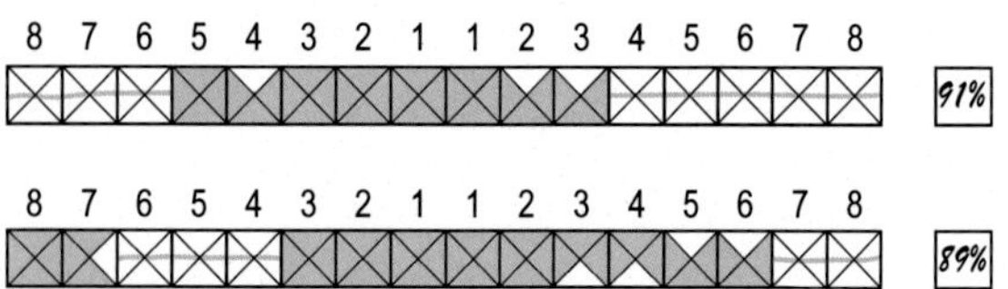

Figure 1.12 Typical plaque chart of a high caries risk patient before oral hygiene instruction and stabilization of caries.

In a caries risk assessment the diet needs to be evaluated. This can either be by patient recollection and appropriate questioning or a diet diary can be kept, in which all that is eaten and drunk for at least three consecutive days is recorded. This should include two working (or school) days and one non-work day because a patient's diet may be completely different on the different days. The diet diary can then be used to highlight the dietary sugar content, including any hidden sugars as well as the frequency of sugar consumption. This enables the practitioner to provide realistic and achievable diet advice. Figure 1.13 shows the diet diary of the patient seen in Figures 1.4 and 1.9. It is clear that there is frequent intake of sugar in coffee and tea, and mint sweets between meals. Either eliminating the sugar completely or using an artificial sugar substitute that is not cariogenic can be advised. At reassessment the diet diary can be repeated to assess compliance with this advice.

Diet diaries are frequently criticized as patients often do not fill them in correctly and can deliberately avoid recording what they know is likely to be the cause of the caries. It can be argued that if they know what not to include, they have the knowledge necessary to prevent their caries and may already be in the process of amending their diet.

Fluoride

Topical fluoride is important in a caries preventive program and information on its use needs to be gathered in a caries risk assessment. Although most European-marketed adult toothpastes contain fluoride at about 1400 ppm, some toothpastes do not contain fluoride, such as some obtained from health food shops and websites; if in doubt, check the list of ingredients. Frequent brushing with a fluoride toothpaste is adequate for lower caries risk individuals, but for those who are higher risk supplemental fluoride should be considered. These can be applied professionally in the surgery/office or by the patient at home. In the surgery/office, a fluoride varnish can be applied to early lesions and susceptible restoration margins. Duraphat varnish (Colgate-Palmolive (UK) Ltd, Guildford, Surrey) contains a 50 mg/ml suspension, which equates to 2.26% (22 600 ppm) of sodium fluoride. This should be avoided in patients who are hypersensitive to colophony, one of its constituents, and for patients with severe asthma who have been admitted to hospital for the condition. Application of fluoride in high doses leads to the formation of calcium fluoride which is relatively soluble and acts as a fluoride reservoir, protecting against further carious attack by inhibition of tooth mineral dissolution when the local pH falls. High dose fluoride toothpastes (Duraphat 2800 ppm F (not recommended for <10 year olds) and Duraphat 5000 ppm F (not recommended for <16 year olds); Colgate-Palmolive (UK) Ltd) are available by prescription and are useful for high-risk patients. Fluoride mouthwashes can be used on a daily (usually around 0.05% sodium fluoride, 227 ppm F) or weekly basis (usually around 0.2% sodium

	Sunday		Monday		Tuesday	
	Time	Items	Time	Items	Time	Items
Before breakfast	9.30	Mug of tea/1 sugar	6.45	Mug of tea/1 sugar		
Breakfast	10.30	Bacon roll Mug of tea/1 sugar	7.15	Bowl of porridge with syrup Mug of tea/1 sugar	7.15	Jam doughnut Mug tea/1 sugar
Morning	11.30 12.15	Mug of coffee/2 sugars, chocolate bar Half a packet of mints through morning	10.30	Mug of coffee/2 sugars, biscuit 3 mints in morning	10.45 12.00	Mug of coffee/2 sugars Mug of coffee/2 sugars
Mid-day meal	2.15	Bowl of soup Can of cola drink	1.00	Egg sandwich, bag crisps, chocolate bar Mug of coffee/2 sugars	1.30	Banana, crisps, chocolate bar Mug of coffee/2 sugars
Afternoon	4.00	Mug of coffee/2 sugars Crisps Half packet mints	3.30	Mug coffee/2 sugars Mints	3.30 6.30	Mints Can of cola drink Mug tea/1 sugar
Evening meal	6.00	Roast chicken, veg, 2 glasses wine	8.30	Spaghetti bolognaise Can of cola drink	8.00	Prawns, salad, potatoes, water
Evening	8.00 10.00	Mug coffee/2 sugars Hot chocolate			9.30	Mug coffee/2 sugars

Figure 1.13 Diet diary of patient seen in Figures 1.4 and 1.9 at initial assessment.

fluoride, 909 ppm F) depending upon patient choice and what suits their lifestyle best. Note that formulations and fluoride content of mouthwashes may differ between countries.

Saliva

Saliva is extremely important for oral health and function. In its absence, there can be devastating effects, which include difficulty with mastication, swallowing and speech, loss of taste, oral soreness, a feeling of thirst and widespread rampant caries. The feeling of a dry mouth, or xerostomia, is usually a result of hyposalivation or oral dryness. It is a side effect of commonly prescribed drugs such as antihypertensives, diuretics, antidepressants, antipsychotics, antispasmodics and some antihistamines. Other causes of dry mouth include autoimmune diseases such as Sjögren's syndrome, diabetes, radiotherapy to the head and neck, and the use of recreational drugs such as caffeine, alcohol and amfetamines.

Clinically, a dry mouth can be obvious and an examination difficult as the dental mirror sticks to the oral mucosa. The amount of saliva production can also be measured under either unstimulated or stimulated conditions. The normal unstimulated and paraffin-wax-stimulated flow rates are given in Table 1.2, together with those for patients diagnosed as having hyposalivation.

Saliva and its constituents have many important properties which are illustrated in Figure 1.14. When providing patients with advanced operative dentistry it is important to bear in mind that these restorations have to be maintained throughout life and changes in a patient's medical history (e.g. medication causing a dry mouth) may increase their caries risk and hence the level of maintenance required in the future.

Table 1.2 Unstimulated and paraffin-wax-stimulated whole saliva for a normal patient and one with hyposalivation

SALIVA FLOW	UNSTIMULATED ml/min	STIMULATED ml/min
Normal	0.3	1.5
Dry mouth	≤0.1	≤0.5♀ : 0.7♂

A patient with a dry mouth will want to take frequent sips of liquid. It is obviously important for this liquid not to contain sugar due to the reduced oral clearance. Plain water should be advised. Some patients also suck on sweets, especially those with a bitter taste, to stimulate some salivary flow. Again this should be avoided and sugar-free sweets or sugar-free chewing gum can be suggested as a good alternative. Even then care must be taken as some artificial sugars such as sorbitol can be metabolized by plaque in some subjects and this could be of

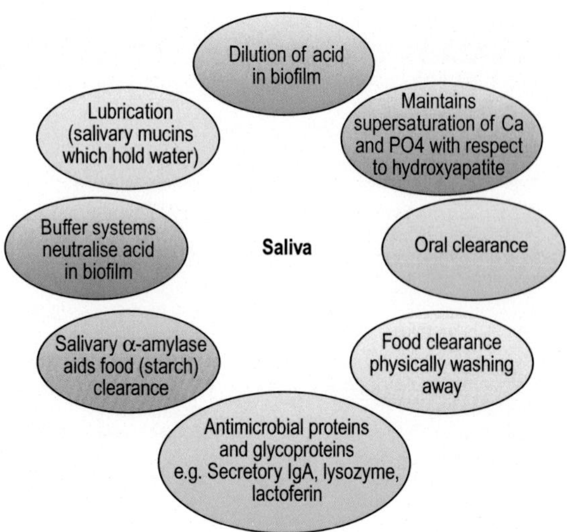

Figure 1.14 Important constituents and properties of saliva.

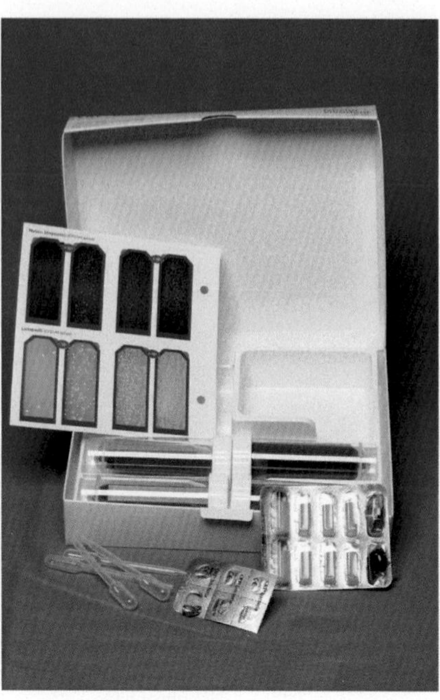

Figure 1.15 Commercially available kit to measure the counts of organisms within saliva (CRT Bacteria, Ivoclar Vivadent, Schaan, Liechtenstein).

concern for some xerostomic patients. For some patients, artificial saliva may give relief from the symptoms of dry mouth, but it is important to ensure that the pH is not acidic which could cause erosion in the dentate patient. Referral to an oral medicine specialist should also be considered for a patient with a dry mouth as a result of radiotherapy or Sjögren's syndrome. If there is sufficient functional glandular tissue remaining, prescription of pilocarpine can be considered to stimulate salivary flow.

Saliva microbiology

Salivary tests for mutans streptococci and lactobacilli have been used for many years and commercially available kits have been produced to measure the counts of both organisms within saliva. It is assumed that if the levels of these cariogenic organisms are high in the dental biofilm on the surface of the tooth or within active carious lesions, the levels will also be high in the saliva. Indeed, a number of studies have found associations with these two organisms in saliva and the caries experience of individuals. More recent evidence suggests that these salivary counts are not good in predicting future caries; however, they may be useful in assessing patients' compliance with dietary advice, for as the level and frequency of sugar in the diet reduces, the ensuing modification in the local oral environment is reflected in a reduced count of both species. This can serve as a tangible reward to a compliant patient and spur on their efforts in changing their dietary lifestyle.

Figure 1.15 illustrates one such kit (CRT Bacteria, Ivoclar Vivadent, Schaan, Liechtenstein). In this a sample of stimulated mixed saliva is collected and applied, at the chairside, to selective culture plates. Following incubation at 37°C for 48 hours, the numbers of colony forming units (CFUs) are estimated by comparing the cultures to a chart (Figure 1.16). Figures 1.17 and 1.18 illustrate this for a high caries risk patient and one of low risk.

The various caries risk factors described are subjectively drawn together for each patient, with the outcome influencing the patient's treatment plan. A more formal and objective way of assessing this is by using a computer-based caries risk model. The Cariogram is such a system which was developed in Malmö Dental School by Douglass Bratthall and co-workers. Information is gathered from the patient about caries risk, clinical and radiographic findings, and the results from various salivary tests. This information is given a score of 0–3 (or in some cases 0–2). These scores are then entered into the Cariogram program, from where information is weighted according to its impact on caries risk. The program evaluates the data and then presents it as a pie chart with a clear indication of future caries risk expressed as a 'Chance to avoid caries'. The various risk factors described above and those evaluated in the Cariogram and the corresponding scores given are detailed in Table 1.3. Table 1.3 also summarizes actions that can be taken to address each factor positively, with an aim to change the patient's caries risk. Figures 1.19 and 1.20 show what the Cariogram would look like for a low- and a high-risk patient, respectively.

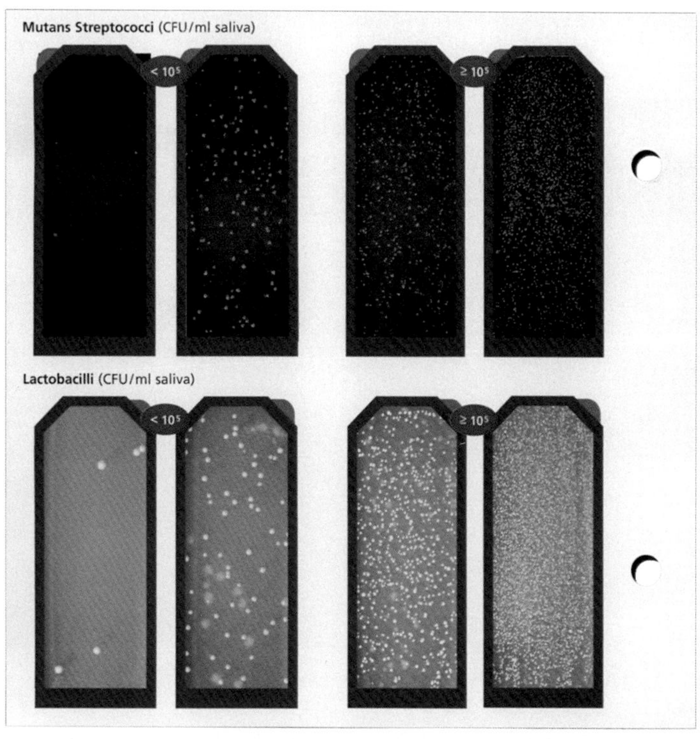

Figure 1.16 Chart enabling the number of colony forming units (CFUs) for mutans streptococci and lactobacilli to be estimated.

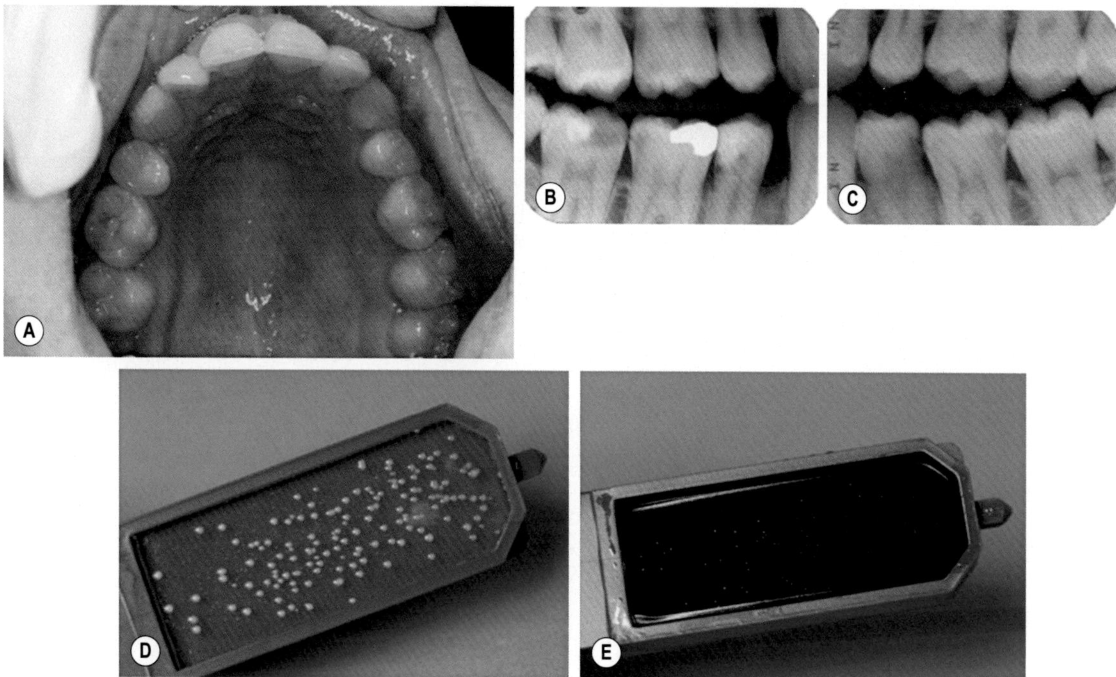

Figure 1.17 Clinical image of upper arch and bitewing radiographs of a high caries risk patient together with their lactobacilli and mutans streptococci counts.

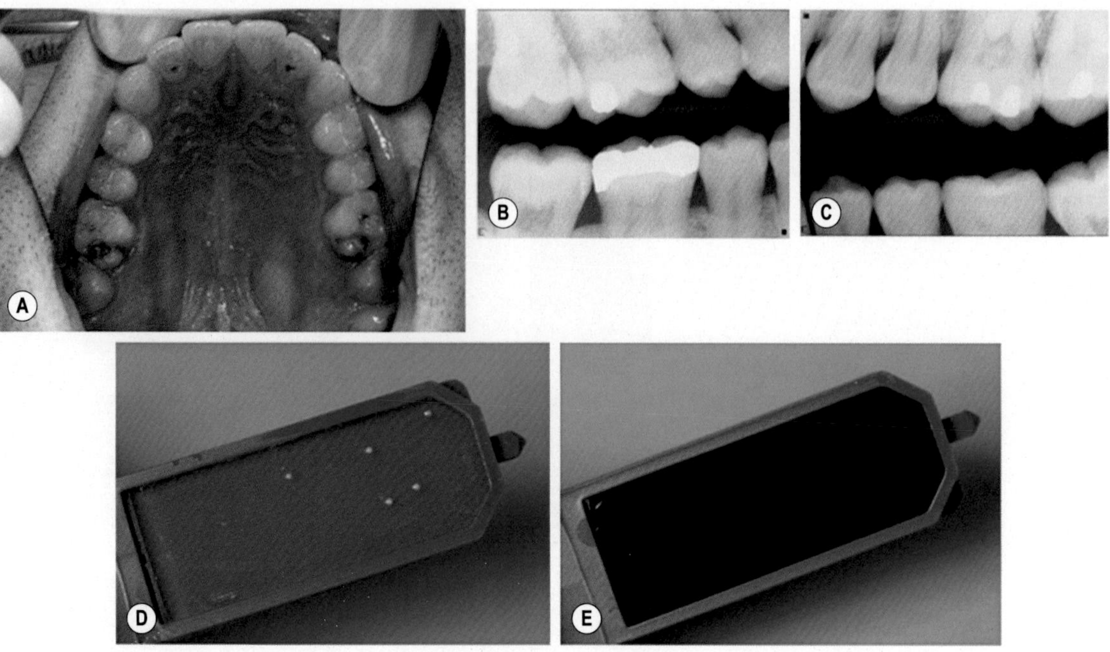

Figure 1.18 Clinical image of upper arch and bitewing radiographs of a low caries risk patient together with their lactobacilli and mutans streptococci counts.

Table 1.3 Examples of various caries risk factors, how they can be assessed, the score they would be given in a caries risk model (the Cariogram) and how that risk factor can be modified

FACTOR	INFORMATION TO BE COLLECTED	CARIOGRAM SCORE	ADVICE AND MANAGEMENT
Caries experience	Decayed/Missing/Filled Teeth (DMFT), Decayed/Missing/Filled Surfaces (DMFS), new caries in last year	0: No caries, no fillings 1: Better than normal for age group 2: Normal for age group 3: Worse than normal for age group	All of the below
Related general diseases	Medical history and medications	0: Healthy 1: Illness that contributes moderately to caries risk 2: Serious illness with strong influence on caries	Liaise with medical practitioner – avoid medication with sugar or causes dry mouth where possible
Diet content	Diet history (or *Lactobacillus* test), quality of diet	0: Very low sugar content (LC $\leq$1000) 1: Low sugar content (LC 10^4) 2: Moderate sugar content (LC 10^5) 3: High sugar content (LC $\geq 10^6$)	Reduce sugar consumption Suggest safe snacks and drinks Artificial sweeteners
Diet frequency	Diet history – mean number of meals/ snacks per day	0: Maximum 3 meals/day 1: Maximum 5 meals/day 2: Maximum 7 meals/day 3: More than 7 meals/day	Advice on reduced frequency of sugar intake Sugar with main meal Safe snacks

(Continued)

Table 1.3 Examples of various caries risk factors, how they can be assessed, the score they would be given in a caries risk model (the Cariogram) and how that risk factor can be modified—cont'd

FACTOR	INFORMATION TO BE COLLECTED	CARIOGRAM SCORE	ADVICE AND MANAGEMENT
Amount of plaque	Silness–Löe plaque index	0: No plaque visible 1: Plaque visible on a probe 2: Plaque visible with the naked eye 3: Plaque visible all around tooth	Disclose, oral hygiene instruction, toothbrush technique, electric toothbrush with oscillating head, interdental aids (interdental brushes and floss)
Streptococcus mutans	Salivary mutans streptococci counts	0: *S. mutans* <104/ml saliva 1: *S. mutans* <106/ml saliva 2: *S. mutans* <107/ml saliva 3: *S. mutans* >107/ml saliva	Improved oral hygiene (see above)
Fluoride programme	Estimation of extent of fluoride exposure	0: Maximum fluoride exposure 1: Additional fluoride measure (other than toothpaste) but infrequent application 2: Fluoride toothpaste only 3: Avoidance of fluorides (e.g. no fluoride exposure)	Ensure brush at least 2–3 times per day with at least 1400 ppm fluoride toothpaste High-risk supplement with professional application of fluoride varnish, high-dose fluoride toothpaste or fluoride mouthwash
Saliva secretion rate	Stimulated saliva flow rate	0: ≥0.7 ml saliva/min 1: 0.3–0.7 ml saliva/min 2: ≤0.3 ml saliva/min	Liaise with medical practitioner – consider alternative medication (less of a dry mouth side effect) if possible Dietary advice – sugar-free drinks, chewing gum, sweets Artificial saliva Oral Medicine referral? Prescription of pilocarpine
Saliva buffering capacity	Buffer kit – Dentobuff	0: Adequate, saliva pH >6.0 1: Reduced, saliva pH 4.5–5.5 2: Low, saliva pH <4.0	

Table generated from Alian et al. (2006), Bratthall et al. (2001) and Ruiz Miravet et al. (2007) LC, Lactobacillus Counts.

SUMMARY AND PRINCIPLES OF TREATMENT PLANNING FOR A HIGH CARIES RISK PATIENT

Early caries detection and caries risk assessment are important to target prevention for those patients that are at risk of developing new caries. Monitoring of caries is essential to determine the success of preventive care. When this primary prevention has not been instituted or has failed, a clinical outcome such as that described in Figures 1.4 and 1.9 may be observed. History taking, examination, diagnosis and treatment planning for this patient should be structured and staged in the following way and allow re-evaluation prior to complex and advanced restorative dentistry:

- Any emergency treatment should be provided first; this may include extraction or extirpation of a pulp for a tooth with an irreversible pulpitis.
- Assessment of risk factors.
- Appropriate preventive advice and treatment should be given as outlined in Table 1.3 based upon the individual's risk factor.
- Stabilization of disease. In relation to gross caries, a quadrant at a time may be taken and caries removed from all teeth in that quadrant and provisionally restored. For deep carious lesions, stepwise excavation can be considered (see Ricketts, 2001). If root canal treatment is needed for any teeth, the first stage of treatment (e.g. pulpal extirpation) can be carried out and the tooth provisionally restored.
- Each tooth can then be carefully and definitively restored, ensuring good adaptation, cavity seal and

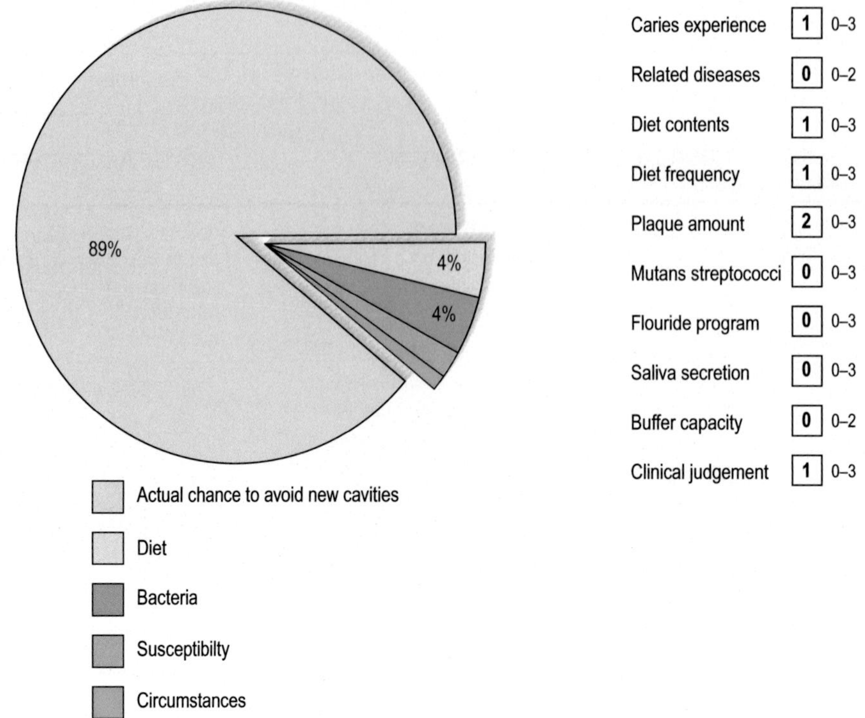

Figure 1.19 Cariogram of a low caries risk individual with a high (89%) chance of avoiding new caries.

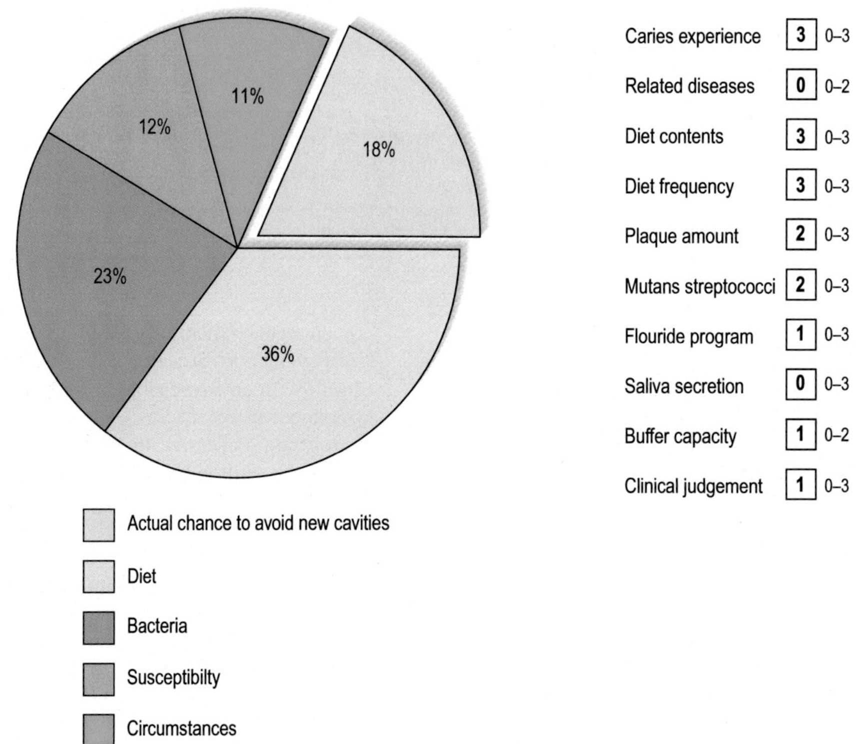

Figure 1.20 Cariogram of a high caries risk individual with a low (18%) chance of avoiding new caries.

contour of the restorative material chosen. Initial stabilization will ensure that other lesions do not progress whilst this protracted stage of the treatment plan is being carried out – continued preventive advice and support should be conducted throughout.

- Once all the provisional restorations have been replaced, consideration can be given to endodontic treatment of those teeth that require it.
- Reassessment of caries risk. Re-evaluation of all the risk factors in Table 1.3 should now take place and any new lesions recorded. If the patient appears to have addressed the main risk factors and no new lesions have appeared, consideration can now be given to an advanced stage of the treatment plan, which might include crowns and bridges. If in any doubt as to the patient's caries risk status and compliance with preventive advice, a further period of monitoring would be advised.

FURTHER READING

Alian, A.Y., McNally, M.E., Fure, S., Birkhed, D., 2006. Assessment of caries risk in elderly patients using the Cariogram model. J. Can. Dent. Assoc. 72, 459–463.

Bratthall, D., Stjernswärd, J.R., Petersson, G.H., 2001. Assessment of caries risk in the clinic – a modern approach. In: Wilson, N.H.F., Roulet, J.F., Fuzzi, M. (Eds.), Advances in operative dentistry: challenges of the future. Quintessence Publishing, London, pp. 61–72.

Fejerskov, O., Kidd, E., 2008. Dental caries and its clinical management, second ed. Blackwell, Munksgaard.

Ricketts, D., 2001. Management of the deep carious lesion and the vital pulp dentine complex. Br. Dent. J. 191, 606–610.

Ruiz Miravet, A., Montiel Company, J.M., Almerich Silla, J.M., 2007. Evaluation of caries risk in a young adult population. Med. Oral Patol. Oral Cir. Bucal 12, E412–E418.

Chapter | 2 |

Periodontal disease

Angela Gilbert

CHAPTER CONTENTS

THE NECESSARY ORDER OF THINGS

There is no doubt that screening patients, diagnosing periodontal disease and then effectively treating the disease is an essential part of restorative treatment. It is crucial that successful periodontal management, demonstrated over a period of time, precedes provision of complex fixed and removable prosthodontics and implants. One analogy of this would be to consider the construction of a new building. It would make no sense to begin building walls or choosing the lighting if the foundations were not sound.

SUSCEPTIBILITY TO PERIODONTAL DISEASE

It is clear from many studies that there is considerable variation in individual susceptibility to periodontal disease. This information has shown that a relatively small percentage of the population (probably less than 15%) suffer from severe or advanced disease and are highly susceptible. A similar percentage appears to be disease resistant and have a very low susceptibility, while the remaining 70% show some susceptibility demonstrated by moderate disease progression.

It is essential to have some understanding of an individual patient's susceptibility to periodontal disease as several things flow from this. If a patient has a high susceptibility their periodontal treatment may need to be protracted and complex if stability is to be achieved, their recall times will have to be shorter and their periodontal prognosis is reduced. For highly susceptible patients, complex fixed and removable prosthodontics can be undertaken, but *only* when both periodontal stability and adequate plaque control have been demonstrated over time – usually at least a few months. Conversely, for patients with low susceptibility, the treatment needs are usually simple, the recall times can be longer and the periodontal prognosis is good. In these patients, the decision to provide complex fixed and removable prosthodontics is much more straightforward.

Susceptibility of an individual patient is determined by relating three things:

- the age of the patient
- the plaque control
- the severity of periodontal disease

A young patient with severe disease whose plaque control is good would be regarded as having a high susceptibility whilst an elderly patient with poor plaque control and little evidence of disease would be regarded as having a low susceptibility. Susceptibility is thus a very individual concept relating to each patient. It must be appreciated that a patient's innate susceptibility cannot be changed as this is partly genetically determined. Recognition of this has led to the realization that risk recognition and control forms an essential part of periodontal management, particularly in patients with higher susceptibility.

THE CONCEPT OF RISK

It is known that the presence of risk factors will increase the chance that periodontal disease will occur. Local risk factors are essentially plaque retentive features such as restoration overhangs. These factors must be corrected before commencing periodontal treatment. Systemic risk factors may be genetic (e.g. Down's syndrome), haematological (e.g. cyclic neutropenia), behavioural (e.g. smoking, poor oral hygiene), environmental (e.g. effects of drugs, HIV), endocrine/metabolic (e.g. poorly controlled diabetes) or lifestyle (e.g. stress, poor nutrition). Factors such as smoking are modifiable whilst others, such as genetic predisposition, are not. In susceptible patients, recognition of the risks and control of the modifiable risk factors is essential if periodontal therapy is to be successful. This is particularly true if provision of more complex fixed and removable prosthodontics is envisaged.

Risk recognition begins at the stage of taking thorough histories from patients.

TAKING HISTORIES FROM PATIENTS WITH PERIODONTAL DISEASE

Taking thorough histories is an essential part of a patient's oral health care and is particularly relevant to periodontal therapy. This takes time but should not be ignored or truncated as the information derived is essential if appropriate decisions regarding treatment planning, provision of periodontal therapy and maintenance are to be made. This again is particularly important when periodontal management precedes and is integrated into treatment plans that involve complex fixed and removable prosthodontics.

There are four main histories to be taken. These are Medical, Dental, Social and Family histories, and aspects of relevance to periodontal disease are highlighted here.

Medical history

This serves three main functions:

1. It may explain, at least in part, the severity and extent of periodontal disease encountered. An example would be the increased disease which may be seen in some patients with poorly controlled diabetes. If control is not improved, the chance of producing a successful periodontal treatment outcome is reduced, thus making the later provision of complex restorative work unlikely.
2. It may alert the clinician to precautions which should be taken to safeguard the patient. This may include provision of steroid cover or highlight the need for treatment in a specialist or hospital setting. These complications may also make the provision of complex restorative work less likely.
3. It may alert the clinician to potential risks posed by a patient to staff and subsequent patients in the surgery. Standard cross-infection procedures should be operated for all patients but it would be wrong, for example, to use an ultrasonic scaler in a patient carrying a known infective risk. Ultimately, however, provided periodontal stability has been achieved, there should be no reason not to proceed with complex restorative work if this was the desired outcome.

Dental history

It is clear that patients who attend the dentist irregularly are not candidates for advanced restorative treatment plans. In addition to the standard parts of a dental history, particular aspects that should be assessed in relation to periodontal health are as follows:

- *Plaque control regime used.* If there is active periodontal disease in the mouth, plaque control is, by definition, 'inadequate' and must be modified. It is usually very straightforward to recommend appropriate changes to the techniques and frequencies employed; however, it must also be recognized that plaque will potentially cause caries. This means that even if plaque control is sufficient to control the periodontal condition, it may not be sufficient to prevent damage to the teeth themselves. If plaque control is not subsequently improved, the provision of complex restorative treatment would not be indicated.
- *Wearing a removable appliance.* Use of an appliance such as a denture is relevant as numerous studies have shown that this increases plaque retention, which in turn may be sufficient to take the plaque levels above the patient's individual disease threshold. Adequate denture hygiene and advice to remove the appliance at night are essential.
- *A previous history of periodontal disease.* This is the best indicator of future risk because the innate susceptibility has not changed. As stated previously, provided periodontal stability is demonstrated over time, and provided the plaque regime is adequate to control both caries and periodontal disease, provision of complex operative care should not be withheld. It must be recognized, however, that the patient is not 'cured' and it is worthwhile considering that the disease may reactivate.
- *A history of previous periodontal treatment.* This may indicate both the patient's attitude to treatment and the degree of difficulty encountered in treating their previous disease. If it has proven difficult to stabilize the periodontal condition in the past (repeated root surface instrumentation, periodontal surgery, use of antimicrobials, etc.), this suggests a high susceptibility and increased chance of subsequent periodontal breakdown. If complex restorative work was being considered in such circumstances it would be wise to delay this until periodontal stability had been demonstrated over several months at least. Short recall times would also be needed for a substantial period after placement.

Social history

There are three particular aspects of the social history that are relevant to periodontal disease. The single most important factor is a history of smoking. Recent research suggests that smoking accounts for up to 50% of cases of chronic periodontitis and it has been established that the incidence and severity of periodontal disease increase with increasing tobacco exposure. Tobacco exposure should be quantified as 'pack years' and this is calculated as the number of packs of 20 cigarettes smoked per day multiplied by the number of years for which the patient has smoked. For example, smoking 20 cigarettes per day for 10 years would equate to 10 pack years. This provides a better indicator of total nicotine exposure than knowing that someone smokes 20 cigarettes per day but without knowing for how long they have had the habit. Some patients do not smoke standard cigarettes and for them it is possible to convert to 'pack years' by assuming that 1 g of pipe tobacco is equivalent to one cigarette, one small cigar is equivalent to 3 cigarettes and 1 standard cigar is equivalent to 5 cigarettes. The impact of 'pack years' is also relevant to implant assessment as it is widely accepted that smoking reduces the success of osseointegration.

The other two factors that are thought to influence periodontal disease, but to a lesser extent, are alcohol consumption and stress. Several sources, including the Third National Health and Nutrition Examination Survey (NHANES), United States, have found a moderate but consistent dose-dependent relationship between alcohol consumption and periodontal disease. The recommended maximum number of units of alcohol per week for a woman is 14 and for a man it is 21. In times of stress, amongst other things, a patient's oral hygiene and oral health care may deteriorate, their nutrition may suffer, their salivary flow decreases, immune function is depressed, and plaque becomes stickier and thicker. Stress is not easy to measure, however, and although regarded as a risk factor, its single impact on dental care is difficult to determine.

Family history

The genetic links associated with aggressive periodontitis (AgP) are much stronger than with chronic periodontitis. It is important to know if there is a family history of periodontal disease, particularly involving early loss of teeth, as this may be significant in making the periodontal diagnosis. AgP, as the name suggests, is characterized by a very rapid loss of periodontal support and referral to a specialist periodontist is often indicated. Clearly, there should be no provision of complex restorative work until the periodontal condition is stabilized. Fortunately, many AgP cases 'burn out' and when stability is subsequently demonstrated over time, advanced restorative care can be considered.

It should also be noted that siblings or children of AgP patients should be regularly screened for the disease.

ASSESSMENT OF PERIODONTAL DISEASE

A clinical examination and where necessary sensitivity testing, will inform the clinician as to whether radiographic examination is required and if so which views are required in order to produce a diagnosis and treatment plan.

The clinical assessment

The basic periodontal examination (BPE)

The BPE (Table 2.1) is a screening tool to enable practitioners to determine whether or not their patient has significant periodontal disease. This examination should be used to screen:

- all new patients
- all those patients who have not had a periodontal examination of any kind in the past year.

The BPE can only be performed using a WHO probe and the probing force applied should be 20–25 g. There are two common variants of the WHO probe in use: the WHO-E (epidemiological) type probe and the WHO-C (clinical) type probe (Figure 2.1). The key elements to note on each are a ball-shaped probe tip of diameter 0.5 mm and a coloured band extending from 3.5 to 5.5 mm. The WHO-C probe has, in addition, a second coloured band extending from 8.5 to 11.5 mm.

To carry out a BPE, the dentition is divided into sextants (first premolar to second molar and canine to canine). The probe tip is gently placed in the base of the gingival crevice/pocket and 'walked' around all the teeth in the entire sextant. One code is assigned per sextant and this is the highest encountered anywhere within it. Table 2.1 shows the criteria used for assigning the BPE codes and the corresponding management for each sextant.

Third molars are not included in the BPE and at least two teeth must be present in a sextant for it to be coded. If there is only one tooth in a sextant this is included in the adjacent sextant and if there are no teeth present in a sextant this is denoted on the completed chart as 'X'.

An example of a completed BPE chart is shown below:

X	4	3
*	1	2

Table 2.1 BPE codes, together with the description, a clinical example and appropriate management

BPE CODE	DESCRIPTION	CLINICAL PICTURE	MANAGEMENT
0	The coloured band (3.5–5.5 mm) is completely visible and there is *no* bleeding on probing from the base of the pocket		No treatment required
1	The coloured band (3.5–5.5 mm) is completely visible plus there *is* bleeding on probing from the base of the pocket		Oral hygiene instruction (OHI)
2	The coloured band (3.5–5.5 mm) is completely visible plus either calculus (supra or subgingival) or a defective restoration is present		OHI plus removal of calculus ± correction of plaque retentive margins of restorations

(Continued)

Table 2.1 BPE codes, together with the description, a clinical example and appropriate management—cont'd

BPE CODE	DESCRIPTION	CLINICAL PICTURE	MANAGEMENT
3	The coloured band (3.5–5.5 mm) is only partly visible	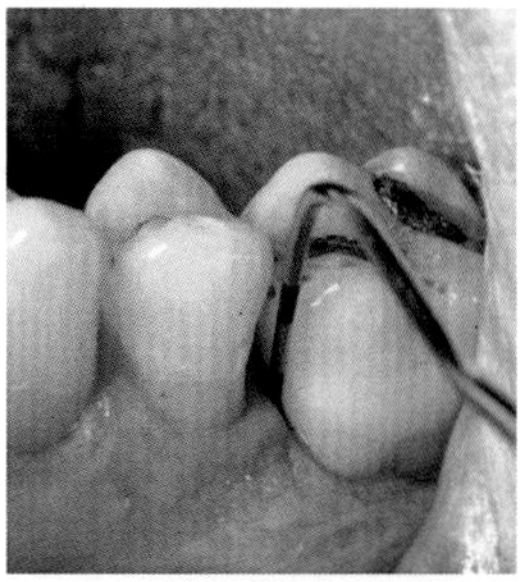	Full charts required at start and finish of treatment. OHI plus calculus removal, correction of defective margins of restorations and root surface instrumentation (RSI) as required
4	The coloured band (3.5–5.5 mm) is completely hidden	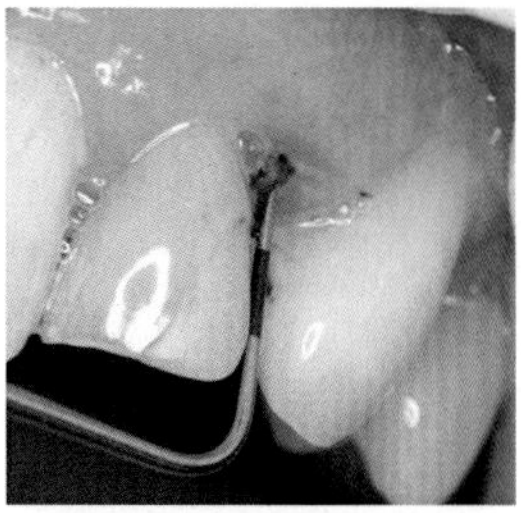	Full charts required at start and finish of treatment, including note of furcation involvements and any other relevant clinical findings. OHI plus calculus removal, restoration margin correction and RSI as appropriate. Surgery may be needed and consideration should be given to referring the patient to a periodontal specialist
*	Loss of attachment of ≥7 mm	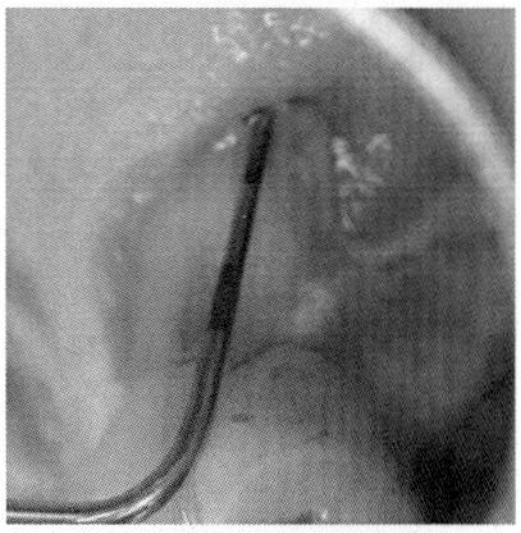	
*	Furcation involvement	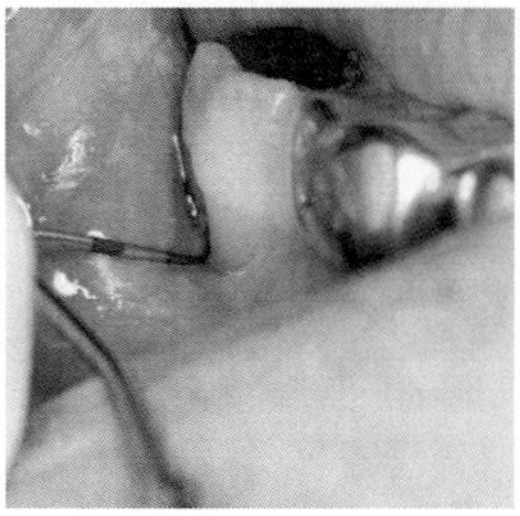	

Should significant disease be found (BPE Codes 3, 4 or *), a more detailed periodontal, clinical and possibly radiographic examination is required (see later).

As with any system, the BPE has both advantages and disadvantages (Table 2.2) and the reader should be aware of these if the system is to be correctly applied and interpreted.

Clinical examination

For all patients who have BPE codes 3, 4 or *, a full periodontal examination is required. This needs to be performed at all sites in the mouth as there may be variation in the severity of disease at different sites and at different times. This is because periodontal disease is

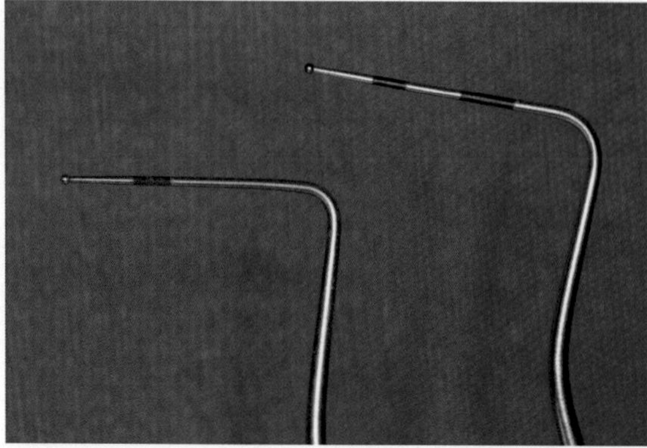

Figure 2.1 WHO-E (epidemiological) type probe (left) and the WHO-C (clinical) type probe (right).

recognized as being both site specific and episodic in nature.

The five essential clinical assessments required to determine extent and severity of periodontal disease are as follows:

- *Probing (pocket) depth.* This is measured from the gingival margin to the base of the pocket. Pocket depths deeper than 3 mm are regarded as being significant as patients cannot efficiently clean them. Reduction of pockets to this depth is thus one of the principal aims of therapy.
- *Loss of attachment.* This is measured from the amelo-cemental junction (ACJ) to the base of the pocket. This represents the sum of all the episodes of disease which have taken place at a particular site since the tooth erupted, though it does not indicate how many episodes of disease have occurred or when they occurred. A completed pocket/loss of attachment chart (Figure 2.2) is particularly useful in determining the severity of periodontitis and aiding treatment planning in terms of sites that may require root surface instrumentation (RSI). The chart will also differentiate between true and false pockets and make identification of sites with recession/tissue shrinkage and/or gingival overgrowth clear.

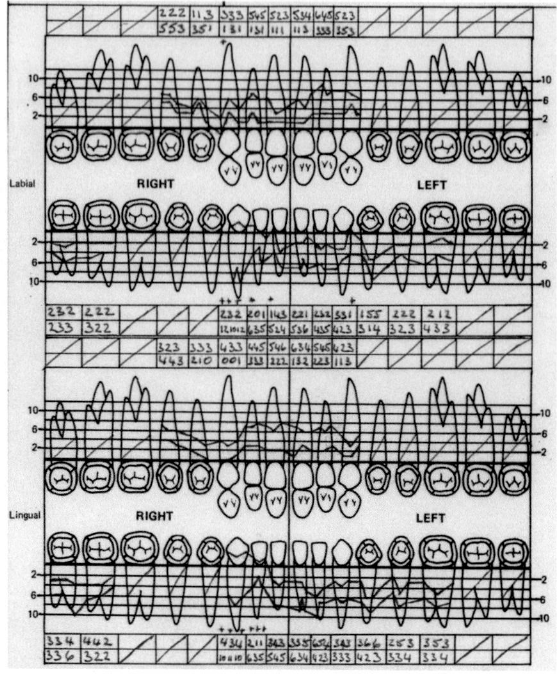

Figure 2.2 Completed pocket/loss of attachment chart.

- *Lack of bleeding on probing (BOP) from the base of the pocket.* This indicates a lack of disease activity at a site at a particular time. Virtually all sites not showing BOP will not go on to lose attachment. Previously, sites which did show BOP were regarded as a positive indicator of disease activity, but unfortunately only

Table 2.2 Advantages and disadvantages of the BPE

ADVANTAGES	DISADVANTAGES
• It is a screening system which detects individuals requiring a more detailed periodontal assessment • It is recognized internationally • It is quick and easy to carry out and the required equipment is inexpensive • It encourages examination of the periodontium in general dental practice • It summarizes the periodontium in a readily communicable form • It gives an indication of treatment requirements and who should treat the patient – should the patient be referred to a specialist?	• It lacks detail within sextants • It cannot be used to monitor disease • It requires a special probe • It does not distinguish between true and false pockets. • It lacks information on disease activity. bleeding on probing (BOP) is only mentioned in Code 0 (where it is not present) and in Code 1 (where it is present) • It lacks detailed information on loss of attachment (LOA). LOA is mentioned in Code * alone • It lacks detailed information about furcation involvement

30% of sites showing BOP will go on to lose attachment. Using lack of bleeding is thus a much more robust assessment. A bleeding chart (Figure 2.3) may be used to illustrate this. Both gingivitis and periodontitis can be said to occur only if bleeding is present. This chart is particularly useful in determining the distribution of disease, i.e. whether it is localized or generalized (see later in section on diagnosis).

- *Furcation involvement*. This should be assessed in all multirooted teeth. Involvement is significant because affected teeth have a reduced prognosis. This is partly because these sites are often extremely difficult for both dentist and patient to clean and partly because the affected teeth may lose vitality. Curved furcation probes (Figure 2.4) are useful to facilitate this part of the examination (Figure 2.5). When reporting furcation involvement, the clinician should note specifically which tooth is affected, which furcation is affected and the severity of the involvement at affected sites. There are several furcation severity grading systems in use but the one suggested by Hamp et al. (1975) shown in Table 2.3 is particularly helpful. Lastly, every tooth with furcation involvement should be sensitivity tested. This should be done with cold stimulation and an electric pulp tester to minimize the possibility of obtaining both false-positive and false-negative results (see Chapter 3). If a tooth has a true combined (perio-endo) lesion, the endodontic treatment must be carried out first. If furcations are exposed in teeth that are planned for crowns and bridges, special care needs to be taken in tooth preparation and restoration contour to avoid positive ledges in the furcation area.
- *Tooth mobility*. There are several dental causes of tooth mobility of which periodontal disease is only one. Other common dental causes include occlusal trauma and periradicular disease. It is essential to establish both the cause(s) of the observed mobility and its severity. Grading the degree of mobility should be done using two instrument handles to check for movement and it is important to use a suitable index to reduce the subjectivity of the assessment. One such index is Miller's Index which is described

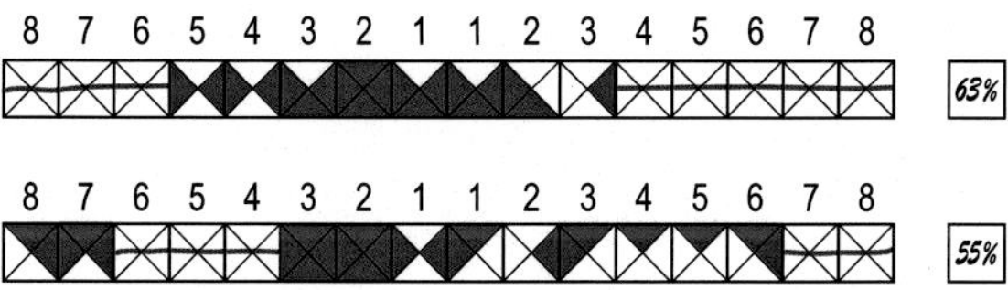

Figure 2.3 Bleeding chart. As for the plaque chart, the circumference of the gingiva around the tooth is divided into quarters, and the site(s) where bleeding occurs recorded. A percentage bleeding score can then be calculated.

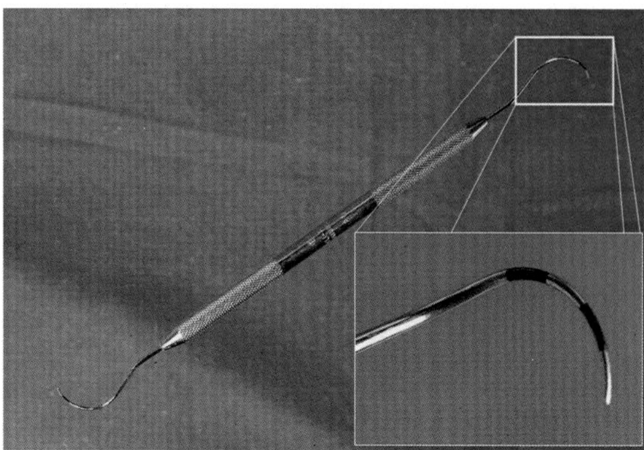

Figure 2.4 Furcation probe (main image) with head magnified (inset).

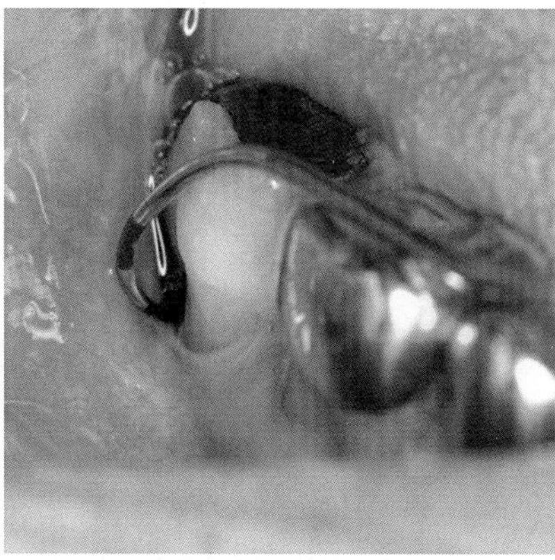

Figure 2.5 Furcation probe demonstrating buccal furcation in the lower right second molar tooth.

Table 2.3 Furcation classification described by Hamp et al. (1975)

FURCATION CLASSIFICATION	DESCRIPTION
1	Horizontal loss of periodontal support ≤1/3 of the width of the tooth
2	Horizontal loss of periodontal support >1/3 but not encompassing the total width of the tooth
3	Horizontal 'through and through' destruction of the periodontal tissues in the furcation area

Based on Hamp S, Nyman S, Lindhe J. Periodontal treatment of multirooted teeth. Results after 5 years. J Clin Periodontol 1975;2:126–135.

in Table 2.4. It is important to note that failure to elucidate the reason(s) for tooth mobility precludes effective treatment. The distribution and severity of tooth mobility may also be recorded on a chart (Figure 2.6).

It will be noted that an assessment of plaque control is not included in the assessment of disease. This is because there is no direct link between the amount of plaque and the presence, severity and activity of periodontal disease (see above for discussion of susceptibility). It will of course be assessed separately after the above examinations are completed and a plaque chart may be useful in this regard (Figure 2.7). This chart records the presence of plaque only and makes no attempt to quantify it. If plaque control is inadequate (i.e. there is active periodontal disease and/or caries), this chart identifies the sites the patient is not cleaning and appropriate targeted oral hygiene instruction may be given.

There may or may not be an obvious correlation between sites with bleeding and sites with plaque in the same mouth. Although correlation will depend upon the innate susceptibility of the patient, it must be recognized that plaque varies greatly in composition and thus pathogenicity. It is also true that plaque scores taken on the day of presentation may not be representative of the usual plaque control exercised by patients who may clean unusually well before their appointment. However, even with all these considerations it is possible to gain some insight into the susceptibility by comparison of the two charts. This is especially the case if the plaque scores are high and the bleeding scores are low, implying a low susceptibility to disease.

In addition to these parameters it is often useful to know whether the patient is suffering from problems with hypersensitivity (see Chapter 4 for the management of dentine sensitivity), inadequate function or an aesthetic problem such as tooth migration.

Completion of these examinations establishes the presence, location and severity of any periodontal disease, and it is only at this juncture that the clinician can establish whether a radiographic examination is required and, if so, which radiographs are appropriate.

Table 2.4 Miller's index for tooth mobility

MOBILITY CLASSIFICATION	DESCRIPTION
0	Horizontal movement up to 0.2 mm
1	Horizontal movement of >0.2 mm but ≤1 mm
2	Horizontal movement of >1 mm
3	Movement in both horizontal and vertical planes

Based on Miller SC. Textbook of periodontia. Philadelphia: Blakiston, 1938.

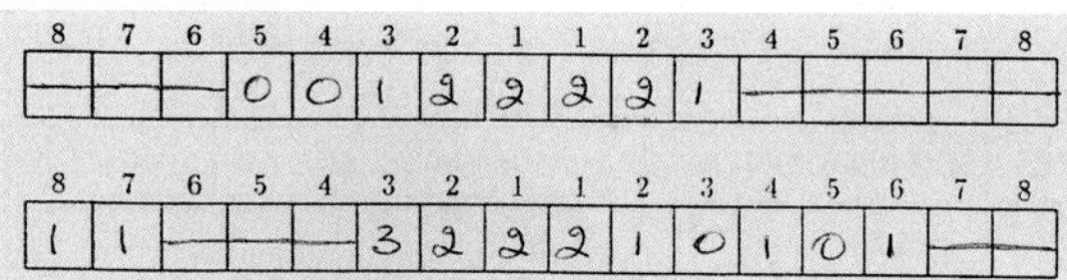

Figure 2.6 Mobility chart.

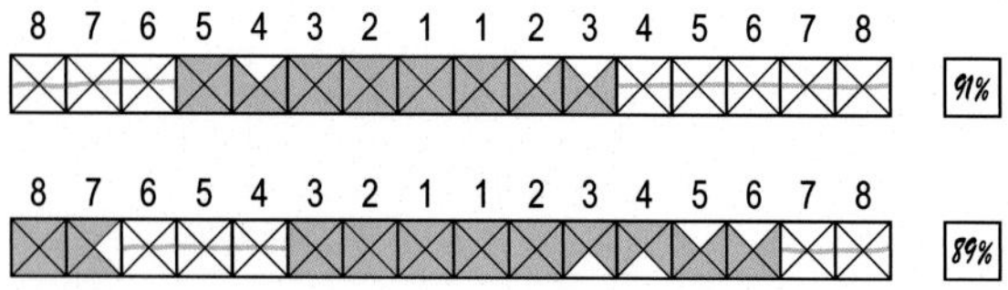

Figure 2.7 Plaque chart. Each tooth is divided into quadrants and the presence of plaque recorded in each quadrant. The percentage surface coverage in plaque can be calculated.

The radiographic examination

A radiographic examination, if required, is a useful adjunct to the clinical examination and not an alternative. At all times a balance is needed between the diagnostic yield from the radiograph and the amount of radiation to which the patient is exposed. It is mandatory that the radiation exposure is kept to the minimum for the diagnostic purpose.

Which radiographs?

There are published guidelines about which radiographs to use in particular situations, and although these are useful, there are often individual considerations to ponder. It is important not to take radiographs if there is no definite clinical indication to do so. An example of this would be in cases of chronic gingivitis – irrespective of whether the condition is localized or generalized, there will be no useful diagnostic yield.

In periodontology three main radiograph types are employed: dental panoramic tomograms (DPTs), peri-apicals, and both vertical and horizontal bitewings. The choice depends on the results of the individual clinical examination. Horizontal bitewing radiographs have very limited use in periodontology as furcation areas and even the alveolar bone crest may not be visible, depending upon the severity of the bone loss. Vertical bitewings have their advocates as a greater proportion of each tooth is seen, but relatively few teeth are shown per radiograph and the apical areas are not consistently visible.

The quality of DPT radiographs has greatly improved in recent years and these can give an excellent overview of the jaws. However, the detail is not as good as that produced by peri-apicals and this is particularly true in the anterior region where there is often superimposition of the cervical spine (Figure 2.8). If fine detail of the entire dentition is required it is often wise to take peri-apical radiographs at the outset. This would be appropriate if there was severe periodontal disease and/or the teeth were heavily restored. In such cases it is necessary to see apical areas, bone support and furcation areas clearly. It may be tempting to take a DPT first and supplement this later with additional peri-apicals; however, if several such peri-apicals are taken, the total radiation associated may exceed that which would have been required for full mouth peri-apicals at the outset (Figure 2.9). If detailed examination of specific areas only is required, then only the appropriate and minimum number of radiographs should be taken.

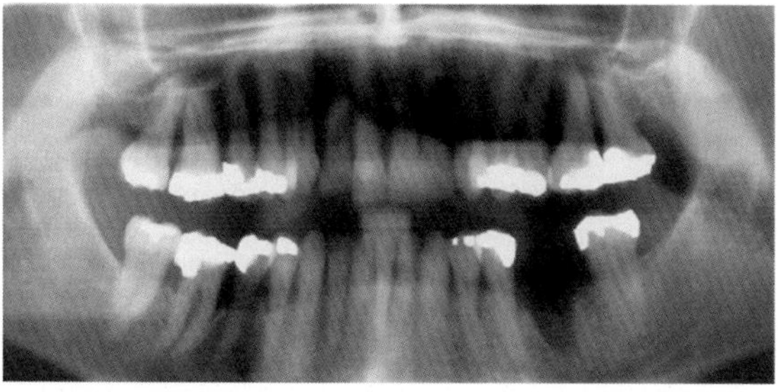

Figure 2.8 DPT radiograph of patient with moderate to severe chronic periodontitis. Note the image in the upper arch, especially in the anterior region, is unclear.

The radiographic report

Completing the radiographic report as soon as possible is an essential discipline if the diagnostic yield is to be maximized. The information gleaned invaluably informs diagnosis and treatment planning. Of particular relevance to periodontal disease, a note should be made of the presence of restoration overhangs/deficiencies that will make plaque removal impossible; such defects must be corrected if periodontal therapy is to be successful. Radiographs should be checked for the presence of calculus 'wings' although these are seen only on proximal surfaces and only if the calculus is sufficiently mineralized. Dark triangular 'arrowhead' lesions seen between the roots of multirooted teeth suggest the presence of furcation involvement though this must always be confirmed clinically. Periradicular lesions should also be noted.

Presence of periodontal bone loss can only be evaluated by looking at interproximal bone. This is because the teeth are so radio-opaque that buccal or lingual bone overlying them is obscured. Bone loss should be described under three headings: the distribution (whether localized or generalized), the pattern (whether horizontal or vertical) and the severity. Bone loss is localized if up to and including 30% of sites are affected; it is generalized if more than 30% of sites are affected. There are several methods of assessing severity but it is probably best to look at the percentage bone loss in relation to the root length.

The radiographic findings are critical not only from a periodontal point of view but also give an idea of the long-term prognosis of the tooth/teeth and suitability for use in more complex treatment plans involving indirect restorations. This having been said, it is important to remember that radiographs have distinct limitations. They give no information about soft tissues and so are not helpful when assessing pocket depth, loss of attachment, disease activity (lack of bleeding on probing) or tooth mobility. They also give no indication of the duration

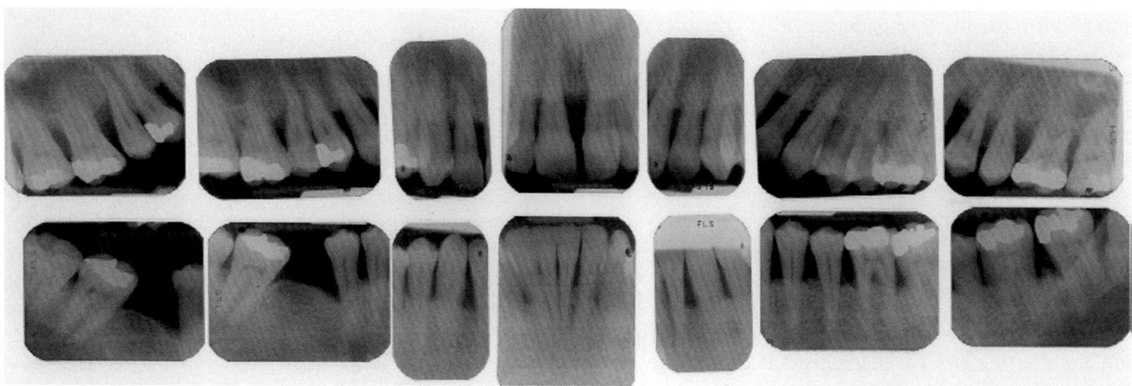

Figure 2.9 Full mouth periapical radiographs of a young patient with aggressive periodontitis. More detail is provided for each tooth compared to that obtained from a DPT. The radiation involved is justified due to the severity of the periodontal disease.

of the periodontal disease, the number of periodontal disease episodes or the timing of these episodes.

MAKING A PERIODONTAL DIAGNOSIS

A periodontal diagnosis should be formulated for all new patients, and also at all scheduled recall and any unscheduled appointments should an acute periodontal condition arise. An individual diagnosis is useful in its own right on a given day as well as being useful in a comparative way over a period of time. If a patient originally had a 'localized moderate chronic periodontitis' but over a time this had changed to become a 'generalized severe chronic periodontitis', this would highlight that the disease had become both more widespread and more severe. Again, if such changes took place over a known period of time, the rate of change would also be known. If there had been a high rate of change, advanced operative procedures would be contraindicated. This would affect treatment planning and may prompt further investigations should an underlying pathogenesis such as a systemic disease be suspected.

Periodontal diagnosis is often regarded as being a complex and difficult subject, but the reality is that there are really only three basic periodontal diagnoses. These can be modified and applied to any given situation. There has been general agreement on the classification of periodontal disease using the 1999 World Workshop system and the reader is advised to consult this for reference. The three basic diagnoses are as follows.

Periodontal stability

This is the diagnosis when two conditions are satisfied: (1) there is a lack of bleeding upon probing, implying a lack of disease activity; and (2) there are no pockets greater than 3 mm in depth (pockets shallow enough for the patient to maintain). This is the desirable situation and is more likely in patients with a low susceptibility to periodontal disease. It is also seen in successfully treated periodontal patients with higher susceptibility but it must be remembered that such patients are not cured and that recurrence of disease is possible. This is the ideal situation in which to begin planned complex restorative work provided the stability is demonstrable over a period of time.

Gingivitis

This is the diagnosis when there is bleeding on probing and there is no loss of attachment. If this is the case, two descriptors need to be applied to complete the diagnosis – namely whether the disease is localized (up to and including 30% of sites affected) or generalized (greater than 30% of sites affected). It is also important to name the type of gingivitis present. By far the most common is chronic gingivitis though the reader should consult the 1999 Classification of Periodontal Disease to see the other possibilities.

A diagnosis can then be constructed (e.g. generalized chronic gingivitis). Should localized gingivitis be present, the sites affected should be highlighted (e.g. localized chronic gingivitis affecting lower incisors and canines). There is no need to apply any description of severity of gingivitis as there is no loss of attachment. Gingivitis should not be ignored, however, as it is the precursor for periodontitis in susceptible patients which is irreversible.

Periodontitis

This is the diagnosis when two conditions are satisfied: (1) there is bleeding on probing; and (2) there is loss of attachment. If this is the case, three descriptors need to be applied to complete the diagnosis. These are:

- whether the disease is localized or generalized (assessed in the same way as for gingivitis)
- the severity of the periodontitis (based on loss of attachment (LOA); a LOA of 1–2 mm is defined as 'slight or mild', LOA of 3–4 mm is defined as 'moderate' and LOA of 5+ mm is defined as 'severe')
- the type of periodontitis (while chronic periodontitis is the most common type of periodontitis, the reader is again directed to the 1999 classification system to see other recognized conditions, including aggressive periodontitis).

In a similar way to gingivitis, a diagnosis can then be constructed (e.g. generalized moderate chronic periodontitis). Further refinements can be made to describe any given situation accurately (e.g. generalized moderate chronic periodontitis with localized severe chronic periodontitis affecting lower incisors and canines).

Aggressive periodontitis

It is worth making special mention of this particular form of periodontitis. This is not because it is very common (it affects only ~0.1–0.2% of caucasians and 2.6% of black populations.) but because there is often a strong family history in this disease and, if present, it can cause rapid irreversible loss of periodontal support leading ultimately, in some cases, to loss of teeth. It must be diagnosed as early as possible and treated effectively. There are recognized radiographic and clinical features of the condition (some of which are illustrated in Figures 2.9 and 2.10, respectively) and clinicians should be familiar with these (see Clerehugh 2004). In general, prompt referral to a specialist periodontist follows diagnosis of this condition. It is likely that treatment will involve both physical hands-on

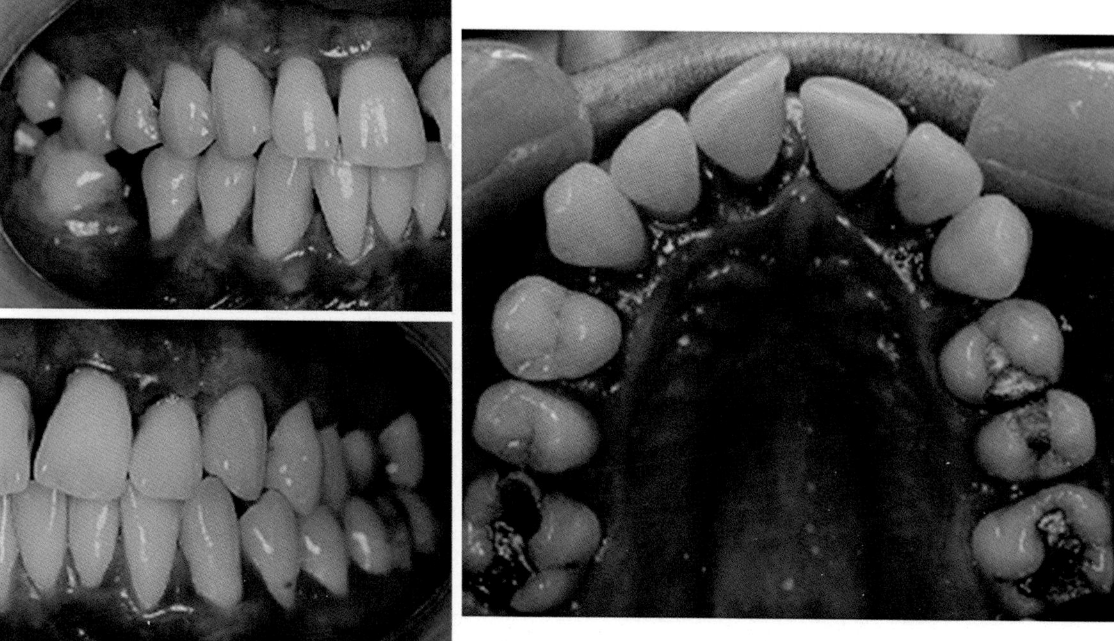

Figure 2.10 Clinical images of the patient seen in Figure 2.9. Note that plaque control is good. There is migration of both the upper right central incisor and canine. It would be easy to greatly underestimate the severity of periodontal destruction using clinical visual assessment alone.

periodontal therapy (with or without surgical access) plus prescription of systemic antimicrobials. In the past, the drug choice would have been oral tetracycline 250 mg four times per day for 2–3 weeks. Unfortunately, increasing bacterial resistance means that this is no longer as effective in some patients as it once was and a new drug regimen has been recommended. This is oral metronidazole 400 mg *plus* oral amoxicillin 250 mg, both three times per day for 1 week.

PERIODONTAL TREATMENT PLANNING

Periodontal treatment planning is straightforward and the following section gives a logical outline for the clinician to follow. It can be infinitely adapted to the requirements of individual patients, with inclusion of different permutations of the elements being necessary in some cases but not in others. There is no single complete blueprint for periodontal therapy that can be applied indiscriminately to all patients as the overall disease experienced, susceptibility and attendant risk factors vary between individuals.

The five phases of treatment planning

It is useful to consider the complete treatment plan within this framework. Whilst in this chapter there is focus on periodontal treatment planning, the same principles can be applied to other conditions such as caries and tooth wear, and a multidisciplinary treatment plan can be constructed.

Phase 1 – Relief of pain and initial examination

It is relatively unusual for periodontal disease to cause pain, but should this be the case investigation, diagnosis and relief of this is an absolute priority. The cause of the discomfort may or may not be periodontal in origin. At this point, history taking and examination of the periodontium along the lines discussed earlier would be undertaken so that a provisional diagnosis and treatment plan can be formulated.

Phase 2 – Cause-related therapy

The primary purpose of this stage is essentially to control risks. If the radiographic examination revealed caries, presence of overhangs, suggestion of furcation involvement, presence of periradicular areas, etc., these should be confirmed clinically and appropriate treatment prescribed. Treatment elements here will include whichever of the following are relevant to the patient:

- Clinical evaluation of caries, plaque retentive factors, possible furcation involvements and sensitivity testing of appropriate teeth
- Oral hygiene instruction. The plaque chart will show whether smooth surface (tooth brushing) and/or interproximal instruction is required. Where possible, interproximal cleaning is best achieved by TePe brushes of the correct size (Figure 2.11)
- Removal of plaque-retentive factors such as overhangs
- Smoking cessation advice
- Alcohol reduction advice
- Extraction of teeth of hopeless prognosis
- Scaling and polishing of teeth
- Root surface instrumentation (RSI) of sites with true pockets ≥4 mm in depth which also show BOP and where the patient has achieved excellent plaque control
- Dietary advice. This may be required if caries or erosion has been found in the mouth. A diet diary may be useful to highlight both sugar and acid sources and consumption frequency (see Chapters 1 and 4)
- Stabilization of caries if necessary.

Phase 3 – Re-examination

This stage is absolutely essential and should be timed for a minimum of 6–8 weeks after the last RSI has taken place. This time is the minimum required for healing to occur. It is hoped that completion of Phase 2 will achieve control of the periodontal disease but this is not certain. Clinical re-examination at this time (preferably with completion of new periodontal charts if they were used at the beginning of therapy) will reveal whether disease is controlled or not.

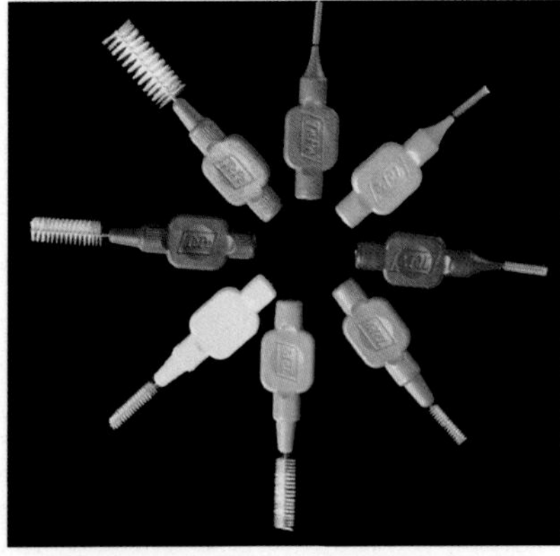

Figure 2.11 TePe brushes for interdental cleaning.

It is also at this stage that for the first time it will be possible to assess both the tissue response to treatment and patient compliance. This aspect of care is important. The time needed for re-examination is necessary to determine whether periodontal stability has been achieved or not. Complex prosthodontic treatment cannot be considered until it has.

Three outcomes are possible at this time:

- *Clear treatment success*. This is the outcome if periodontal stability has been achieved. This is the desirable outcome but it must be remembered that the patient is not 'cured'. Patients with this outcome progress directly to Phase 5 – Maintenance or supportive periodontal therapy (SPT). It is only when this outcome has been achieved should more complex operative intervention such as crowns and bridges be considered, and even then only when this stability is maintained successfully for some time – perhaps up to 6 months or even more.
- *Clear treatment failure*. This will be apparent as persistence of BOP and continued presence of pockets too deep for the patient to maintain. At this point it is essential to establish why failure has occurred and whether the reason(s) can be controlled. If this is not established, further treatment is likely to fail. Although the most common cause for failure is inadequate plaque control, there are others that include inadequate debridement, incorrect diagnosis of the condition (e.g. presence of an undetected endodontic lesion or root fracture) or the patient having a refractory response to treatment (fortunately a very rare scenario).

  If it is possible to correct the reason(s) for failure, the patient progresses to Phase 4 – Definitive treatment, with reasonable hope that a positive outcome may be achieved. If, however, it is not possible to correct the reason(s) for failure, thus leading to persistence of disease (e.g. the patient is unable or unwilling to achieve adequate plaque control), palliative care is recommended. The aim of palliative care is to keep the patient comfortable and to maintain a functioning dentition for as long as reasonably possible. Treatment will be simple – often scaling and polishing every 3 months. It is essential that the patient understands this situation and details must be entered in the patient records to avoid any future medico-legal complications should extractions become necessary. Patients on palliative care are not good candidates for provision of complicated restorative work, partly as the foundation of the dentition is compromised and partly as placement of any structures which further compromise plaque removal is likely to hasten the demise of the remaining dentition.
- *Intermediate result*. In this case there is no BOP (and thus no disease activity) but there are still some

periodontal pockets which are too deep for the patient to maintain. This outcome is common and may represent sites which are healing more slowly. As there is no disease activity, further RSI at these sites would be contraindicated. Equally, however, deep pockets which cannot be maintained by patients may become active again. At this stage RSI must *not* be undertaken. The way to deal with this apparent conundrum is to give any necessary oral hygiene instruction and perform any required scaling and polishing, and then review the patient again in approximately 1 month. At this time healing may have progressed and the patient can move into the maintenance phase (Phase 5); alternatively, the involved sites may have become active once more (BOP is present) and the probing depths are still too deep for the patient to maintain themselves. If this latter situation pertains, the patient should be managed as for 'clear failure' as described above. As always, the clinician should not proceed with advanced restorative work until stability has been achieved and maintained for sufficient time. Premature complex treatment may result in reactivation of the periodontal disease and ultimate failure of the overall treatment. Patience is rewarded!

Phase 4 – Definitive treatment

This often includes re-root surface instrumentation of sites. Should this prove ineffective, and the conditions for surgical intervention are satisfied, periodontal surgery may be undertaken. The planning of the type and extent of the surgery cannot be judged until this stage has been reached.

Only once stability has been achieved does the patient progress to Phase 5.

Phase 5 – Maintenance or SPT

This is basically a recall system that patients only commence once periodontal stability has been achieved and that aims to keep them in this stable condition. There are many factors to consider when setting the recall times but in general they will start being short (certainly no more than a couple of months if RSI was required as part of the treatment) and will lengthen only when stability is demonstrated over time.

Reaching Phase 5 does not mean that the patient remains in it in perpetuity. Should disease recurrence occur, the patient will have to re-enter the earlier phases of treatment and reach Phase 5 again only once stability has been regained. Patients thus enter, leave and re-enter Phase 5 as dictated by their disease activity. Advanced operative procedures should not be undertaken until Phase 5 has been reached and maintained for an acceptable period.

PERIODONTAL CONSIDERATIONS IN RELATION TO ADVANCED OPERATIVE DENTISTRY

Should active periodontal disease recur during or after provision of advanced operative dentistry, this must be recognized as early as possible. Failure to do this may result in rapid deterioration of the periodontal condition that may become progressively more difficult to treat. It is essential that the patient is regularly examined during this time and, if necessary, a rapid referral for advice/treatment to a specialist periodontist may be warranted.

Margin placement

It is much easier to get good impressions and thus well-fitting fixed and/or removable prosthodontics if the periodontium is healthy. The gingival margins should be stable and the tissue of good quality. This means that there should be no or limited bleeding when impressions are taken for indirect restorations such as crowns. Limited gingival retraction may be required and methods to achieve this are detailed in Chapter 13. If the tissue is healthy there should be little or no need for gingival electrosurgery.

Margin placement is of great importance and there is no doubt that, where possible, it should be supragingival. It may be tempting to place margins on visible labial surfaces subgingivally in an attempt to maximize aesthetics. This is ultimately futile as this complicates and often compromises the impression-taking process, makes checking and fitting of margins more difficult, and often results in marginal plaque accumulation. This will result in some degree of gingival inflammation that in turn results in an aesthetic deficit and often activation of ongoing periodontal disease. Gingival swelling or shrinkage may then result and, in the latter case, the margin placed subgingivally may become supragingival. It must be better to place restoration margins on visible labial surfaces just within the gingival crevice.

Temporary cover

Well constructed temporary cover is important (see Chapter 14). Poorly fitting margins, with or without cement overflow, will almost inevitably result in gingival inflammation. This increases the difficulties associated with taking impressions and fitting of final restorations. It is also true that in susceptible patients periodontal disease may be initiated or show recurrence in such circumstances, with all the ensuing potential problems of treatment at that time. In such cases the aesthetics of the final restorations may also be compromised.

Choice of advanced restorations

In the past, it was often assumed that patients with a positive history of periodontal disease were unsuitable for advanced operative dentistry. This is not true. Provided the periodontal condition has been successfully stabilized and the patient is able to maintain this, provision of well-planned and carefully executed fixed restorative work and/or implants should be considered where justified (Figure 2.12); provision of a removable prosthesis may simply compromise periodontal health.

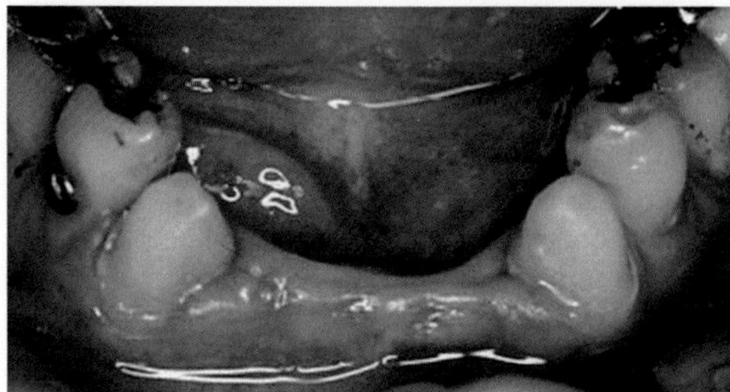

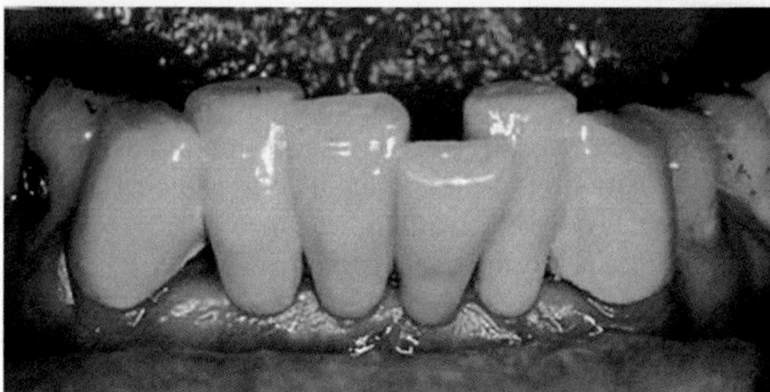

Figure 2.12 Fixed conventional bridge in a patient who has lost lower incisors due to periodontal disease. Successful stabilization of the periodontal disease has enabled fixed prosthodontic treatment. Note supragingival margins on lower canines to ensure maintenance of periodontal health.

Occlusion and the periodontium

If the periodontium is stable, application of even abnormal occlusal forces may cause teeth to become mobile but the changes which occur do not affect the supracrestal periodontal tissues. This means that occlusal trauma alone cannot initiate gingivitis or periodontitis. However, application of normal or abnormal occlusal forces to teeth which already have plaque-induced periodontal disease may result in exacerbation of the periodontal disease.

It must also be remembered that teeth with reduced periodontal support (loss of attachment, bone loss, etc., even if the disease has been controlled and is no longer active) will show signs of occlusal trauma as a result of smaller occlusal loads than would teeth with non-reduced periodontal support. It is essential in these cases in particular to carefully plan and execute restorations which will spread occlusal load efficiently throughout the dentition as much as possible and avoid high pressure on individual elements. Care must also be taken to ensure that there is consideration of the effect of the occlusion in all excursions of the mandible, including right and left lateral and protrusion. This is true at all stages of construction, including temporary coverage.

Signs of occlusal trauma may be clinical or radiographic. Clinically, by far the most important sign is progressive increase in mobility over months or weeks. Other clinical signs include migration of teeth, hypertrophy and hypertonicity of the muscles of mastication, and even signs of temporomandibular disorders (see Chapter 6). Radiographic signs include widening of the periodontal ligament space, funnel-like bone resorption of the crestal bone or loss of definition of the *lamina dura* (Figure 2.13), though this last element should be interpreted with great caution.

If teeth exhibit mobility, occlusal adjustment by spot grinding etc. will be effective in reducing this only if there is widening of the periodontal ligament. If tooth mobility is related to reduced periodontal support and/or periradicular disease, occlusal adjustment will be ineffective.

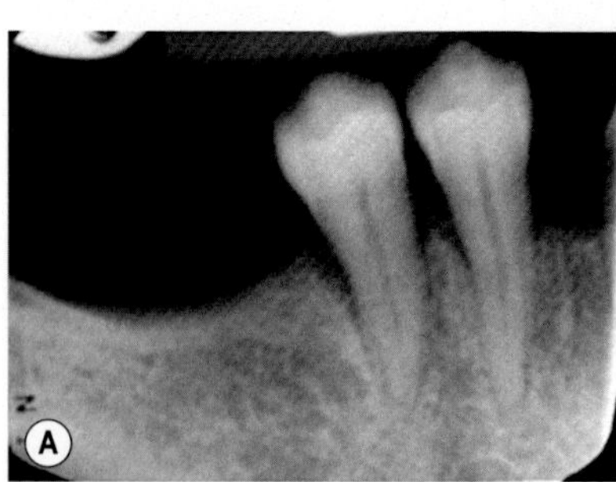

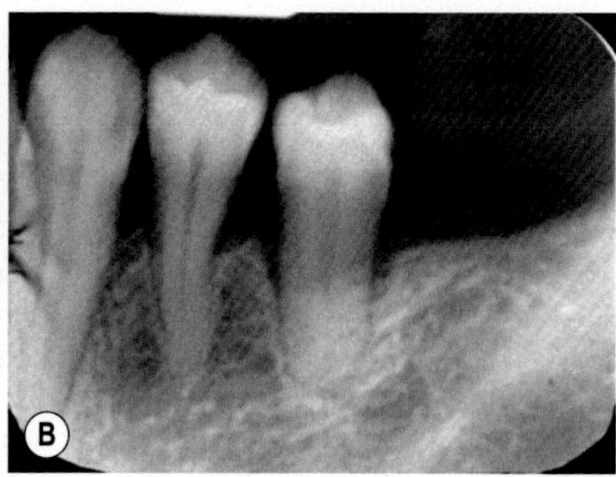

Figure 2.13 Funnel-shaped loss of crestal bone and loss of definition of the lamina dura affecting mandibular premolars as a result of occlusal trauma.

SUMMARY

This chapter has highlighted the importance of establishing periodontal health prior to advanced operative dentistry. To achieve this, a detailed examination, special tests, diagnosis and phased treatment of the periodontium has been discussed. Such a methodical and meticulous approach underpins the success and lays down the foundations for the restorations described in this textbook.

FURTHER READING

Croucher, R., 2005. Why and how to get patients to stop smoking. Dent. Update 32, 143–149.

Tezal, M., Grossi, S.G., Ho, A.W., Genco, R.J., 2004. Alcohol consumption and periodontal disease. The Third National Health and Nutrition Examination Survey. J. Clin. Periodontol. 31, 484–488.

1999 World Workshop system. In: Wiebe, C.B., Putnins, E.E., 2000. The periodontal disease classification system of the American Academy of Periodontology – an update. J. Can. Dent. Assoc. 66, 594–597.

Aggressive periodontitis

Clerehugh, V., 2004. Periodontal diagnosis in young patients. In: Wilson, N.H.F. (Ed.), Periodontal management of children, adolescents and young adults. Quintessence Publishing, London, pp. 86–89.

Hamp, S.E., Nyman, S., Lindhe, J., 1975. Periodontal treatment of multirooted teeth. Results after 5 years. J. Clin. Periodontol. 2, 126–135.

Chapter 3

Endodontic problems in advanced operative dentistry

William Saunders

CHAPTER CONTENTS

ENDODONTIC HEALTH

The health of the pulp and periradicular tissues is of paramount concern when undertaking operative and fixed prosthodontic procedures. Maintaining the health of the dental pulp is an ideal that should be realized if at all possible and consideration always given to the dental pulp when embarking upon operative care for a patient. Should the pulpal tissue become irreversibly damaged, then steps must be taken to prevent disease spreading to the periradicular tissues, or permit healing of those tissues if they are already diseased. Unfortunately, it is well known that operative procedures may cause damage to the pulp and this may be exacerbated by previous interventions. They may also cause disruption of the tooth surface, allowing subsequent entry of micro-organisms into the tooth. Pulpal disease is microbial in aetiology and it is important to prevent microbial elements reaching the dental pulp in such concentrations that irreversible damage occurs.

GENERAL ANATOMICAL AND PHYSIOLOGICAL CONSIDERATIONS

The dentine pulp complex

The dental pulp is encased within the hard tissue structure consisting of the enamel and dentine. As the dental pulp and the dentine are so inter-related it is better to consider them together as the dentine–pulp complex and hence to consider dentine as a vital tissue.

The dentine is derived from complex cells, the odontoblasts, that form a layer at the periphery of the dental pulp (Figure 3.1). The dentine forms a tubular structure, each tubule filled with an odontoblastic process. The tubules are more highly concentrated at the pulp surface than at the enamel–dentine junction. There is a diffusion gradient across the dentine that is related to the number of tubules and the thickness of the dentine. The response of the pulp to progressive injury is by the deposition of dentine (reactionary or tertiary dentine) from the intact odontoblasts and also mineralization within the dentinal tubules (peritubular dentine), thereby reducing their diameter and their ability to allow diffusion through them (Figure 3.2). Thus, the tissue has modulating effects on restorative procedures and that, combined with inherent neutralizing capabilities of tissue fluids from the pulp for both acids and alkalis, means that the amount of residual dentine thickness, after tooth preparation, is inversely proportional to the damage that may occur to the pulp after chemical application to the dentine surface. This is important when considering the use of filling materials, including temporary dressings, and bonding techniques, where an acid is applied to the dentine surface.

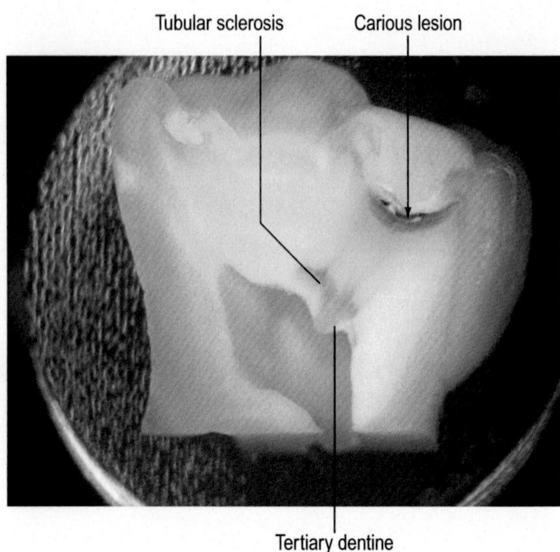

Figure 3.2 A hemisected tooth showing a carious lesion and dentine–pulp complex reactions.
(Courtesy of Dr Chris Longbottom)

Dentine is laid down throughout the life of the tooth: primary dentine as the tooth develops, secondary dentine after eruption of the tooth and tertiary dentine as a result of some insult to the tooth which may result in invasion of the dentine by bacteria or their toxic products. The aetiology of the last is usually dental caries or tooth wear, but may be induced by a restorative procedure (Figures 3.2 and 3.3). Odontoblasts are post-mitotic cells and may easily be damaged during restorative procedures. If this

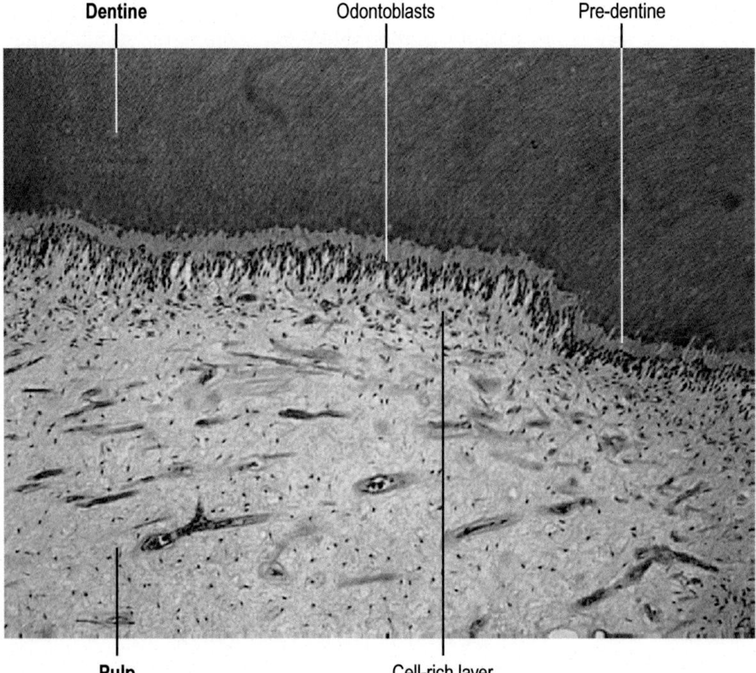

Figure 3.1 Decalcified section showing normal dentine pulp complex.

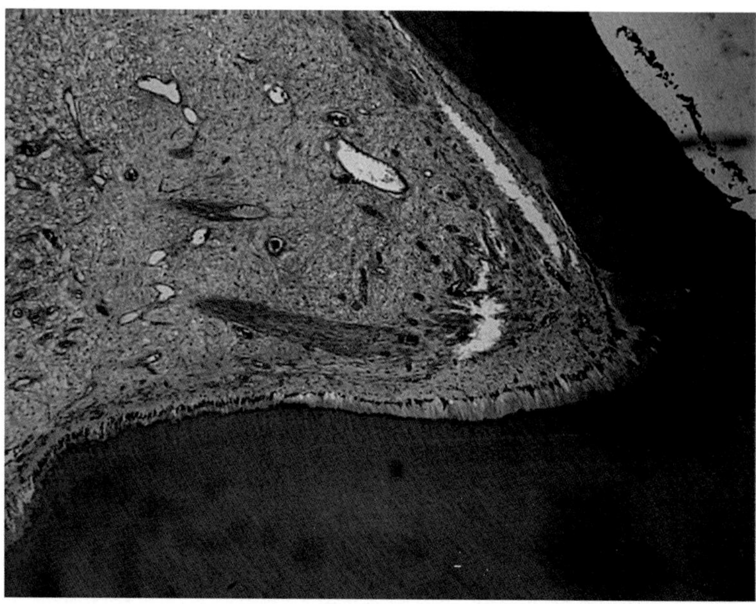

Figure 3.3 A decalcified section showing a carious lesion (top right corner) and tertiary dentine formation. The caries is likely to have been rapidly progressing as the tertiary dentine formation is less regular and has lost its tubular structure. Note the pulp is inflamed with an increased number of blood vessels and inflammatory cells.

occurs, they are replaced by stem cells from the pulp that differentiate into odontoblast-like cells and lay down mineralized tissue at the injury site. The quality of tertiary dentine is dependent upon the intensity of the insult to the pulp: in general terms, the greater the intensity of the insult (e.g. rapidly progressing caries), the more rapid the formation and the poorer the quality (Figure 3.3). Tertiary dentine is often porous, which makes it susceptible to invasion by micro-organisms and toxins. Therefore, once tertiary dentine is exposed by tooth wear or caries there is a greater risk of subsequent pulp pathology.

Nerves in the pulp

The principal elements of the dental pulp consist of stromal cells, fibroblasts, and an extensive network of nerves, blood vessels and lymphatics (see Figure 3.1). The nerves of the pulp conduct pain sensation. They consist of two main types: myelinated Aδ-fibres that conduct rapid, sharp pain sensation, and unmyelinated C-fibres that transmit the dull aching sensation that is typical of 'toothache'. In addition, nerves of the autonomic nervous system are also present. Various vasoactive neuropeptides are contained within these nerves. They are produced in the cell bodies of the trigeminal ganglion and are stored in the terminals of the nerves in the pulp. Release of these peptides causes a number of tissue reactions including changes in pulpal blood flow, blood vessel permeability and recruitment of immunocompetent cells as part of the inflammatory reaction. This is known as *neurogenic inflammation*, which may be damaging to the dental pulp. There are also effects on the growth of cells in the pulp, including fibroblasts and odontoblasts, where release of neuropeptides such as calcitonin gene-related peptide may cause the expression of bone morphogenetic protein-2 transcripts which results in more dentine formation. Recently it has been shown that fibroblasts in the pulp may also release these peptides, particularly substance P.

Pulp vasculature

The pulp shows a complex vascularity with a capillary bed adjacent to the odontoblast layer. The coronal part of the pulp has a more concentrated distribution of blood vessels than the radicular pulp. The pulp has a positive pressure compared with the outer surface of the tooth and this allows movement of fluid into the dentinal tubules. When the tubules are cut, and the tubule is patent, the outer cut surface of the dentine becomes wet as tissue fluid wells out. This provides a defensive mechanism, diluting toxic products that may enter the tubule and delivering immunocompetent cells and immunoglobulins to the surface. Unfortunately, this mechanism is usually insufficient to prevent penetration by micro-organisms, especially if the surface is heavily contaminated.

The dental pulp is often referred to as a low compliant tissue. This means that any increases in tissue pressure in the pulp – for example, by vasodilation of blood vessels during acute inflammation – may have devastating effects on the tissue because it is encased within a rigid hard tissue framework. It is essential that pathophysiological mechanisms are present to minimize such damaging effects on the pulp. Specific arteriovenous shunts may be opened to reduce damage to the capillary network and it is believed that lymphatic drainage has an important role in the reduction of tissue pressure.

Pulpal blood flow is higher than for other tissues in the oral region and is controlled by neuropeptide release and also the action of the autonomic nervous system. A transient increase in pulpal blood flow can be produced by various noxious stimuli when applied not just to the tooth in question but also adjacent teeth and adjacent tissues. This demonstrates the complexity of the nerve distribution in the oral cavity.

Pulpal defence mechanisms

The dental pulp is a complex structure that demonstrates various strategies to protect itself from injury. It has been shown to have good powers of healing through the deposition of tertiary dentine and mineralization of the peritubular dentine, even in the presence of bacterial contamination. The peritubular sclerosis gives rise to the histological appearance of translucent dentine (seen in ground sections; Figure 3.2) and the dentine in this region becomes more resistant to diffusion of bacteria and their noxious products. If, however, the damage is so severe that odontoblasts adjacent to the region of irritation die, then the tubules are left empty and are much less resistant to ingress of toxins and bacteria. These tubules are known as dead tracts.

Restorative intervention may cause damage to the pulp and it is important that the clinician is aware of this when undertaking operative procedures on the teeth and knows how best to minimize these effects.

THE EFFECT OF RESTORATIVE PROCEDURES ON THE DENTAL PULP

The effect that a restorative procedure has on the dental pulp is related to many factors. These are not only complex but also unpredictable, especially in terms of clinical outcome. They include the health of the pulp when the procedure is performed, the nature and amount of dentine remaining, the materials used for restoration, and the subsequent leakage of micro-organisms and toxins at the interface between the tooth and the restoration – a phenomenon termed microleakage.

Health of the pulp

Clinically it is difficult to tell the health of the dental pulp, especially if there are no outward clinical signs and symptoms. Previously restored teeth that require further clinical intervention may be at risk. Abou-Rass, in 1982, coined the term 'the stressed pulp'. This was a pulp that was neither healthy nor diseased but one that might be compromised to such an extent that further operative intervention would lead to irreversible damage. Taking a careful history from the patient regarding previous symptoms from, and treatment to, the tooth should be taken.

Nevertheless, the dental pulp may be injured during operative procedures on the tooth.

Preparation of the tooth

The most common method of tooth preparation is using rotating instruments in either an airotor, rotating at speeds up to 450 000 rpm, or in a slow speed handpiece that can be varied in speed from 1000 rpm to over 100 000 rpm. Cutting tooth tissue produces a smear layer, an amorphous mixture of inorganic and organic debris that blocks the cut dentinal tubules. Although the smear layer is inconsistent in thickness and distribution, it provides a barrier to bacteria, certainly in the short term. Many restorative procedures involve the removal of the smear layer, leaving open dentinal tubules which may make the pulp more vulnerable to damage by penetration of toxins and bacteria. Odontoblastic processes may also be cut during the preparation which may lead to subsequent irreversible damage to the pulp.

Frictional heat

The heat generated during tooth preparation for a restoration may cause irreversible damage to the pulp. The trauma damages the adjacent odontoblast layer and these cells can be sucked into their respective tubules. This is termed odontoblast aspiration and results in death of the cells and formation of a dead tract. These tracts are more susceptible to bacterial invasion as there is no protective outflow of tissue fluid or ability of the pulp tissue adjacent to the damaged area to form tertiary dentine quickly enough to prevent further damage to the pulp from the bacterial invasion. The microvasculature of the pulp is severely affected with plasma extravasation and a reduction in pulpal blood flow. In some cases the preparation may be so traumatic that haemorrhage occurs into the dental tubules and the pulp is irreversibly damaged immediately adjacent to the affected cut surface. If the tooth does not become non-vital then there may be an increased likelihood of internal root resorption taking place because of the local severe trauma.

Frictional heat occurs more readily with the following conditions:

- *Rotational speed on the bur*. The quicker the speed, the more damage is likely to take place.
- *Cooling the bur*. Cooling the bur, particularly with a jet of water, prevents damage to the pulp. The water must play on the whole cutting surface and for this reason a 'showerhead' water source from the handpiece is preferred. Most modern airotors have at least three water exits but it is essential that these are not blocked and sufficient water flow is present (Figure 3.4).
- *Efficiency of the bur*. A new bur should be used for the preparation of either intracoronal or extracoronal restorations. Diamond-coated burs become clogged with debris and it may be necessary to replace a bur

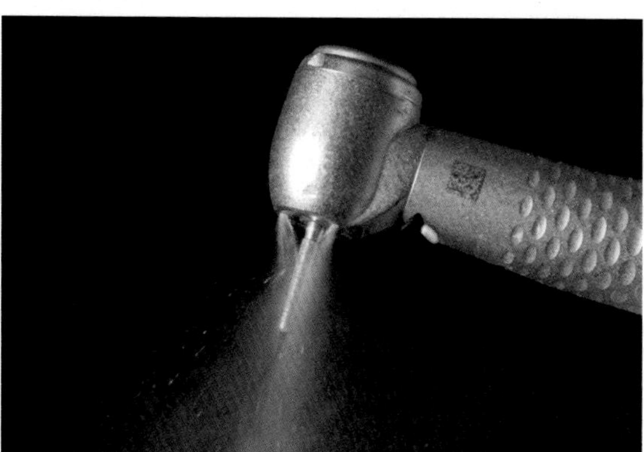

Figure 3.4 A high speed airotor with three jets of water directed to a tapered diamond bur. Good water coolant is necessary during tooth preparation.

during, for example, a full crown preparation. If the bur is blunt there is a tendency to use more force to achieve adequate cutting and the quality of modern handpieces is so good that stalling is unlikely to take place. This results in heat generation and injury.

- *Vibration*. It is believed that vibration of the tooth, especially at the frequencies generated by misaligned bearings in an airotor, may cause release of neuropeptides and induce neurogenic inflammation. It is important to check the handpiece to ensure the bur is running concentrically.

The effects of local anaesthetic

The use of laser Doppler flowmetry has shown that the delivery of local anaesthetic containing adrenaline adjacent to a tooth causes a reduction in or complete cessation of blood flow in the dental pulp. This may result in stagnation of the blood and a catastrophic fall in oxygen tension in the tissues. This does not result in irreversible damage to the pulp in most cases as the effect is present only for a short period during the duration of the local anaesthetic. However, the effects of overheating during tooth preparation are even more critical. In addition, multiple procedures on a tooth may place the pulp at risk. There is an argument to suggest that impressions using a rubber- or silicone-based material should not be undertaken at the same appointment that the preparation has been carried out on a tooth that has been anaesthetized in this way.

The effects of dental materials on the dental pulp

Following tooth preparation for indirect restorations, a temporary restoration is placed to protect the prepared tooth structure and prevent movement of the tooth. A number of temporary cements, especially those containing zinc oxide and eugenol, provide an obtundent effect on the pulp although eugenol has been shown to have toxic effects on the pulp, especially if placed in direct contact. The obtundent effect of eugenol on the dental pulp is attributed to its antinociceptive effects via the capsaicin receptor although there is some action on capsaicin-insensitive dental primary afferent neurones. In addition, eugenol has been shown to act like a local anaesthetic by inhibiting voltage-gated sodium channels and high-voltage activated calcium channel currents, and activating transient receptor potential vanilloid subtype 1. Eugenol also possesses antimicrobial properties; thus a zinc oxide–eugenol temporary dressing has sufficient free eugenol to prevent bacterial leakage. Some temporary filling materials consist of a paste-like composite-based material that hardens in the presence of fluid. This setting process may injure the underlying odontoblasts by dehydration and are thus not recommended in vital teeth.

Overall, the effects on the dental pulp of the most commonly used restorative materials is usually only mild and short-lived when there is no microbial contamination at the interface between the tooth and the material. There is evidence, however, that some inflammatory changes occur in the dental pulp in more than 50% of cases. Clinically, this reaction is probably not of consequence but it does add weight to the argument of the 'stressed pulp' condition.

Crown cementation

An informative review by Lam and Wilson (1999) concluded that sealing of the dentinal tubules after crown preparation and prior to cementation may be beneficial. Dentine bonding agents reduce dentinal fluid flow and therefore may prevent pulpal damage.

Marginal microleakage

Achieving a marginal seal at the interface between the restoration and the tooth has long been regarded as an important goal for the clinician. The presence of bacteria within this interface is associated with inflammation in the pulp. If this leakage is kept at a low level, the pulp responds defensively, with a reduction in dentine permeability and production of tertiary dentine. Nevertheless, much research has focussed on developing materials that bond to tooth structure in an attempt to reduce microleakage. Bonding to enamel is well known but there are concerns about long-term bonding to dentine. Nanoleakage arising from incomplete bonding in the hybrid layer allows penetration by fluids with subsequent degradation by hydrolysis. This will eventually allow bacterial penetration into the dentinal tubules and possible damage to the pulp.

It is important, therefore, to protect exposed dentine from bacterial penetration. The more dentine that becomes uncovered, the more dangerous it is, and the more likely that damage to the pulp will occur. A preparation for a full crown is at much more risk than a shallow cavity in an occlusal pit or fissure.

It is clear that there are risks to the dental pulp during advanced operative procedures on teeth. This damage may manifest itself in the short term with the development of symptoms of acute pulpitis with sensitivity. This may be reversible or irreversible. The latter is particularly embarrassing for the practitioner as further, often complicated treatment is required, involving time and expense, on a tooth that was previously symptomless. Root canal treatment will be required, with access to the root canal system gained through the new restoration at best, but at worst following removal of the new restoration for improved access and vision.

There is evidence to show that advanced operative treatment may cause pulpal demise in the long term. A number of studies have shown the incidence of periradicular disease in crowned teeth not previously root-canal treated to be in the region of 10–18%. Most of these lesions are symptomless and are only discovered on incidental radiological examination.

Pulpal survival is linked to the type of restoration. The pulps in teeth with single ceramic fused to metal crowns perform better than those in teeth supporting a bridge retainer (Figure 3.5). Cheung et al. (2005) showed in their clinical study that the 10-year survival for the pulp was 84.4% for crowns and 70.8% for bridge retainers. This decreased to 81.2% for the crowns and 66.2% for the bridge retainers after 15 years. The reason for the difference between single units and bridgework may be the tendency to overcut teeth for bridge retainers to ensure parallelism. This causes more operative trauma to the tooth.

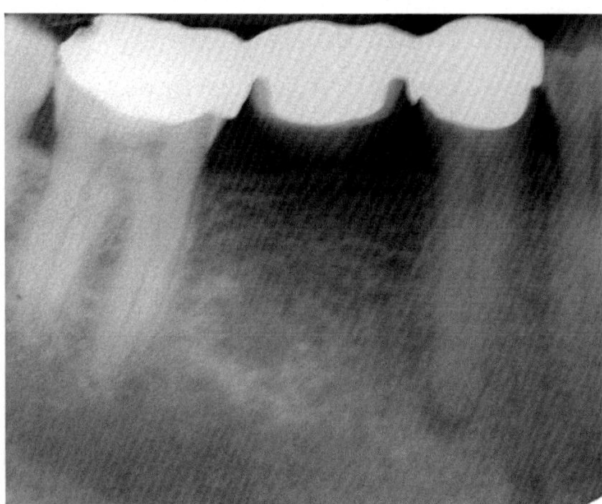

Figure 3.5 Periapical radiograph of lower right second premolar and molar teeth which have been prepared for a three unit fixed–fixed conventional bridge. The premolar tooth has a periradicular radiolucency and the distal root of the molar tooth is showing signs of root resorption.

It is important to note that the presence and quality of a coronal restoration is linked to the incidence of periradicular disease; teeth that are well restored are less likely to have periradicular disease because there is an improved coronal seal.

DIAGNOSING THE STATE OF THE DENTAL PULP

Testing pulp sensitivity

It is very difficult to diagnose the pathology of the dental pulp from diagnostic tests because direct inspection cannot be used. Indirect tests are usually employed and these generally test the sensitivity of the pulpal nerves using heat, cold (Figure 3.6) or electrical stimulation (Figure 3.7). This test is used to indicate pulpal necrosis. However, pulp vitality depends solely on blood supply and irreversible pulp damage may still be present despite a positive nerve response. More recently more sophisticated testing apparatus, using laser Doppler flowmetry or pulse oximetry, which determine blood flow and oxygen saturation levels, respectively, have also been used in research but no reliable product has been produced commercially for routine use in clinical practice.

Reliability of sensitivity testing

Although it is impossible to find a diagnostic test that provides 100% reliability all of the time, it is important to know how accurate a particular test might be. A useful study carried out by Petersson et al. and published in 1999, compared sensitivity testing with cold (ethyl chloride), heat (hot gutta-percha) and electricity (using a proprietary electric pulp tester). The results showed that the probability of obtaining a nil response in a case with a necrotic pulp was 89% with the cold test, 48% with the heat test and 88% with the electrical test. Conversely, the

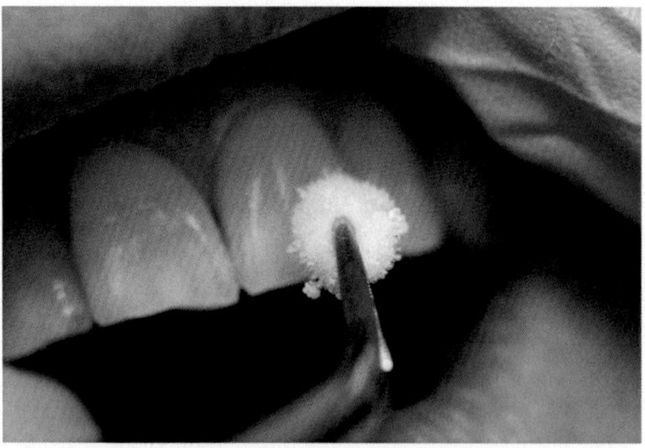

Figure 3.6 Sensitivity testing with ethyl chloride.

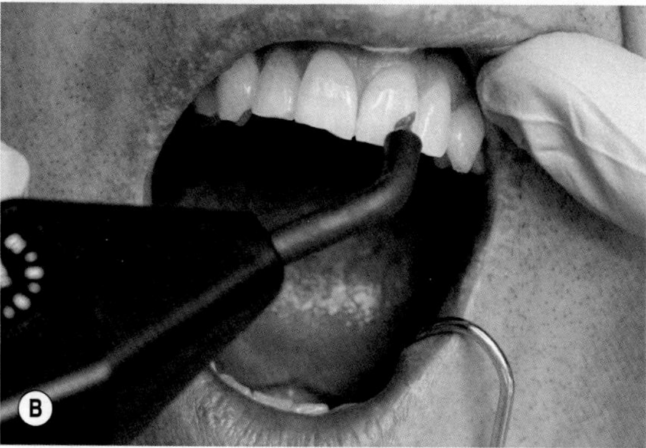

Figure 3.7 Sensitivity testing with an electrical pulp tester.

probability of a positive (sensitive) reaction representing a vital pulp was 90% with the cold test, 83% with the heat test and 84% with the electrical test. This study showed a relatively high probability that teeth not reacting to cold would have a necrotic pulp. In another study (Hyman & Cohen, 1984), however, this figure was less than a 50:50 probability. This may be because of the effect of having few teeth with extensive restorations and obliterated pulp chambers in the Petersson study. It is important to take note of how the presence of restorative materials may affect this test. A ceramic restoration provides excellent insulation but metal restorations are good conductors. Finally, the response from the patient is very subjective. For this reason it is best to test the contralateral tooth in addition to the tooth in question.

Tests using heat

A gutta-percha stick is heated and placed on the surface of the tooth. It is best to place a thin layer of petroleum jelly on the surface to prevent the gutta-percha sticking; it would be distressing for the patient if an extreme positive response was accompanied by the inability to remove the gutta-percha quickly from the tooth. In general, the heat test is not reliable and should be used only in combination with other tests.

Tests using cold

There are a number of ways cold can be applied to the tooth. Cold air, cold water or an ice stick affects fluid flow in the dentinal tubules and stimulates pulpal nerves. The most common method is the use of a cotton wool ball held in tweezers, sprayed with ethyl chloride (see Figure 3.6). As the chemical evaporates it cools rapidly to give a temperature of approximately −5°C. There is very little evidence to show that one material is better than another. When use of a dry ice stick has been compared with a refrigerant spray, 1,1,1,2-tetrafluoroethane, both have been found to be equivalent in eliciting a response, regardless of tooth type and presence of a restoration. However, the response with refrigerant spray is quicker. The use of refrigerant sprays is said to predispose to cracking of enamel because of the rapid fall in temperature, but there is no evidence for this. These sprays reduce the temperature to approximately −50°C.

Electrical testing

Proprietary electrical pulp testers are available. These send a weak electrical current through the tooth, stimulating the nerve and eliciting a pain response. There is a rheostat that allows an increasing current to be sent but there is no correlation between the reading and the state of the pulp (see Figure 3.7). Hyperaemic pulps may respond earlier than normal pulps. A bipolar device is presumed to be more accurate because the current is confined to the coronal pulp. Electrical pulp testing stimulates both Aδ and C fibres.

Clinical technique for electric pulp testing

The purpose of the test should be explained to the patient. The tooth should be dry and isolated with cotton wool rolls or a rubber dam to prevent salivary contamination. If an electrical device is being used, then a conducting medium should be placed on the probe tip (see Figure 3.7). This can be a fluoride gel or prophylactic paste. If possible, the application should be made at the incisal edge or as close to the pulp horn for maximum efficiency. Where the reaction is unclear, consider redoing the test with another device and testing teeth in a different order.

False-positive and false-negative responses to sensitivity testing can occur in a number of instances.

False-positive responses

- The use of sensitivity testing in multirooted teeth is unreliable, where a positive reaction may be elicited despite irreversible damage to the tooth. At least one root may contain vital tissue but the other roots may be necrotic.
- Improper technique (e.g. poor isolation). This could lead to contamination with superficial saliva and in the case of electric pulp testing, conduction of the electric current to an adjacent tooth or gingiva and stimulating these instead of the tooth being tested.

- An anxious patient may have a heightened perception or anticipation of a positive response.
- C-fibres may respond for a short period following loss of vitality.

False-negative responses

- Traumatized teeth. Following trauma a tooth may be concussed and not respond to sensitivity tests.
- Situations in which there is excess secondary and tertiary dentine formation (e.g. heavily restored teeth or teeth with extensive tooth wear).
- Patients with a high pain threshold.

The use of radiographs

The routine radiological image taken for examining the periradicular tissues of a tooth is the intraoral periapical radiograph. This should always be taken using a paralleling technique and with a beam-aiming device to minimize distortion of the resultant image. It is obvious that the health of the pulp cannot be seen on the radiograph; however, in a tooth with irreversible pulpitis, as the inflammation spreads through the root canal system, changes in the periradicular tissues lead to bone resorption. This is seen initially as loss of lamina dura. As the cortical plate is eroded, a radiolucency will be detected, but it may take up to 14 days for these changes to be seen radiographically. When the periradicular tissues are acutely inflamed, the tooth is usually tender to percussion and there may be tenderness on palpation in the buccal sulcus. Ultimately, if the tooth is untreated, the pulp may become necrotic and the periradicular lesion may become larger (Figure 3.8). At this stage there are usually no symptoms and a chronic periradicular periodontitis is diagnosed.

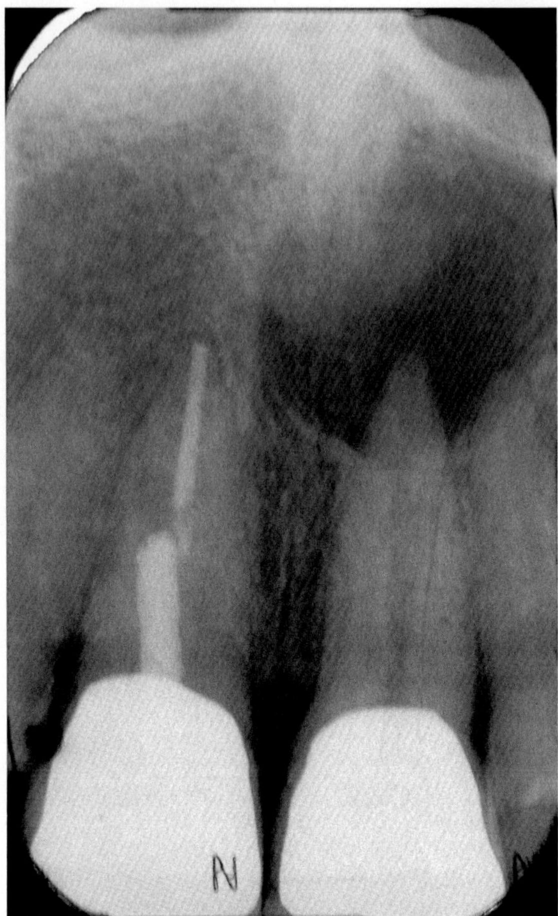

Figure 3.8 The crowned upper left central incisor has lost vitality and has a large periradicular radiolucency.

Linking symptoms to pulpal status

Symptoms of pain will also provide clues as to the state of the pulp but, unfortunately, these are not always reliable. Indeed, in the majority of cases, necrosis of the pulp occurs without symptoms. Conversely, a sharp pain that occurs spontaneously and perhaps disturbs sleep may not be easily attributed to a particular tooth, especially if a number of teeth on that side of the mouth are heavily restored or carious. There is some evidence to indicate that symptoms of pain increase as the histopathology of the dental pulp worsens. Patients presenting with intense or referred pain usually give a history of previous pain. The amount of pathology in the dental pulp can usually be determined by asking about a previous history of pain, and this may also help in determining the source of the pain in cases of referred pain.

Sharp pain

Sharp pain to cold stimuli that lasts only as long as the stimulus is present is linked to stimulation of Aδ-fibres. In these cases the pulp is usually reversibly inflamed. This pain is sometimes referred to as hypersensitivity and occurs when there are exposed dentinal tubules. Teeth affected by repeated bouts of these symptoms may develop an irreversibly damaged pulp. Hypersensitivity is related to teeth with exposed dentine and is typically seen in patients with the effects from erosion and abrasion and in teeth with gingival recession such as treated periodontal disease.

Lingering pain

Pain to hot stimuli, and occasionally cold, that lingers for minutes or hours after the stimulus is removed, is indicative of an irreversibly inflamed dental pulp, known as irreversible pulpitis (Figure 3.9). In these cases there is stimulation of the unmyelinated C-fibres, which generate neurogenic inflammation. Sometimes the pain is relieved by cold but again this is probably irreversible pulpitis.

Spontaneous pain which usually prevents the patient from sleeping is associated with severe inflammation of the pulp and irreversible pulpitis.

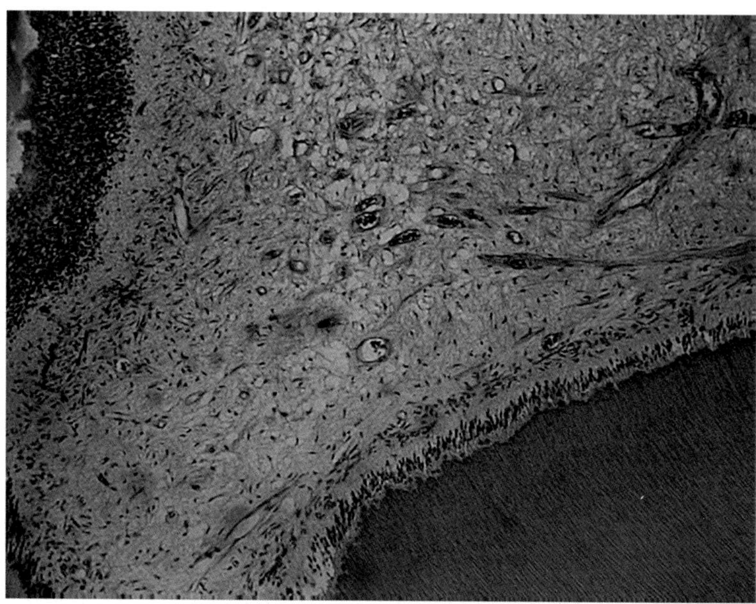

Figure 3.9 A decalcified section of a carious tooth which had symptoms of an irreversible pulpitis. Note the dense inflammatory infiltrate, top left.

Pain is a subjective emotion and pain thresholds vary from patient to patient. It is essential that a full history is taken, as well as appropriate special tests, prior to making a diagnosis of pulpitis. Acute symptomatic pulpitis progresses either to chronic pulpitis, which is usually painless, or to acute periradicular (periapical) periodontitis where the tooth becomes tender to tap, when an acute inflammatory reaction occurs in the periodontal ligament. Up until that time it may be difficult to diagnose which tooth is causing the problem.

TREATMENT FOR PULPAL INFLAMMATION

It is clear that the pulp has good reparative powers if the assault on the tissue is neither too severe nor prolonged. Teeth diagnosed with reversible pulpitis should have the pulp protected by blocking the tubule openings with a proprietary material. Those teeth with a clear irreversible pulpitis should be root-canal treated, or perhaps extracted if endodontics is not feasible, the tooth is unrestorable or is not strategic.

ASSESSING TEETH WITH PULP AND PERIRADICULAR DISEASE

Prior to treating irreversible pulpitis a clear indication of the quality of the remaining tooth structure must be made. As well as determining the presence of dental caries and the marginal integrity of the existing restoration, the clinician should carefully examine the tooth structure for cracks. This full examination cannot be done unless the restoration is removed (Figure 3.10). A study by Abbott (2004) showed that in 245 restored teeth from 220 patients referred for root canal treatment, 19.25% of the teeth had caries, 23.3% had cracks and 39.2% had marginal breakdown. However, when the restorations were removed, the incidence went up to 86.1%, 60% and 99.6%, respectively. Of these teeth, over 90% had more than one of these factors.

It is important to ascertain the extent of the remaining tooth tissue prior to embarking upon root canal treatment (Figure 3.10). It is embarrassing to undertake endodontic treatment and find that the tooth is unrestorable at the end of often complex, time-consuming and, inevitably, expensive treatment. Bandlish et al. (2006) have produced a useful system of measurement of remaining tooth structure (Figure 3.11). The crown of the tooth is divided into sextants and a score of 0–3 is given per sextant for the amount of tooth tissue remaining following preparation for the final restoration. Thus a maximum score of 18 is available for a wholly intact crown of the tooth. Consider the tooth in Figure 3.10; once the tooth has been root filled and the buccal cusp reduced for a full gold crown, for example, the restorability index will be low. It is not clear what minimum score is required before the tooth can be considered to be non-saveable and it also requires a vision of the tooth structure that might remain following final preparation. Further study of the longevity of restorations on root-filled teeth, applying these criteria, is required.

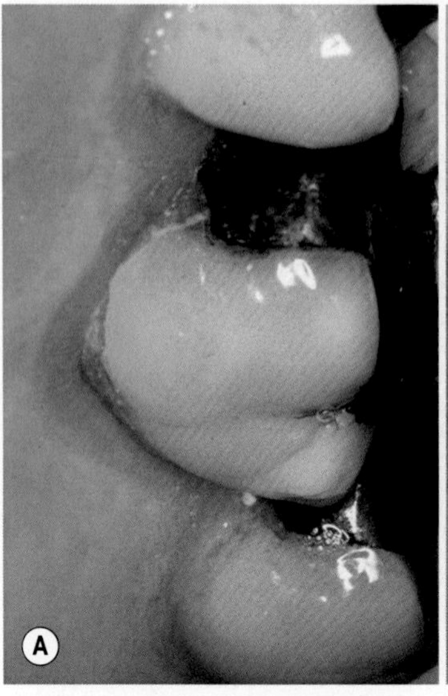

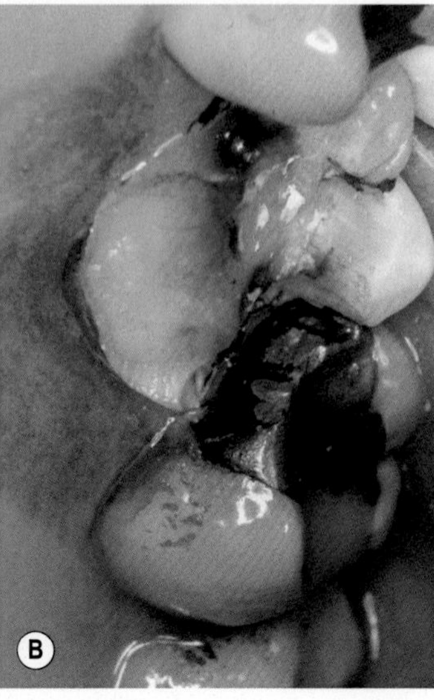

Figure 3.10 A The upper left first molar tooth is heavily restored and requires root canal treatment. It has an obvious crack palatally. The true extent of the crack can only be determined when the restoration has been removed. **B** Once the restoration was removed, the palatal cusp fractured. At this stage the restorability of the tooth can be assessed prior to carrying out root canal treatment.

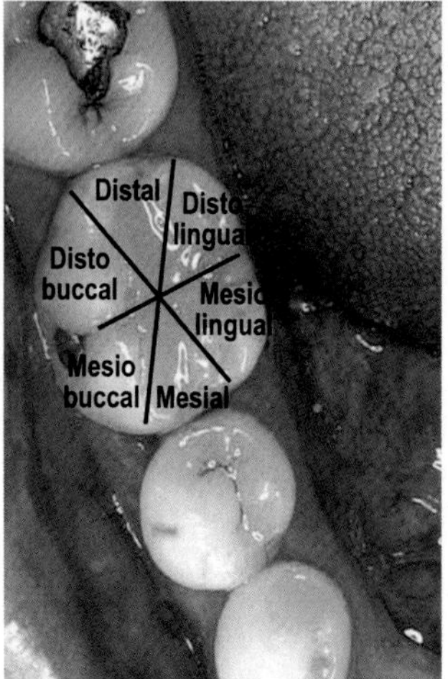

0– **None**
Two thirds or more of sextant, no axial wall of dentin or no height of dentine to support restoration

1– **Inadequate**
Inadequate coronal dentin present but inadequate to contribute to retention (wall < 1.5 mm thick)

2– **Questionable**
More dentin than 1 but cannot be confident that it would contribute to retention/resistance

3– **Adequate**
There is sufficient coronal dentin in terms of height, thickness and distribution to contribute to retention/resistance

Maximum of 18 can be scored for tooth

Figure 3.11 Assessment of the amount of remaining coronal dentine in root-treated teeth.
(Reproduced with permission from Bandlish et al., 2006)

RADIOGRAPHIC ASSESSMENT OF THE ROOT-FILLED TOOTH

If a root-filled tooth is to be restored with an indirect restoration such as a crown, or is to be used as a bridge abutment tooth, a thorough evaluation of previous symptoms is required. A good quality periapical radiograph will provide the following important information:

- *Evidence of a periradicular radiolucency.* If possible, this radiograph should be compared with an image taken immediately after the root canal treatment was completed to compare changes.
- *Quality of the root canal treatment.* The radiograph will reveal the extent of the root filling, the density of the obturation and evidence of iatrogenic damage, including faults in the preparation, perforations and fractured instruments (Figure 3.12).
- *Presence of a post.* An indication of the type of post, its shape and extent can be ascertained (see Figure 3.8).

There is now some evidence to suggest that if a periradicular radiolucency in a root-filled tooth has not reduced in size within 1 year, then the treatment has failed and should be redone, especially if the tooth is to be restored with an extracoronal restoration. Scar tissue represents only about 2% of residual periradicular radiolucencies and can thus be discounted as a reason for the radiolucency. If the root filling is extruded through the apex of the tooth, or is more than 2 mm from the radiographic apex, then the success rate is reduced.

Periapical radiographs provide only a two-dimensional view of a three-dimensional structure. This limits diagnostic reliability, especially in multirooted teeth and in the presence of superimposed anatomical structures. In addition, periapical radiography has been shown to have low sensitivity in determining the presence of a periradicular radiolucency. The recent introduction of cone-beam computed tomography (cone-beam CT) has improved diagnostic capability in endodontic cases immeasurably. Cone-beam CT produces three-dimensional images of the site of interest and these images can then be manipulated using computer software. Periradicular lesions can be detected earlier and

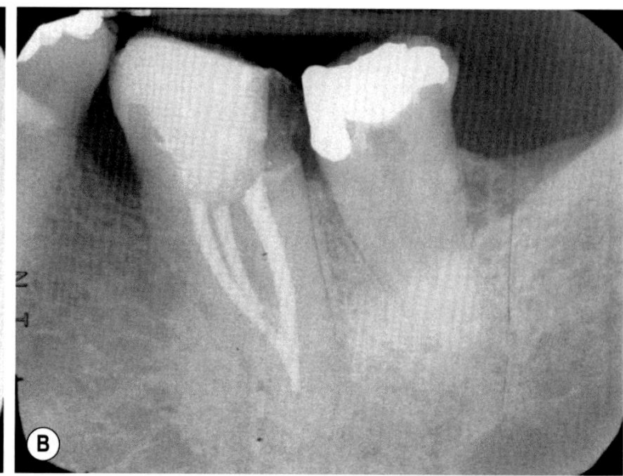

Figure 3.12 **A** Radiograph of lower second molar tooth showing fractured spiral filler in one of the two mesial canals. The obturation in the remaining canals appears to be of satisfactory length. **B** Radiograph of the tooth seen in **A**. The fractured instrument has been removed and root canal re-treatment carried out. The improved preparation and obturation clearly shows that the root canals fuse apically.

with greater consistency than with periapical radiography. Using the smallest field of view necessary it is possible to reduce radiation exposure to those of periapical radiography. Whilst cone-beam CT images are, at this stage, not recommended for all endodontic cases, they can be used in circumstances when diagnosis may otherwise be difficult or where non-surgical or surgical root canal treatment is being considered.

SURVIVAL OF ROOT-CANAL TREATED CROWNED TEETH

Patients may have concerns regarding the longevity of crowned teeth that have been root canal treated. For example, would it be more advantageous to have the tooth extracted and replaced by an implant-retained restoration? A systematic review of studies concerning the survival of root-filled teeth was undertaken by Stavropoulou and Koidis (2007). They were able to find 10 clinical studies that were suitable to be analysed. Root-canal treated teeth with a crown had a 10-year survival rate of 81%, compared with 63% for those root-canal treated teeth with a direct restoration. Other studies have also demonstrated that crowned teeth with good quality root fillings survive as well as crowned teeth that are vital.

So how might a root-canal treated tooth fail and why should carefully restoring such teeth be advantageous?

- *Structural integrity*. Root-canal treated teeth are, in general, compromised structurally. They often have lost a lot of tooth structure already and this, combined with cutting an access cavity and removing the roof of the pulp chamber, makes the tooth weaker. The preparation of the coronal part of the root canal system using rotary instruments, especially Gates Glidden and Peeso burs, may remove excessive amounts of tooth structure if not executed carefully.
- *Microcracks*. The dentine of root-canal treated teeth does not become harder, even 10 years after the treatment, but microcracks have been noted in the tooth structure of root-filled teeth. Occlusal forces may allow these cracks to propagate and lead to catastrophic failure of the tooth whilst in function (Figure 3.13).
- *Occlusal forces*. It has been shown that root-filled teeth are able to tolerate up to twice the occlusal load compared with vital teeth. This indicates that proprioceptive nerves fibres are almost certainly present in the pulp which sense occlusal forces that are applied and help prevent overload.
- *Chemical changes in the dentine*. It is known that some root canal sealers containing zinc oxide and eugenol have an effect on the physical properties of dentine. Zinc has been shown to migrate into dentine at the expense of calcium but the effect on the mechanical properties of the dentine is unknown. Eugenol also has an effect, increasing the hardness of the dentine but this reaches a maximum in 3 weeks.
- *Irrigants*. Irrigants used in root canal treatment also have been shown to have a negative effect on the mechanical properties of dentine. Sodium hypochlorite has been shown in some studies to have an effect and chelating agents such as citric acid and ethylene diamine tetra acetic acid (EDTA) remove the mineralized component of the dentine.

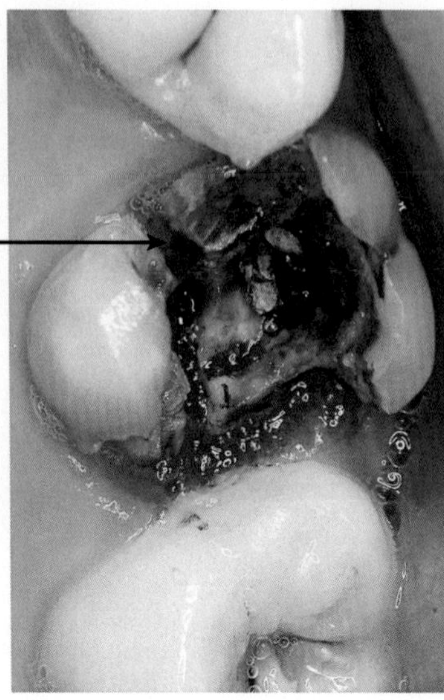

Figure 3.13 Vertical root fracture of a root filled molar tooth (arrowed). The loss of both mesial and distal marginal ridges, combined with removal of the roof of the pulp chamber, has weakened the tooth catastrophically.

- *Microbial action on dentine*. The interaction of microbes and food substrate, releasing acid, may also have an effect on the mechanical properties of the root dentine and, of course, dental caries at the root face will have a serious negative effect on tooth strength.
- *Microbial leakage*. Coronal leakage of micro-organisms, their by-products and nutrients has been shown to have a deleterious effect on the prognosis of root-filled teeth. All root canal filling materials leak and research has shown that gutta-percha, the most commonly used root canal filling material, does not resist leakage at its interface with the sealer. In addition, the dentinal tubules may be invaded by micro-organisms when the interface between the sealer and the root canal wall is disrupted. These bacteria then provide a reservoir for reinfection of the apical part of the root canal system which may cause the persistence or redevelopment of periradicular disease. Prevention or at least reduction of coronal leakage may be achieved by ensuring that a well-fitting, leak-proof restoration is placed after root canal treatment is completed. A base placed across the floor of the pulp chamber and the openings to the root canals has been shown to delay the initiation of periradicular disease and reduce the severity of inflammation in the periradicular tissues should periradicular periodontitis develop.

SUMMARY

It is clear that every effort should be made to prevent damage to the dental pulp during operative procedures. This relies, to a large extent, on the skill and knowledge of the practitioner. Care to protect the pulp during the preparation and subsequent restoration of the tooth is essential, bearing in mind the number of iatrogenic causes of pulp damage. This is particularly important in teeth that have been restored previously. Bacterial microleakage at the interface between the tooth and the restoration must be reduced and this is achieved by ensuring that the restoration adapts well to the tooth and, if possible, some micromechanical bonding of the restoration to the tooth structure is achieved, using specific techniques.

Should the pulp of the tooth become irreversibly damaged then the treatment options are either extraction or root canal treatment. The longevity of root-filled teeth depends on many factors but a proper restoration that protects both the remaining tooth structure and the root filling is essential.

FURTHER READING

Abbott, P.V., 2004. Assessing restored teeth with pulp and periapical diseases for the presence of cracks, caries and marginal breakdown. Aust. Dent. J. 49, 33–39.

Abou-Rass, M., 1982. The stressed pulp condition: an endodontic–restorative diagnostic concept. J. Prosthet. Dent. 48, 264–267.

Bandlish, R.B., McDonald, A.V., Setchell, D.J., 2006. Assessment of the amount of remaining coronal dentine in root-treated teeth. J. Dent. 34, 699–708.

Cheung, G.S., Lai, S.C., Ng, R.P., 2005. Fate of vital pulps beneath a metal–ceramic crown or a bridge retainer. Int. Endod. J. 38, 521–530.

Hargreaves, K.M., Goodis, H.E. (Eds.), 2002. Seltzer and Bender's dental pulp. Quintessence Books, Chicago.

Hyman, J.J., Cohen, M.E., 1984. The predictive value of endodontic diagnostic tests. Oral Surg. Oral Med. Oral Pathol. 58, 343–346.

Lam, C.W., Wilson, P.R., 1999. Crown cementation and pulpal health. Int. Endod. J. 32, 249–256.

Petersson, K., Soderstrom, C., Kiani-Anaraki, M., Levy, G., 1999. Evaluation of the ability of thermal and electrical tests to register pulp vitality. Endod. Dent. Traumatol. 15, 127–131.

Stavropoulou, A.F., Koidis, P.T., 2007. A systematic review of single crowns on endodontically treated teeth. J. Dent. 35, 761–767.

Chapter | 4 |

Tooth wear

David Bartlett

CHAPTER CONTENTS

INTRODUCTION

Tooth wear is a common clinical finding and may cause diagnostic and management challenges. The early signs of tooth wear are almost universally present in adults but the more severe forms probably affect around 10% of the population. Essential to planning the long-term care of patients with tooth wear is identifying the cause, when to start prevention and when to intervene with operative management, which in most cases involves advanced restorative techniques.

DEFINITIONS

- *Erosion*. The loss of tooth structure caused by acids and not involving bacterial fermentation is called erosion. Acids demineralize the outer surface of enamel or dentine, increasing its porosity. Optimum concentrations of fluoride and calcium may allow some remineralization; however, if another exposure to acid or other forms of tooth wear attack the surface layer, then tooth tissue will be lost.
- *Abrasion*. Abrasion is the mechanical wear of teeth from forces other than teeth.
- *Attrition*. Attrition is the wear of tooth against tooth. It is uncommon to observe the singular effects of erosion, abrasion or attrition and more commonly it is a combination.
- *Abfraction*. Laboratory studies using finite element analysis have hypothesized that a condition called abfraction might occur. This is based on the fact that excessive lateral occlusal forces on teeth cause microscopic flexure, leading to cyclic stress concentration in the cervical area with resultant loss of tooth tissue (Figure 4.1). Although some researchers claim an association between bruxism and abfraction lesions, this theoretical phenomenon has yet to be proven clinically. The lesions that result cannot be differentiated from those that occur as a result of cervical erosion and abrasion. The multifactorial nature of tooth wear will also hinder proof of this hypothesis clinically.

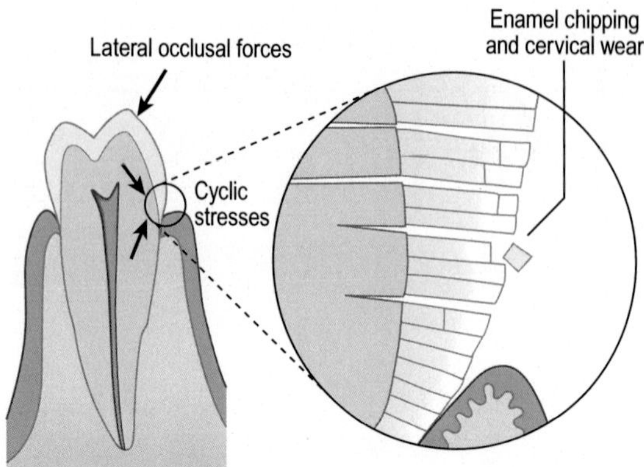

Figure 4.1 Diagrammatic representation of the stresses created at the cervical margin of a premolar tooth due to repeated lateral occlusal forces, leading to chipping and wear of the cervical area.

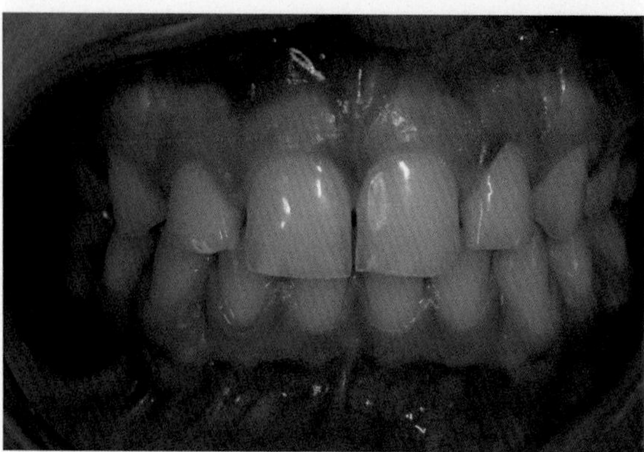

Figure 4.2 In the early stages of wear the anatomical features of the tooth become indistinct and features such as mamelons are worn away.

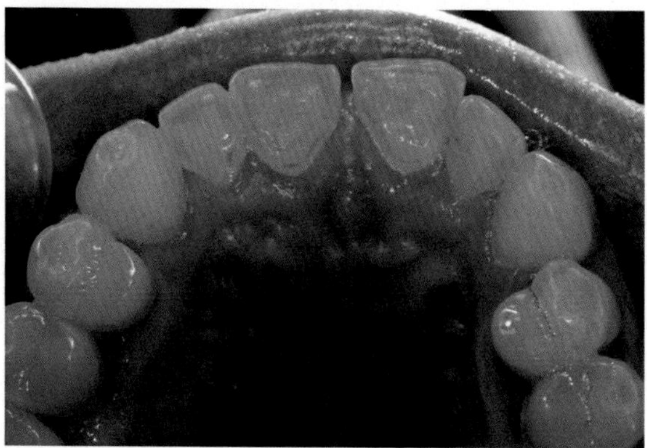

Figure 4.3 The appearance of erosive tooth wear on the palatal surfaces of the upper incisors. Note the exposed dentine centrally and the peripheral rim of enamel.

CLINICAL APPEARANCE

As tooth wear normally presents as a combination of erosion, abrasion and attrition, it is difficult to isolate the impact of the various components. However, there are clinical features which are specific to erosion, abrasion and attrition which can help with the diagnosis.

Anterior teeth

In the early stages of wear the anatomical features of the tooth become indistinct and lose features such as mamelons (Figure 4.2). Erosion results in a glassy appearance, particularly on the facial/buccal surfaces of the upper anterior teeth. As the condition deteriorates, the effects become more pronounced and widespread. Early stages involving enamel wear can be difficult to identify, particularly around the cervical margins of teeth. Localized and extensive lesions limited to enamel will be visible but generalized changes can sometimes be difficult to assess.

Once dentine is exposed, the difference in colour compared with enamel will make the diagnosis clearer. On the palatal surfaces of upper anterior teeth the complete loss of the enamel exposes the dentine, giving the characteristic appearance of perimolysis (Figure 4.3). This is a condition that can arise from chronic vomiting or regurgitation. It is also thought that the rough surface of the dorsum of the tongue may act as an acid reservoir and an abrasive, increasing the tooth wear and producing the characteristic highly 'polished' palatal surfaces with a rim of enamel (Figure 4.3). If the wear process proceeds, the gradual undermining and thinning of the incisal edges of the teeth causes fractures of the enamel and dentine and increases the translucency. The presence of incisal translucency is indicative of a late stage and signifies considerable tooth wear on the palatal surfaces of the upper anterior teeth (Figure 4.4).

Wear along the cervical surfaces of teeth is often mistakenly referred to as abrasion. However, the abrasive nature of modern toothpastes and toothbrushes makes abrasion unlikely. Mechanical wear will occur with overzealous brushing but the formation of V-shaped lesions along the cervical margin (Figure 4.5) is often related to a combination of abrasion and erosion. Historically, textbooks have shown images of rare causes of abrasion, such as that from pipe smoking or where seamstresses have used their teeth to cut thread. However, in today's society, there is a new threat that the dentist needs to be aware of: body piercings. Figure 4.6 shows the amount of tooth wear that has occurred due to the parafunctional chewing of a tongue piercing. Such piercings have also

Figure 4.4 A late stage effect of palatal tooth wear is incisal translucency seen from the labial surface. The loss of palatal enamel and dentine results in thinning of the tooth, increasing its translucency.

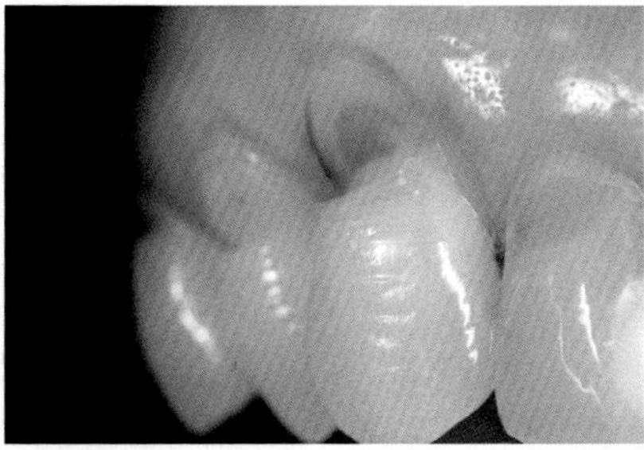

Figure 4.5 Cervical wear is normally found on the buccal surfaces of canines and premolars, producing these characteristic V-shaped lesions.

been the cause of other intraoral complications such as gingival recession.

Frequent acidic challenges may cause dentine sensitivity, particularly following cold stimuli. Dentine sensitivity results from fluid movement within the dentinal tubules which stimulates pulpal nerves – the so-called 'Brännström's hydrodynamic theory' of dentine sensitivity. Tubule fluid movement is caused by expansion and contraction of the fluid as a result of temperature changes or due to changes in osmotic pressure, typically with sweet foods. Normally the dentinal tubules are blocked by smear layer plugs which resist this fluid movement; however, frequent acid attacks can remove these plugs allowing fluid movement and dentine sensitivity.

The presence of staining on enamel or dentine can give an estimation of the progression of erosive tooth wear. A stain-free surface can suggest that any acid erosion is active whilst a stained surface suggests the process is inactive. The successful implementation of dietary controls will have an effect on the progression of erosive tooth wear, with the teeth becoming progressively more stained as the process becomes inactive (Figures 4.7 and 4.8).

Molar teeth

In the early stages discrete circular cavities may appear on the occlusal surfaces of molar and premolar teeth. These cavities, unlike caries, are hard and have a halo of whitened enamel surrounding the deeper yellow of dentine (Figure 4.9). The cause of these lesions is normally associated with erosion but some contribution from abrasion may also be possible. This is often referred to as 'cupping out' of the cusp tips, but may also be seen in relation to the incisal edges of the anterior teeth. If the process deteriorates, the discrete cavities join and the lesion increases in size. If the erosion is rapid and severe, the cusp tips or incisal edges of one or more opposing molar, premolar and/or anterior teeth may appear not to meet on closure into the intercuspal position (Figures 4.10 and 4.11) and, where present, gold, amalgam or composite restorations appear to be proud as the surrounding tooth structure wears at a greater rate than the restoration (Figure 4.12).

If the cause of the wear is predominantly attrition, the occlusal surfaces of either anterior or posterior teeth from

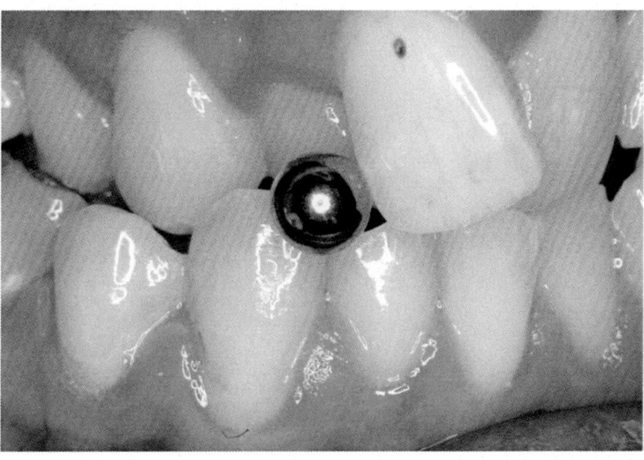

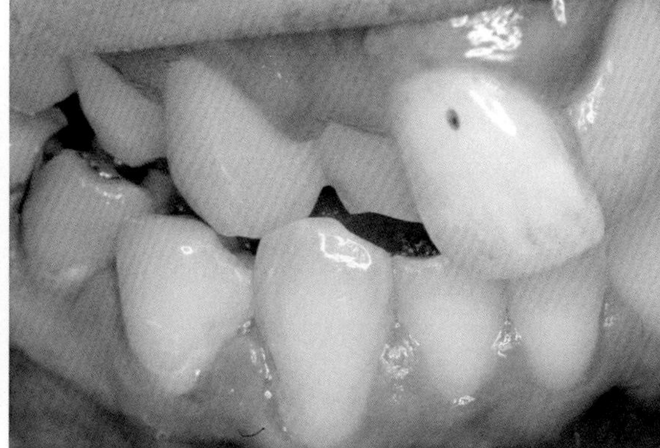

Figure 4.6 Parafunctional chewing of a tongue piercing (left) has led to wear of both upper and lower teeth (right).

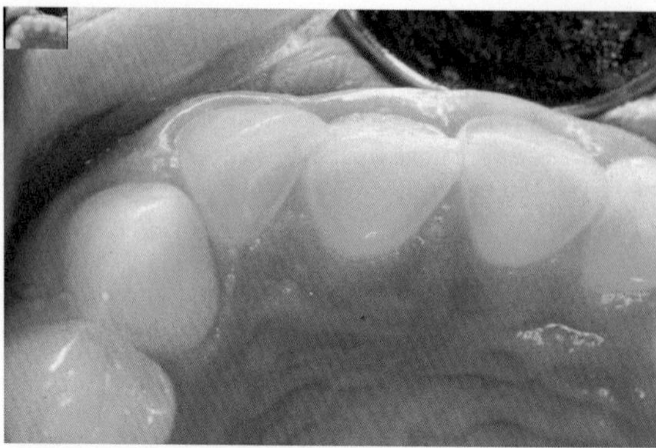

Figure 4.7 The appearance of an unstained tooth surface is suggestive of an active erosive process occurring.

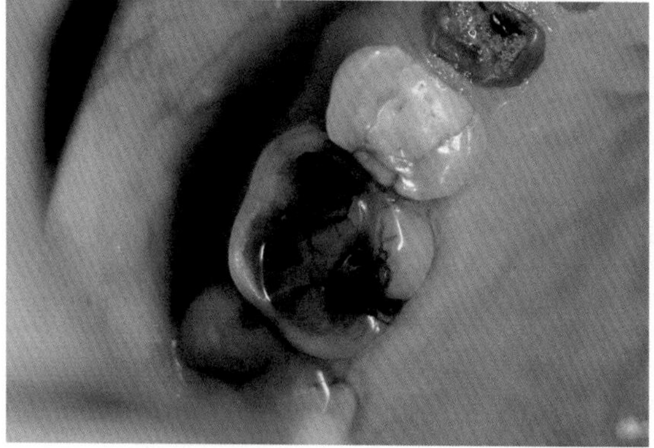

Figure 4.8 When erosion becomes inactive, the teeth become progressively more stained as dietary products accumulate on the tooth surface.

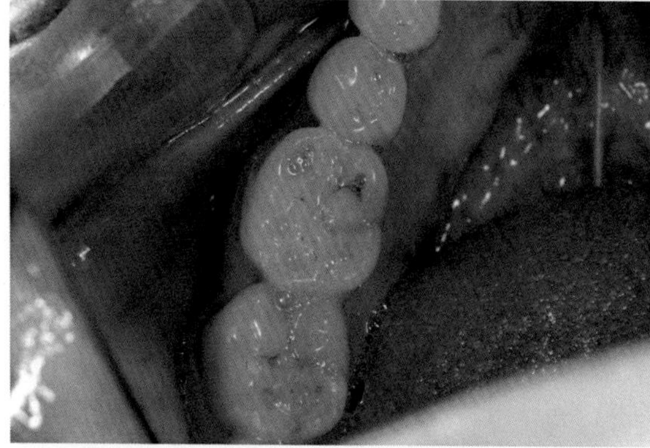

Figure 4.9 Small and discrete cavities formed on the occlusal surfaces of molar and premolar teeth are typically associated with erosion. There may also be an abrasive component, often referred to as 'cupping out' of the cusp tips.

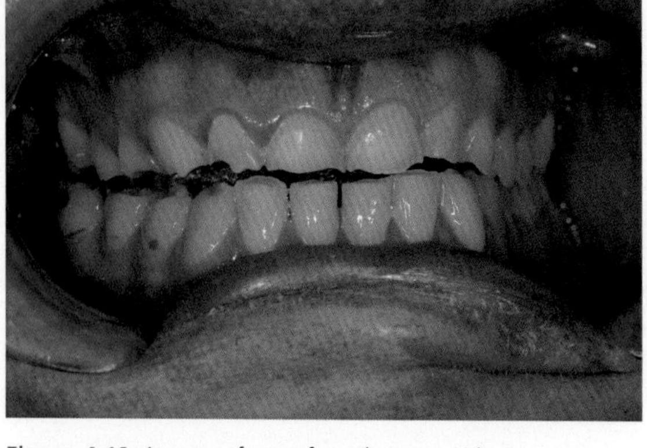

Figure 4.10 A severe form of tooth wear with a predominantly erosive component resulting in the loss of occlusal contact with the opposing teeth. Note only the most posterior teeth are in contact.

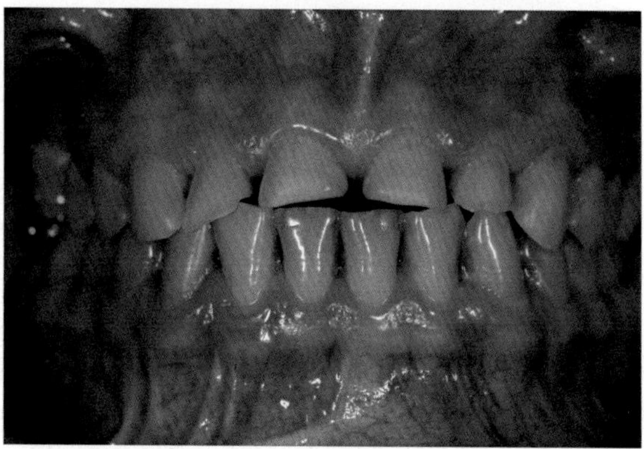

Figure 4.11 When acid erosion is predominant the loss of occlusal or incisal tooth structure will prevent contact between the opposing teeth.

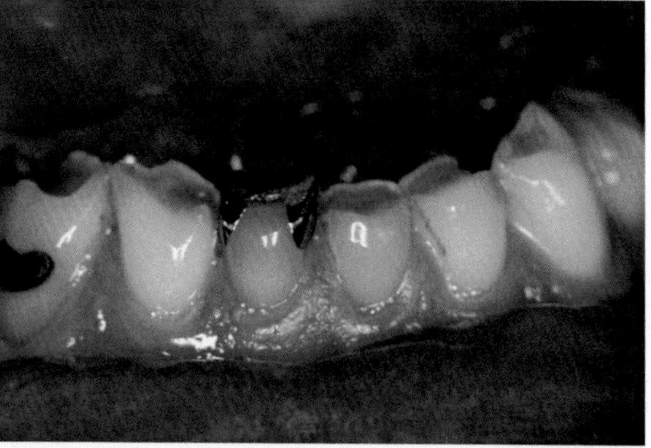

Figure 4.12 The gold restoration on the lower right central incisor tooth now stands proud following a greater differential wear of tooth tissue as a result of erosion and attrition.

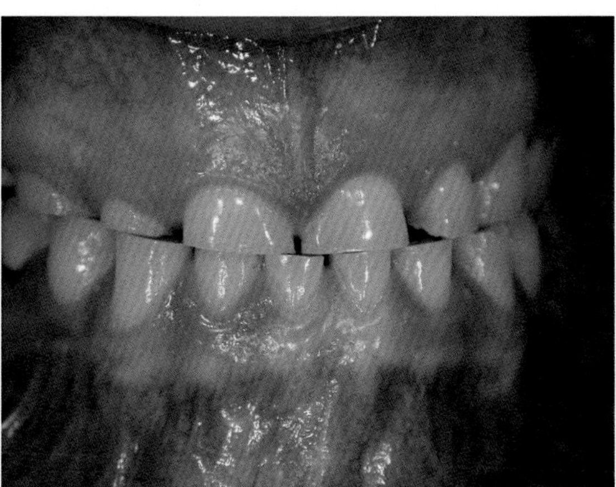

Figure 4.13 Attrition is the wear caused by action of tooth against tooth, and the matched flattening of the incisal edges seen here is characteristic.

both dental arches demonstrate paired wear facets, but in more severe cases they may appear flattened, almost as if they have been filed (Figure 4.13) and the opposing cusps or incisal edges meet and closely interdigitate in the intercuspal position. Typically in severe cases fractured restorations are found following the excessive occlusal loading from the opposing teeth (Figure 4.14).

Sensitivity

Dentine sensitivity is a sign of acid erosion and normally occurs in patients with meticulous oral hygiene. The symptoms are a sharp, short duration pain or sensitivity when cold is applied to the teeth. It normally is most common along the cervical margins of teeth and frequently occurs in association with cervical wear. The aetiology is almost certainly a combination of erosion and abrasion but the role of acids is often ignored. Dentine sensitivity is relatively uncommon on surfaces other than the cervical areas. This is thought to be related to the formation of a smear layer sealing the dentinal tubules, whereas along the cervical margin the frequent removal of the smear layer by tooth brushing increases the risk of sensitivity developing. There are no signs or symptoms to indicate that tooth wear is active apart from the presence or absence of stains on the teeth. Since dentine sensitivity is thought to be an indicator of activity, if it is present alongside a clean, unstained tooth surface particular care should be taken when monitoring progression.

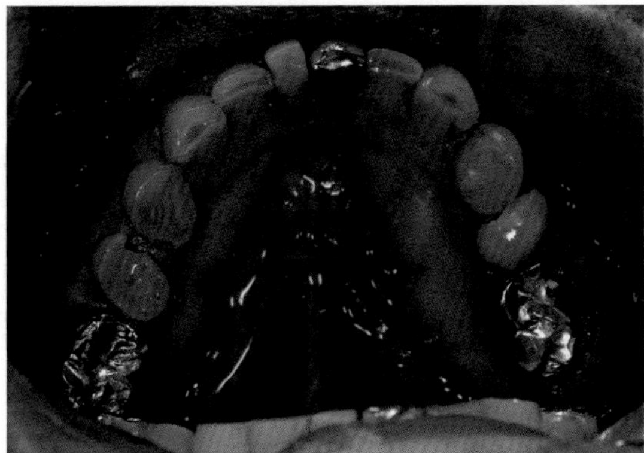

Figure 4.14 The effect of bruxism on the occlusal surfaces of premolar and molar teeth has caused a gradual flattening of the teeth. Often the high occlusal loading causes fracture of restorations which can be seen here on both direct and indirect restorations.

AETIOLOGY

Erosion

The most common cause of erosion is the frequent consumption of acids (extrinsic acids). The strength of the dietary acid is also important. Strong acids with low pH and high titratability will cause demineralization of the hydroxyapatite in the teeth (Table 4.1). The titratability is defined as the volume of alkali needed to neutralize an acid. Common examples of foods which contain strong dietary acids are citrus fruits. Whilst the intake of dietary acids is recognized as being potentially erosive, probably the most important component is the frequency of consumption. Some dietary habits such as sipping acidic drinks or snacking on fruits result in prolonged drops in oral pH which, when combined with other forms of wear such as attrition or abrasion, cause tooth wear. There is an increasing body of evidence to implicate dietary acids (particularly strong acids) in prevalence studies on tooth wear.

Table 4.1 Common dietary acids associated with acid erosion

EROSIVE POTENTIAL	DIETARY SOURCE
High erosive potential (fruit or fruit juices)	Citrus fruits (lemons, grapefruit, oranges, limes) Apples Cranberries Grapes
Medium erosive potential	Cola drinks Vinegar White and red wine
Low erosive potential	Beer Carbonated water

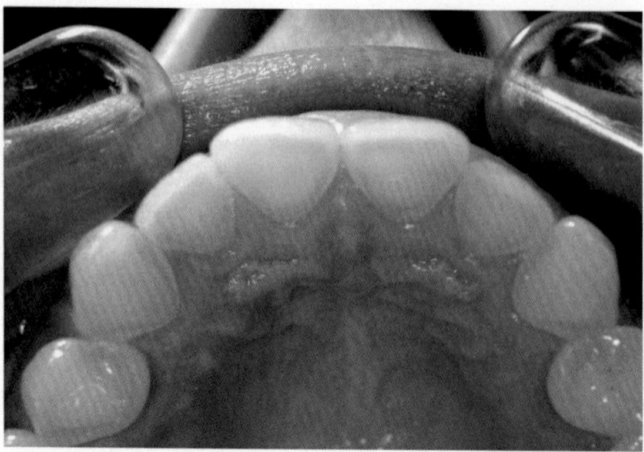

Figure 4.15 The appearance of palatal dental wear caused by gastric regurgitation is typically seen in patients with eating disorders and reflux.

The other major cause of erosion is the effect of gastric acids (intrinsic acids) associated with eating disorders or regurgitation. Anorexia and bulimia nervosa are relatively uncommon disorders predominantly affecting females between the ages of 13 and 20 years old. Sufferers use dietary restriction or vomiting to control their body image. Anorexia is more commonly associated with a low body weight and has other health-related problems such as amenorrhoea, low body mass and low metabolic rates to name but a few, whilst bulimics have a normal body weight but use binge eating and vomiting to control their weight. The distinction between the two conditions may merge, with some anorexics passing through bulimic phases and bulimics entering anorexic periods. The outcome on teeth is palatal dental erosion which is often severe (Figure 4.15).

Regurgitation of gastric juice resulting from an underlying gastro-oesophageal reflux condition is the other major cause of gastric acid passing into the mouth. In some situations the symptoms of reflux (heartburn, epigastric pain, regurgitation) are present but in around 25% there are no symptoms. The outcome on the teeth has an identical appearance to that of patients with an eating disorder. Irrespective of the cause of gastric juice entering the mouth, the outcome on the teeth is generally more severe than that found with dietary erosion. Fortunately, gastric causes of erosion are relatively uncommon but generally the severe cases result in the need for specialist prosthodontic care.

Abrasion

Although the cause of cervical tooth wear has been traditionally associated with overzealous tooth brushing (see Figure 4.5), most of the laboratory studies have shown that normal forces with tooth brushing, with or without toothpastes, is unlikely to cause significant wear on enamel or dentine. However, if excessive force is applied the mechanical action from the tooth brushing may result in wear and this normally appears on the cervical margins of premolar and canine teeth. Concurrent dentine sensitivity can indicate an erosive component to the wear and is successfully managed with dietary advice, together with non-traumatic tooth brushing instruction. The importance of abfraction along the cervical area, predisposing the surface to erosion or abrasion, is unknown.

Attrition

Wear from tooth to tooth contact is a common finding, with facets appearing on teeth used in guidance (e.g. canines and premolars). More severe forms of attrition occur with habits such as bruxism where continual and prolonged loading of teeth causes significant occlusal wear (see Figure 4.13). The reason for a bruxism habit is unknown but some component of stress causing repeated tooth clenching or grinding is acknowledged by most clinicians (see Chapter 6). Others suggest occlusal interferences may trigger the grinding or clenching habits, but since interferences are so common in asymptomatic subjects this association remains unproven.

MANAGEMENT OF TOOTH WEAR

Early detection and monitoring

There is no justification to believe that tooth wear inevitably leads to the total destruction of teeth. In some individuals the extent of the tooth wear may compromise the longevity of the tooth but in most the progression is slow and is part of the ageing process. This is an important factor as the severity of the tooth wear must always be balanced against the patient's age. For example, a degree of tooth wear seen in a 70-year-old patient may be regarded as normal 'wear and tear'; however, if the same amount of wear was seen in a 20-year-old patient, alarm bells might sound.

As with dental caries, the most important aspect to the management of tooth wear is early detection and identification of risk factors. Reducing the effect of these risk factors, which have been discussed previously in this chapter, can prevent further progression of the wear. For many patients whose tooth wear has been identified by their dentist and managed in this manner, monitoring is an effective and acceptable procedure even though there is no attempt to restore the shape and appearance of the teeth. Other patients may present with specific complaints or concerns in relation to the wear of their teeth and it is important to identify what these are and address them. The main issues that arise from tooth wear are:

- Poor appearance
- Poor function
- Sensitivity
- Concerns about continued wear.

One of the main challenges with restoring teeth with wear, which both dentist and patient have to be aware of, is the immediate and long-term cost of care and maintenance. With this in mind most patients presenting with concerns over continued tooth wear will be happy to accept preventive advice and monitoring; the reassurance given that the condition is not deteriorating with time is all that they require. Indeed, many of those concerned about appearance and function will also reflect and accept this advice as the restoration of worn teeth is normally expensive and can require specialist levels of care, mainly because it rarely affects single teeth and more commonly involves sextants, quadrants or even entire arches.

Sensitivity can usually be treated with minimally invasive techniques and changes in dietary habits. Products and techniques used for the management of dentine sensitivity aim to either block the dentinal tubules and so prevent fluid movement or interfere with neural transmission within the pulp. Dentinal tubules can be blocked with agents in toothpaste such as strontium chloride, calcium phosphate or oxalates, or professionally applied dentine bonding agents or adhesive restorations. Topical fluoride application may also promote remineralization within the dentinal tubules. Neural transmission may be affected by potassium salts; potassium is thought to diffuse up the dentinal tubules, altering the membrane potential of pulpal nerves, so decreasing their excitability and neural transmission.

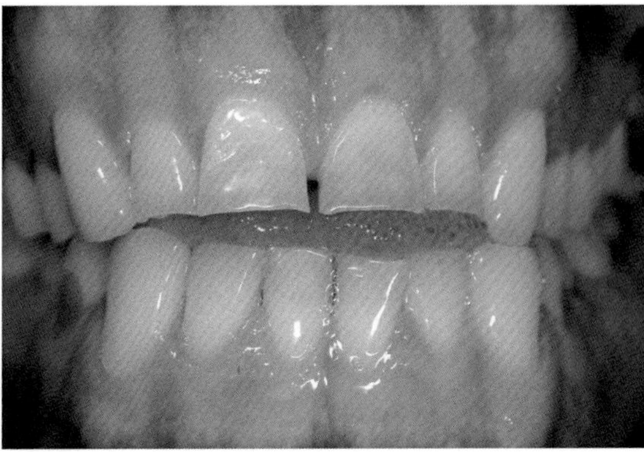

Figure 4.16 Early enamel wear may be predictive of future progression.

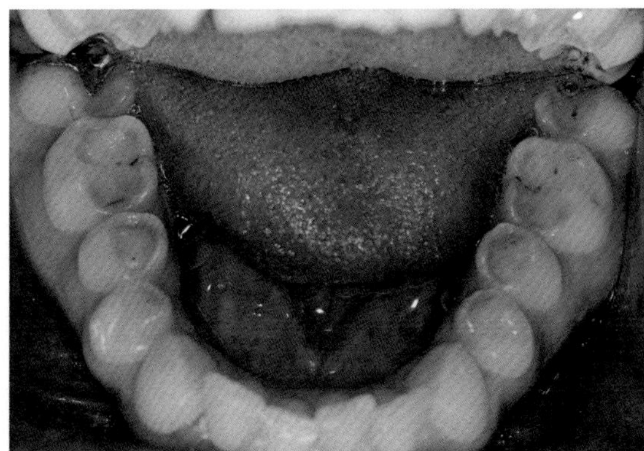

Figure 4.17 Exposure of dentine does not necessarily mean that the wear will continue at the same rate throughout life.

Preventive management

There is some evidence to suggest that if preventive advice is given the rate of tooth wear will reduce and further wear becomes consistent with the ageing process. The role of prevention is often overlooked in favour of operative intervention, but monitoring and having a long-term view on the prognosis of worn teeth is a valuable management technique. Whether the presence of early enamel wear is an indicator of later more severe wear is not known. Prevention of wear, however, particularly that associated with acids, should be considered when the effects of wear are first recognized (Figures 4.16 and 4.17).

The most important aspect to prevention is monitoring the rate of the tooth wear. This is traditionally accomplished by examining sequential study casts or comparing one set, with the date marked, to the patient's teeth. Often it is easier to compare like with like; if sequential study casts are used, an accurate and consistent impression technique is required to record the fine detail of wear (see Chapter 13). As damage to study casts is not uncommon, especially if kept for prolonged periods, it is worthwhile requesting that your technician cast these up in more durable die stone. In a busy clinic storage of models can be problematic and patients often move location. For these reasons it is sensible to give the dated models to the patient to bring with them at subsequent review appointments, taking care to document this in the patient's notes. Some clinicians use matrices to assess how much the wear has progressed but perhaps the simplest method is to use a periodontal probe and measure the height or width of the buccal, incisal/occlusal and palatal tooth surfaces (Figures 4.18 and 4.19).

Dietary advice

If extrinsic acids are thought to be the primary cause of the wear, a diet diary should be carried out like that for dental caries management. Acid content and frequency of intake should be identified and realistic alternatives suggested; for example, replacing juice drinks with water. Eating and drinking habits should also be discussed; for

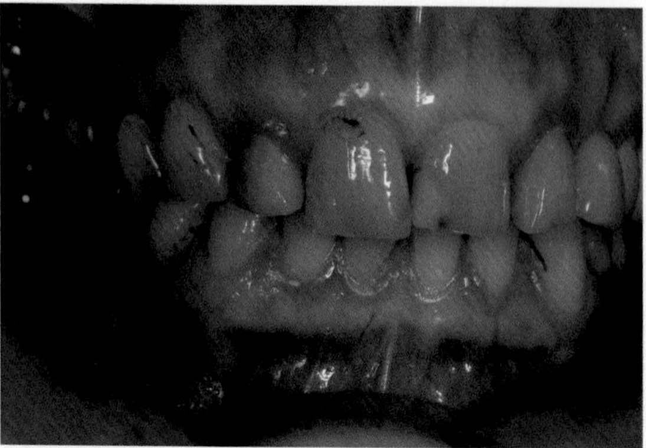

Figure 4.18 Monitoring of tooth wear can be effective. If the rate of tooth wear diminishes and there are undetectable changes, then monitoring can continue.

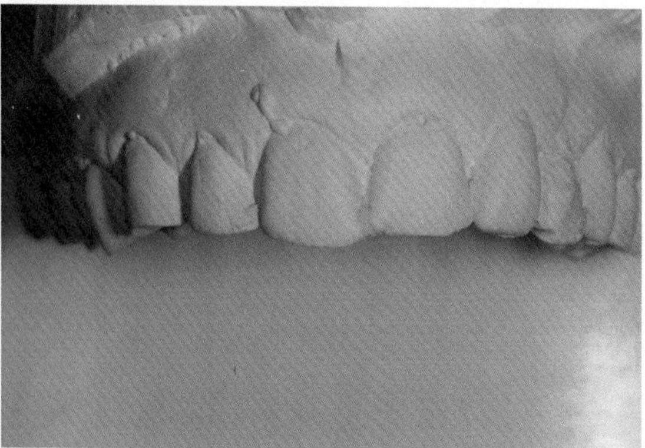

Figure 4.19 The original study cast taken for the patient in Figure 4.18. Comparison to the teeth shows no change over 15 years.

example, holding or swilling drinks in the palatal vault prior to swallowing can exacerbate erosion. Advice on the use of a straw placed toward the back of the mouth and avoidance of bathing the teeth in the beverage should be given if the patient cannot completely cease consumption. Acid drinks should also be avoided last thing at night and patients should be advised not to brush their teeth immediately following an acid drink, but rather rinse with water to clear and dilute the acid.

Fluoride

The role of topical fluoride in the preventive management of dental caries is unequivocally recognized as an effective and efficient modality. The strength of the evidence to support its use in tooth wear is not as well established but the evidence is mounting. There is a good level and varied supply of laboratory evidence to show that fluoride will help to prevent erosion and abrasion. Further evidence, mainly from in situ studies, also supports the preventive action of fluoride; however, there is virtually no clinical patient-based evidence. Nevertheless, based on the current evidence, fluoride is protective for erosive tooth wear.

Fluoride is thought to harden the enamel surface, increasing its resistance to acid dissolution. As acids erode the outer surface of enamel, some penetration of the surface layer is inevitable. This seepage through the enamel surface partly demineralizes and increases the porosity of the tissue, possibly reducing its resistance to further wear. However, if fluoride is freely available it can harden the outer layer and assist in the remineralization of the deeper ones. The effectiveness of fluoride on dentine is understood less but there may be a similar mechanism.

Saliva

The role of saliva in erosion is unclear. Theoretically, an absence should lead to an increase in the severity of erosion but this is not always seen clinically. The reason for this dilemma is not completely understood. It might be that xerostomia results in the severe hypersensitivity to acidic drinks and therefore dietary avoidance. The data from studies comparing saliva to prevalence of tooth wear or erosion are also equivocal, with some studies showing a positive correlation and others not. In principle, the role of saliva should be important in the development of erosive tooth wear.

Dentine bonding agents

Sealant restorations in caries management are well established but in erosive tooth wear there is limited evidence. Using dentine bonding agents to prevent dentine sensitivity is also well established and part of routine care. It is therefore likely that using dentine bonding agents to seal the early erosive lesions would also be effective in prevention of wear. There is some clinical evidence to support the role of dentine bonding agents and their use should be considered in patients where sensitivity is a problem or when ineffective control of the risk factors occurs.

Clinical and laboratory studies have shown that dentine bonding agents can reduce the amount of wear by half over a period of 6 months. However, the bonding agents are thought to be gradually worn away by mechanical action and repeated applications at regular review, particularly on susceptible tooth surfaces, is a preventive and minimally invasive technique.

Splint therapy

The use of full coverage splints will be effective for those patients with mainly a bruxist habit. Their use in patients where erosion is a major contributory factor is probably ineffective. The splints used to prevent bruxism can be made in either a vacuum-formed polyvinyl material or in heat-cured acrylic. Although neither has been shown to be more effective, the durability and longevity of the latter will be better. The use of splints with mandibular dysfunction is a well-recognized treatment but is often forgotten with bruxism and attrition (see Chapter 6) in the haste to provide more interventive restorative treatment.

The use of splints, particularly for those patients with bruxism, can be very effective as crowns and restorations often break under the extreme occlusal loading caused by the habit. A full coverage hard acrylic splint is relatively straightforward to make and simple to fit. Upper and lower impressions should be taken in a silicone material unless an alginate can be poured within 30 minutes. The silicone impressions should be sent to the laboratory with an interocclusal record and a request to make a full coverage upper hard acrylic splint with canine rises in lateral excursions. This is commonly referred to as a 'Michigan splint' (Figure 4.20). On receiving the splint from the laboratory it should be adjusted to ensure that there are even occlusal contacts in the intercuspal position and there is bilateral canine guidance. Providing the laboratory with a facebow recording for mounting of the models on a semi-adjustable articulator will reduce the amount of occlusal adjustment and hence clinical time needed to fit the splint.

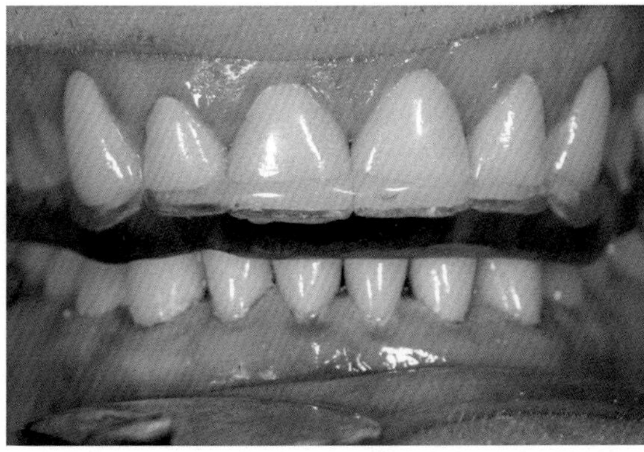

Figure 4.20 A Michigan full coverage maxillary splint used to protect teeth from the effects of bruxism. Normally worn at night, the splint distributes the loading of the clenching or grinding action and protects the teeth and restorations from cracking and fracturing.

When to restore?

The judgement on whether or not to restore worn teeth is in part related to the expectations and wishes of the patient but also to some extent on whether or not the teeth might survive for a lifetime. The main indications which eventually demand restorative treatment of worn teeth are appearance and intractable sensitivity. Another often quoted indication is whether or not the rate of tooth wear will compromise the longevity of the teeth. This judgement is by its very nature an estimate and relies on clinical experience. However, so little is known about the rate of tooth wear and the impact of prevention that the real outcome can never be known. There is a suspicion that tooth wear varies in activity with periods of progression and quiescence. One important assessment in the management of worn teeth, particularly those severely affected by wear, is the ability of the patient to afford the cost of care and maintenance. Since severe wear normally affects more than one tooth, the cost to restore them is high. Whether or not the patient wishes to improve their appearance, if they cannot afford complex care and aftercare, then monitoring with intensive preventive management may be an effective outcome.

SUMMARY

Tooth wear is a multifactorial, complex process that can lead to dramatic defects and loss of tooth structure. Early detection, preventive advice (and treatment) and monitoring the outcome of this form of management is of paramount importance. The need for advanced operative techniques may therefore be avoided. In those patients that present with a late stage of wear or where preventive management fails and there is evidence of continued wear from dated study casts, operative treatment may be indicated. It is important that prior to taking this decision the patient is aware of the complexity and long-term implications of such management and that this is clearly documented in the patient's notes. The operative management of patients with tooth wear will be discussed in Chapter 16.

FURTHER READING

Bartlett, D.W., Shah, P., 2006. A critical review of non-carious cervical (wear) lesions and the role of abfraction, erosion, and abrasion. J. Dent. Res. 85, 306–312.

Bartlett, D.W., Evans, D.F., Anggiansah, A., Smith, B.G.N., 1996. A study of the association between gastrooesophageal reflux and palatal dental erosion. Br. Dent. J. 181, 125–131.

Bartlett, D.W., Palmer, I., Shah, P., 2005. An audit of study casts used to monitor tooth wear in general practice. Br. Dent. J. 199, 143–145.

Harding, M.A., Whelton, H., O'Mullane, D.M., Cronin, M., 2003. Dental erosion in 5-year-old Irish school children and associated factors: a pilot study. Community Dent. Health 20, 165–170.

Sundaram, G., Watson, T., Bartlett, D., 2007. Clinical measurement of palatal tooth wear following coating by a resin sealing system. Oper. Dent. 32, 539–543.

Chapter 5

Aesthetic problems

David Bartlett

CHAPTER CONTENTS

The meaning of an aesthetic problem is vague as perfectly normal looking teeth can appear unacceptable to a patient. So the first stage in any assessment is to determine with the patient what the problem is and to assess what can be done. This chapter details the specific aesthetic problems a patient may present with and some simple solutions to address some of these, such as direct composite additions and vital and non-vital bleaching. Chapter 15 revisits some of the issues raised in this chapter and addresses how optimum aesthetics can be created in indirect restorations and describes in detail aspects such as tooth shaping and correct shade matching.

CAUSES OF AESTHETIC PROBLEMS

The shape and size of teeth

The teeth that are visible for most patients are the upper canines and incisors; however, in some patients, premolar teeth or even molar teeth are visible when the patient talks and smiles. The position of the lips in the extreme natural position of smiling is called 'the smile line' by many prosthodontists. The visible shape of teeth consists of the length, width and their relationship to other teeth. Generally, upper incisors are about 1 cm long and have a width between 0.75 and 0.80 cm (Figure 5.1). Although these dimensions vary considerably, teeth made too wide or too long appear unnatural (Figures 5.1 and 5.2). Therefore, as a base line, knowing the average tooth length and width can be useful in determining what is abnormal and what can be done to teeth in the smile line (see Chapter 15 for creating the ideal aesthetics and average tooth dimensions).

The other important criteria in an assessment of the smile line are the gingival contours, particularly along the margins of the upper anterior teeth. For some patients the smile line is low and the gingival margins are not visible; thus aesthetic anomalies are therefore relatively unimportant. In others, the smile line is high and gingival margins are clearly visible, variations from the norm having a high impact (Figure 5.3). In health, the gingival margins of the canines and central incisors are normally at the same horizontal level and more apical to the lateral incisors (Figure 5.4). The incisal edges of the upper central incisors and the tips of the canines are also usually at

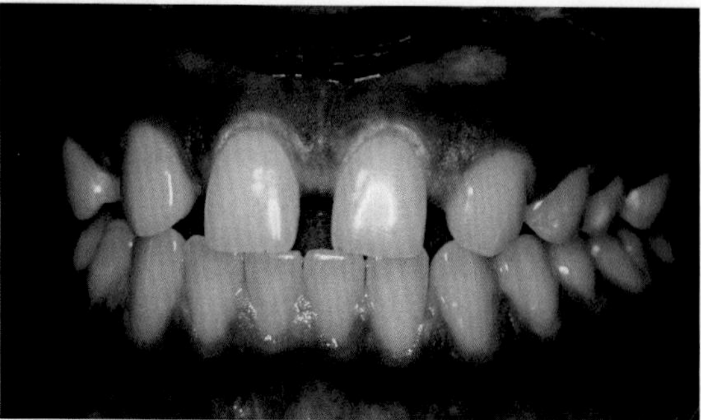

Figure 5.1 Missing upper lateral incisors with a spaced anterior region. The central incisors and canine teeth are already approaching the limit of their width.

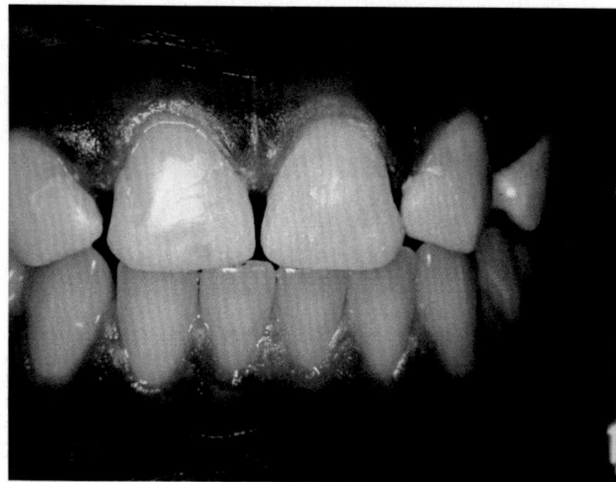

Figure 5.2 The addition of composites to the patient in Figure 5.1 has widened the teeth beyond an acceptable level, leading to less than ideal aesthetics.

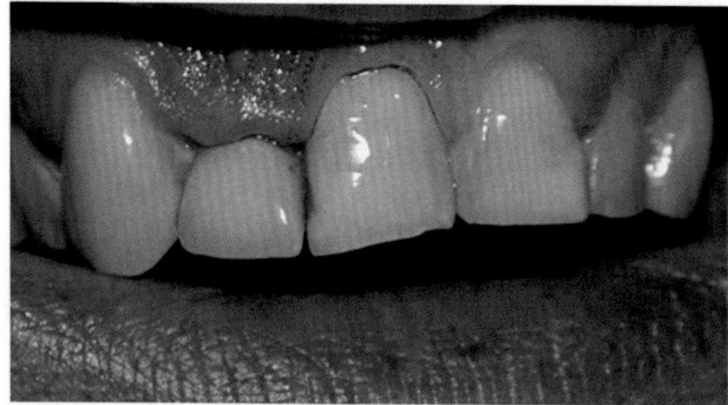

Figure 5.3 The crowned upper right lateral incisor has fractured in the past and overerupted, bringing with it the alveolar tissues, leading to an unsightly appearance at the gingival margin.

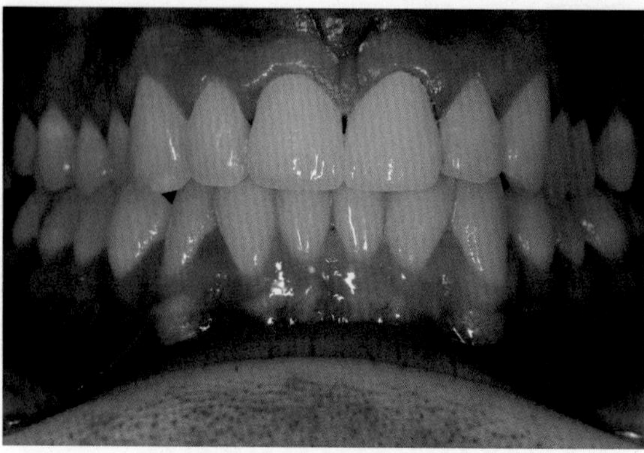

Figure 5.4 The gingival margins of the lateral incisor teeth are placed at a slightly lower position than the centrals and the canines.

the same approximate level but the lateral incisors are normally slightly shorter. The horizontal line along the incisal edges from the incisors to the canines is normally convex and follows the line of the lower lip (Figure 5.5).

Whilst these guides can be helpful they are not prescriptive and individual variation occurs. However, they are worth remembering when trying to assess a patient's smile when problems are present.

Colour of teeth

A frequent patient complaint regarding dental aesthetics is that teeth tend to discolour or darken with increasing age. The reason for this change is believed to be caused by the gradual thinning of enamel from tooth wear. As the

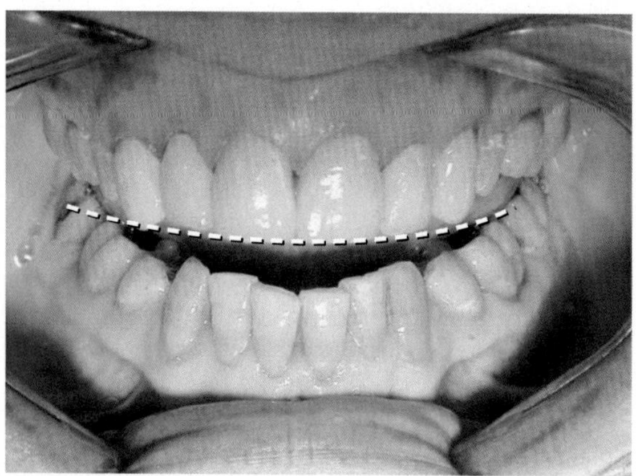

Figure 5.5 The incisal tips of the upper central incisor and canine are at a similar level on the patient's right-hand side but not on the patient's left, where they are more uneven. The ideal relationship is shown on the patient's right side. However, the gingival margins on the left side are present at the most appropriate level, whereas on the right they are not.

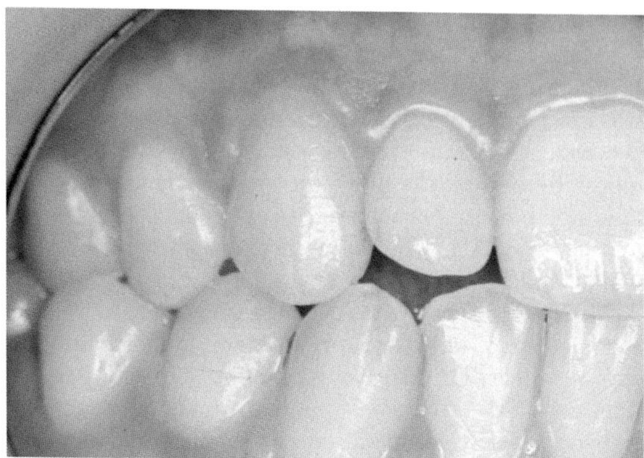

Figure 5.6 The canines are slightly darker than the other teeth. This natural difference between the canines and incisor teeth is sometimes unacceptable to patients and requires bleaching.

enamel wears, the darker dentine shines through and becomes more dominant in the colour of the teeth. An unacceptable colour is personal and subjective. What might appear to be a perfectly normal colour may be unacceptable to a patient. A common example of this is the colour of the canine tooth (Figure 5.6). Naturally, this tooth has a higher saturation of the colour yellow than other incisor teeth and the difference in colour is unacceptable for some patients.

Assessing what is wrong with the colour is challenging and needs careful thought and considered planning time. Generally, if someone wants their teeth to be whiter the treatment options usually at first may appear to be relatively simple. But it is worthwhile taking time to ensure that the colour is the only reason for their dissatisfaction. It is not unusual for patients to focus on one aspect of their appearance while ignoring the others, only to find that after treatment of one problem, the other problems come to the fore. During the assessment of colour it is useful to enquire about previous photographs and use them as a guide to identify the problem.

Occasionally, more serious discolorations of teeth present. This may be a result of fluorosis (Figure 5.7) or tetracycline staining (Figure 5.8). The former can present in patients born overseas where there is a high fluoride content found naturally in spring water, or those given too high a dose of fluoride during tooth development. Our understanding of the action of fluoride is now clearer and the most important preventive effect is from its topical application, systemic fluoride supplements such as drops or tablets are rarely given today due to the disfiguring white and brown mottled defects that can occur (Figure 5.7).

Tetracycline staining is very unlikely to occur to someone born in the UK as the disfiguring side effect of tooth discolouration is well known (Figure 5.8), hence it is rarely given to children during tooth development. For those born outside the UK the chances of developing tetracycline staining will depend on the availability of the drug over-the-counter. In some parts of Asia, for example, drugs which would be prescription delivered in the UK are

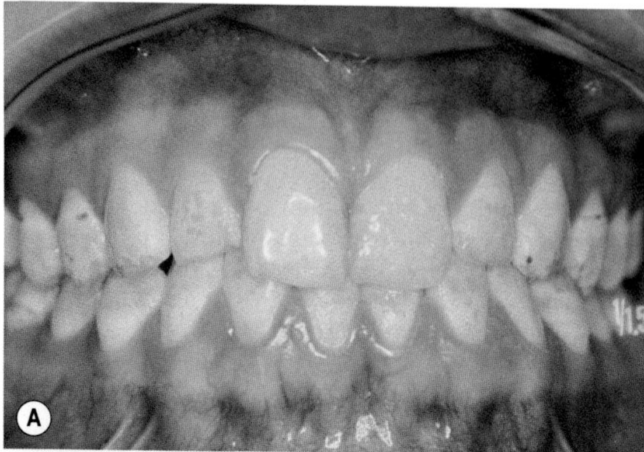

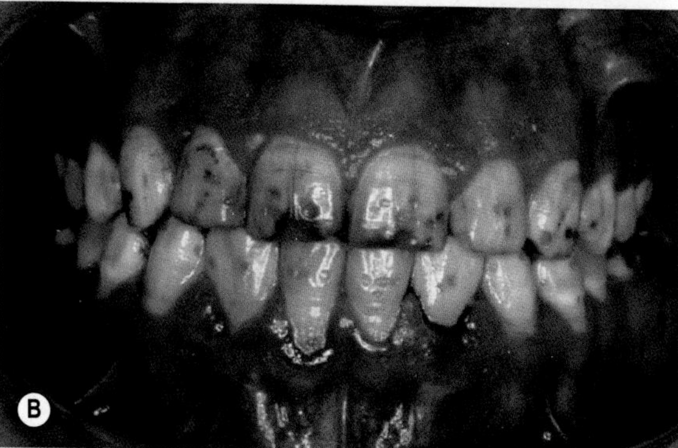

Figure 5.7 **A** Dental fluorosis in this patient has produced an unsightly white and brown mottled appearance. **B** Severe dental fluorosis in this patient has produced an unsightly brown pitted appearance.

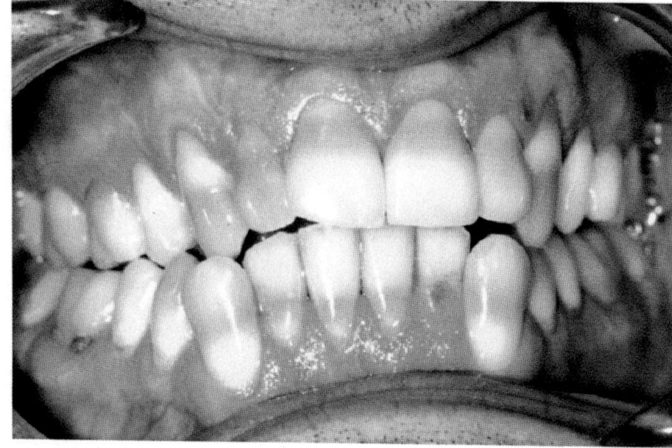

Figure 5.8 Tetracycline staining.

available over-the-counter and this is particularly true of antibiotics. Tetracycline staining can be clearly distinguished as the teeth fluorescence under ultraviolet light.

Genetic disorders such as dentinogenesis and amelogenesis imperfecta also affect tooth development, with both having varying impact upon the teeth. Mild forms of either condition can be difficult to distinguish but more severe forms are characteristic and differentiated by the anatomy of the roots. In dentinogenesis imperfecta there are bulbous roots with root canal obliteration which are visible on radiographs (Figure 5.9), whereas teeth with amelogenesis imperfecta have normal root formation but abnormal enamel development.

Dentinogenesis imperfect (Figure 5.9) is inherited as an autosomal dominant trait, with one parent usually having the condition. The disorder is the result of a defective DSPP (dentine sialophosphoprotein) gene. Three types have been identified: Type I is associated with osteogenesis imperfecta, whilst Type II (some have progressive hearing loss) and Type III are not associated with other inherited disorders and some believe they form a single disorder. It can affect both primary and permanent dentitions. The crowns of teeth affected by dentinogenesis imperfecta appear blue–grey or yellow–brown and translucent; the condition has also been referred to as hereditary opalescent dentine. The defective dentine leads to early loss of the enamel and rapid wear.

Numerous forms of amelogenesis imperfecta have been described based upon the appearance of the teeth and the way in which the disorder is inherited; most cases are inherited as an autosomal dominant trait. Amelogenesis imperfecta results from mutations in the genes that are responsible for the production of proteins that are important in the formation of enamel. It can also affect both primary and permanent dentitions. The teeth are usually discoloured with a pitted or grooved appearance and can

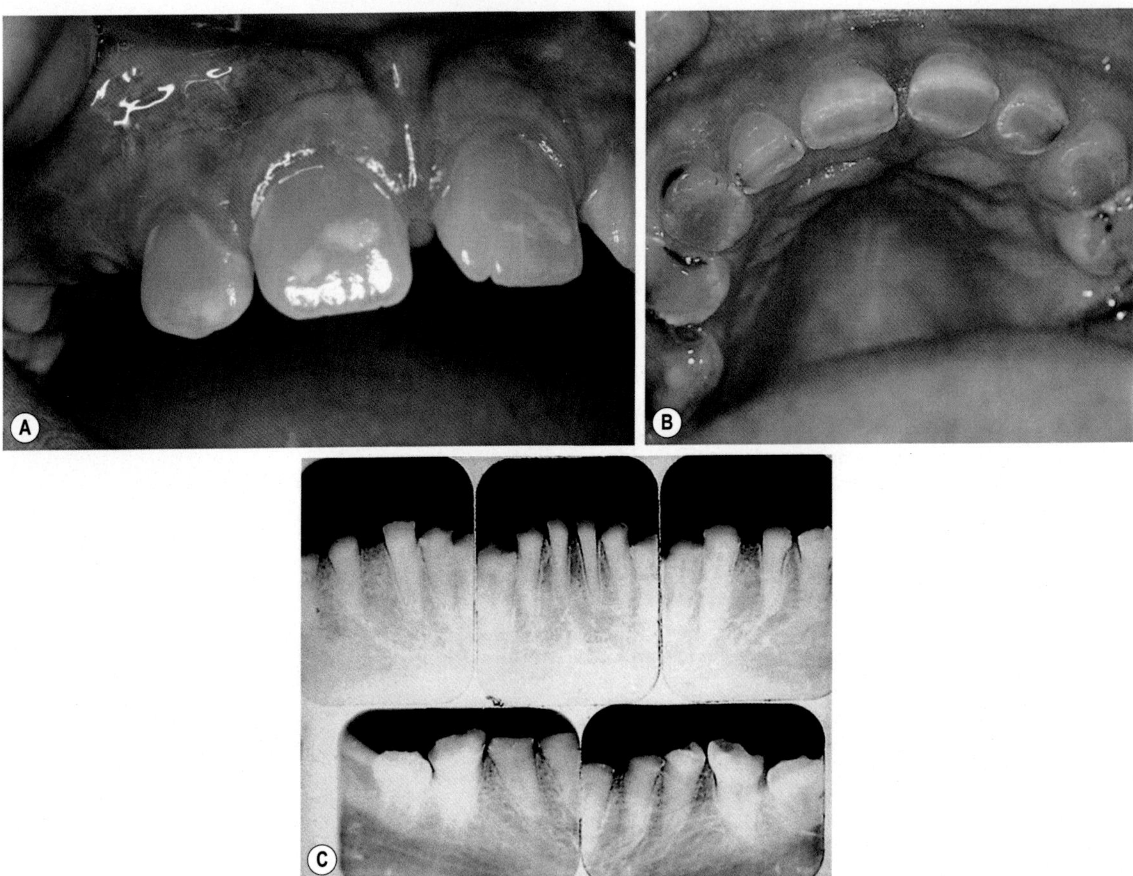

Figure 5.9 Clinical images of a patient with dentinogenesis imperfecta showing yellow–brown discolouration and translucent appearance (A) and the rapid wear in a different patient that can occur due to early loss of enamel (B). The radiographs (C) show bulbous roots with root canal obliteration.

(Courtesy of Scully C, Flint S, Porter SR, Moos K. Oral and maxillofacial diseases, 3rd ed. London: Taylor & Francis, 2004)

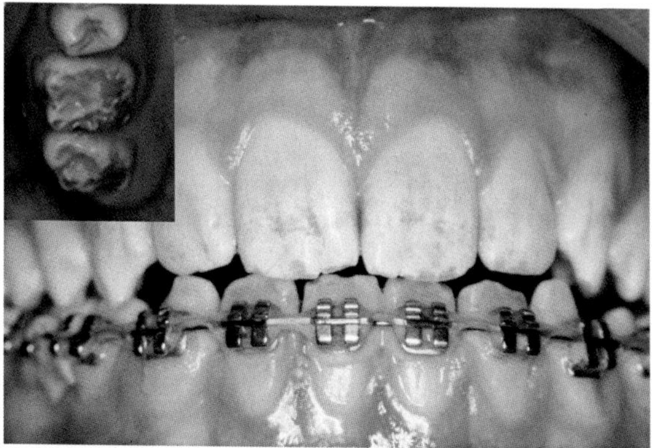

Figure 5.10 This patient has a form of amelogenesis imperfecta leading to rapid wear of the teeth (see inset).

break and wear down rapidly (Figure 5.10). Some forms of amelogenesis imperfecta can be difficult to distinguish from fluorosis (see Figure 5.7), as both conditions can lead to hypoplastic changes to the surface of the enamel.

Due to the often rapid wear of teeth with either dentinogenesis or amelogenesis imperfecta, early intervention with multiple crowns is often required to prevent the teeth from wearing to a degree that would prevent restoration without resorting to removable prosthodontics.

Black triangles

One of the outcomes of periodontal disease is gingival recession. As the gingival margin migrates apically past the widest aspect of the roots (at the crown–root junction), the interdental space takes on a triangular appearance due to the tapering of the roots of anterior and premolar teeth. The crest of the gingiva interdentally will therefore have a wide base and the space between the teeth will have a point towards the contact point – the so-called black triangle (Figure 5.11). A reduction in the extent and position of the interdental papilla is challenging and a suitable solution to address the situation may not be feasible or stable following treatment. Widening the teeth either side of the black triangle to reduce the gap may create teeth with a poor height to width ratio and an unnatural appearance. Another disadvantage of increasing the width of teeth is that the increase in the bulbosity of the tooth at the gingival margin changes the emergence profile and increases the difficulty in cleaning. Continued poor oral hygiene in someone with a history of periodontal disease may increase the risk of further recession and deterioration in any improvements made to the 'black triangle'. Therefore, if changes to the width of teeth are considered it is worthwhile preparing a diagnostic wax-up to assess the planned changes and the impact this will have on the appearance and health of the periodontal tissues.

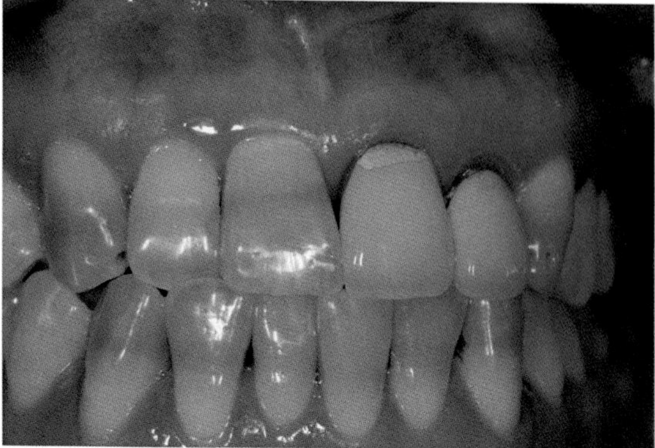

Figure 5.11 The development of some localized periodontal disease and inappropriately shaped upper left central incisor crown has left a black triangle between the two central incisors. This patient also has tetracycline staining.

Tooth position – spacing

Diastemas and generalized spacing between teeth result from a mismatch in tooth and jaw size, which can be unacceptable to patients (Figure 5.12). Closure of diastemas and spaces can be accomplished by orthodontic movement or by restorations. Any orthodontic movement is unlikely to be stable over long periods of time and some degree of retention, using either a removable appliance for night-time wear or a fixed wire retainer, is inevitable.

Restorative intervention can be a useful compromise but the crucial assessment is the width of the teeth. Naturally narrow teeth will accept an increase in width (Figures 5.12 and 5.13) but broader ones may appear to be too wide after any change (see Figure 5.2). A diagnostic wax-up will assist in the preoperative assessment (Figure 5.14) but a composite 'mock-up' may also be useful. Composites can be added to teeth without acid etching and bonding, shaping to a diagnostic wax-up and stent or building up

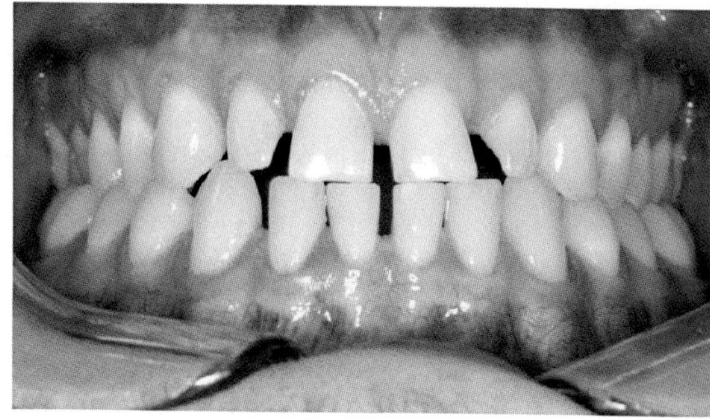

Figure 5.12 Unsightly dental spacing has resulted from relatively small teeth on large dental bases.

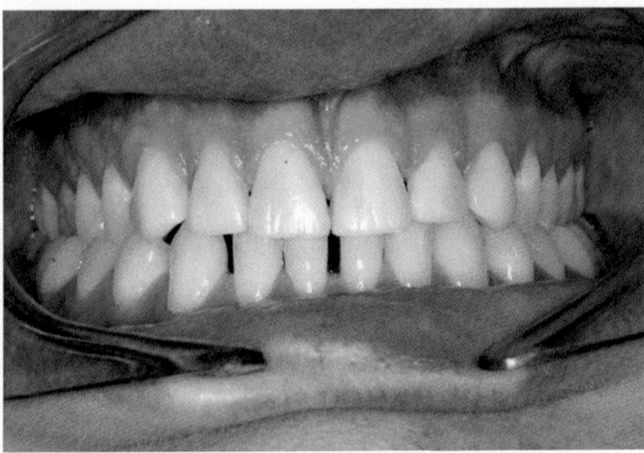

Figure 5.13 The spaces for the patient seen in Figure 5.12 have been successfully closed using composite restorations and no orthodontic treatment was necessary.

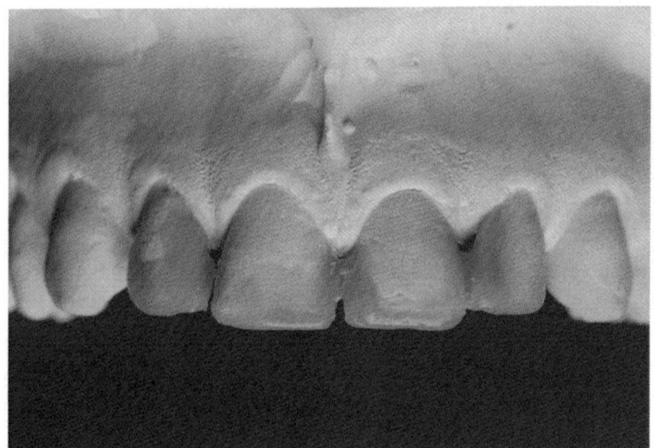

Figure 5.14 Diagnostic wax-up for the patient seen in Figures 5.12 and 5.13.

freehand. This can provide the patient with a realistic opportunity to see the proposed changes to shape and the colour match possible (Figure 5.15). If this is done without a diagnostic wax-up, and the patient is happy with the appearance achieved, an alginate impression of the result should be taken so that it can be copied in the definitive restorations which may be carried out some time later. These composite 'mock-ups' are easily removed once the patient has had sufficient time to assess the changes made by simply using an excavator at the margins of the composite to lever them off the tooth. Care must be taken to avoid the patient swallowing or inhaling the veneers of composite by using high volume suction lingual to the site and using a gauze or Spontex sponge to protect the oropharynx.

When making significant changes with composite it is useful to use a putty stent of a diagnostic wax-up or of a model made from an impression of the composite mock-up. Figure 5.16 shows how this was done for the patient in Figure 5.12.

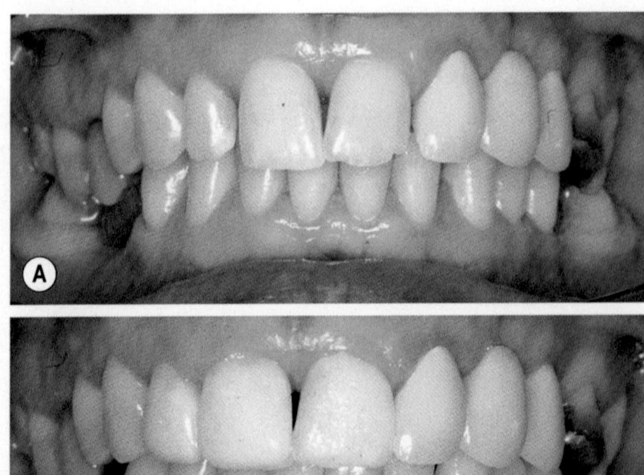

Figure 5.15 This patient was unhappy with the alignment of the upper anterior teeth (A). A composite 'mock-up' (B) without etching the tooth and using bond allows the patient to assess the change in shape and colour possible prior to making a decision as to whether to proceed with the definitive composite additions.

Orthodontic treatment is indicated for more severe changes to the normal position of teeth. The patient must fully appreciate that orthodontics is the ideal treatment for moving teeth and that restorative intervention is often a significant compromise and generally involves at least composite build-ups, veneers or crowns. The irreversible nature of restorative treatment means that the patient must be fully committed and understand the risks involved with the proposals.

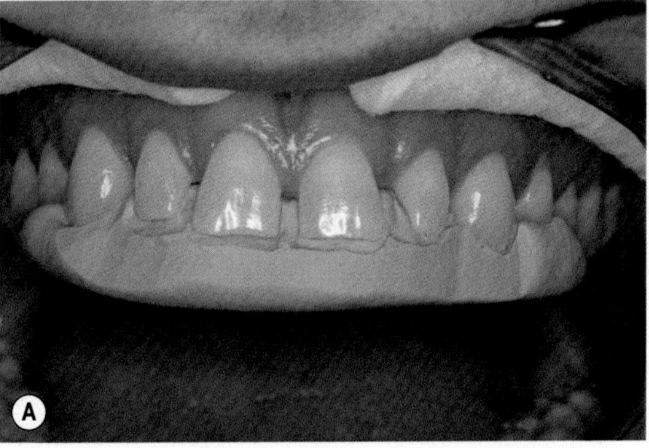

Figure 5.16A Addition cured polyvinyl siloxane putty impression taken of the palatal surface of the diagnostic wax-up seen in Figure 5.14. The putty stent is cut with a scalpel along the incisal edges of the teeth. This is then inserted into the patient's mouth and acts as a guide for the composite additions.

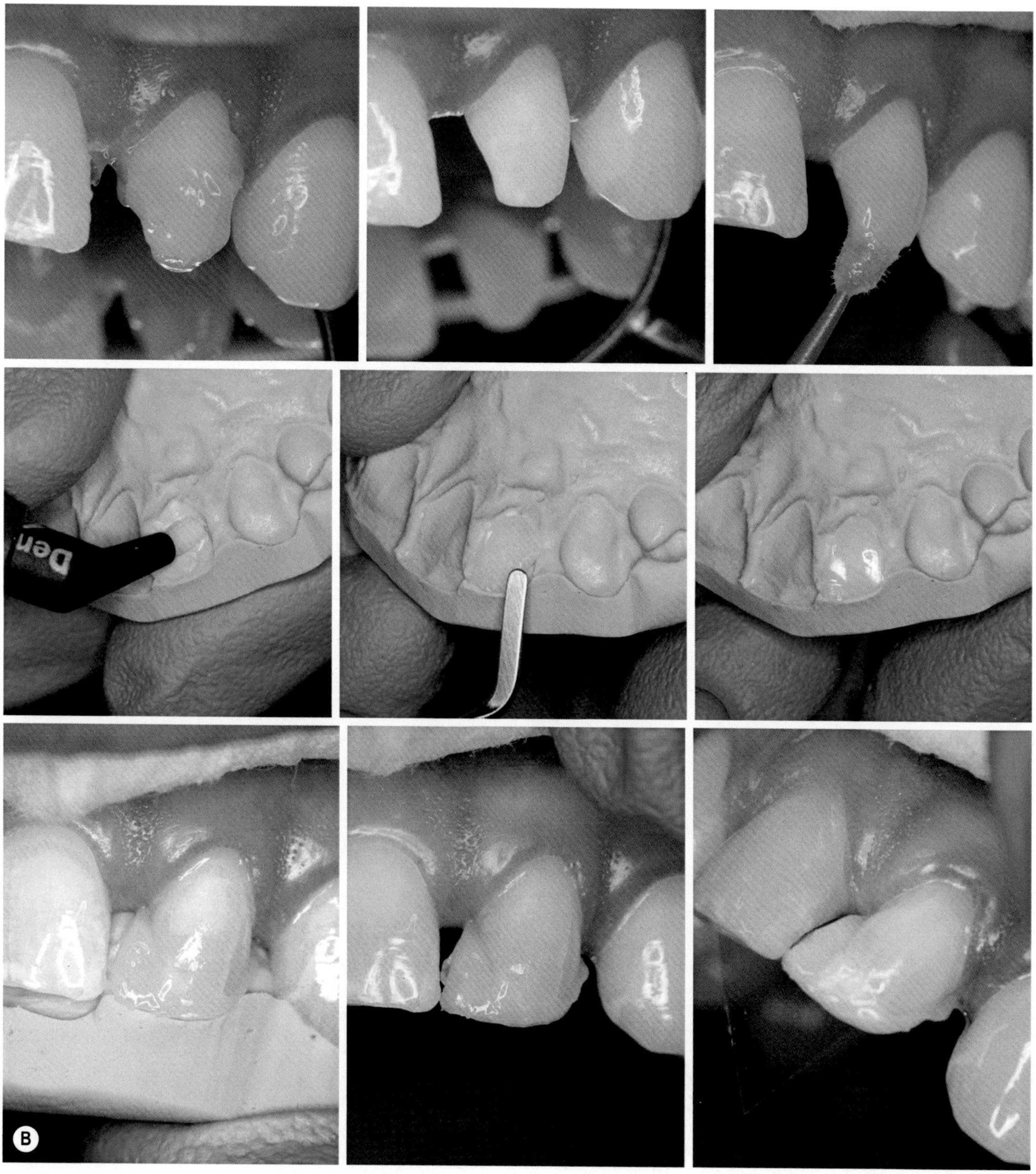

Figure 5.16B From top left to right: peg lateral all surfaces acid etched, rinsed and dried to give frosty appearance and bond applied. Composite added to stent and adapted with a flat plastic instrument. Stent reseated intraorally, ensuring composite adapted palatally and not contacting the adjacent teeth, the composite is now light cured – with stent removed cellulose strip inserted to allow proximal surface to be built up – labial face can now be completed (Figure 5.13).

Malformed teeth

It is relatively uncommon to find malformed teeth, particularly in the upper anterior region. Trauma to the deciduous teeth may result in a malformed permanent successor crown which only becomes visible once the tooth has erupted. Peg laterals are more common and may present with other alignment problems which may form part of an overall orthodontic treatment. Restorative management can be with either composite or porcelain veneers or occasionally crowns.

Missing lateral incisors

Hypodontia is relatively common, particularly missing third molar teeth, but the most commonly affected tooth which affects the appearance is the lateral incisor. This is normally recognized early in the adolescent's development and orthodontic treatment is used either to close the space, masking the canine shape with composite, or to create sufficient space for a replacement lateral incisor using either a minimal preparation bridge or an implant. More severe forms of hypodontia, with multiple missing teeth, create more restorative challenges which are outwith the scope of this book.

THE PREOPERATIVE ASSESSMENT

The first stage in addressing a patient's concern over appearance is to assess whether restorative treatment only is the ideal option. In many instances, particularly those involving tooth positions, orthodontic management may be the preferred option with or without subsequent restorative treatment. When restorative treatment is planned, routine caries and periodontal treatment and other disease control needs to be completed and followed by a reasonable period of stabilization to ensure that there is no new disease (these issues have been addressed in the preceding chapters). This period is not fixed and will to some extent depend on the severity of the problem, but at least 6 months without new disease and evidence of good oral hygiene and compliance may be sufficient.

Following disease control the next stage is to assess which restorative option is acceptable to the patient. A diagnostic wax-up is an invaluable tool to show patients the planned treatment and might be linked to a composite 'mock-up'. If a combined orthodontic restorative approach is considered, a Kessling set-up can be carried out, where teeth are sectioned from a model and moved into the anticipated position that orthodontic treatment could achieve and any restorative work being produced in wax or acrylic teeth (Figure 5.17). In most circumstances the diagnostic wax-up is simple and needs a single set of models; however, in more complex cases where the end result is not easily envisaged, more than one diagnostic wax-up is made to show the patient various options (Figure 5.18). This may also be linked to provisional restorations, preferably before the definitive treatment is provided.

When the only complaint is colour in unrestored teeth, the treatment can be a straightforward case of providing bleaching. For more extensively restored teeth or very discoloured teeth, veneers (see Chapter 12) or crowns are

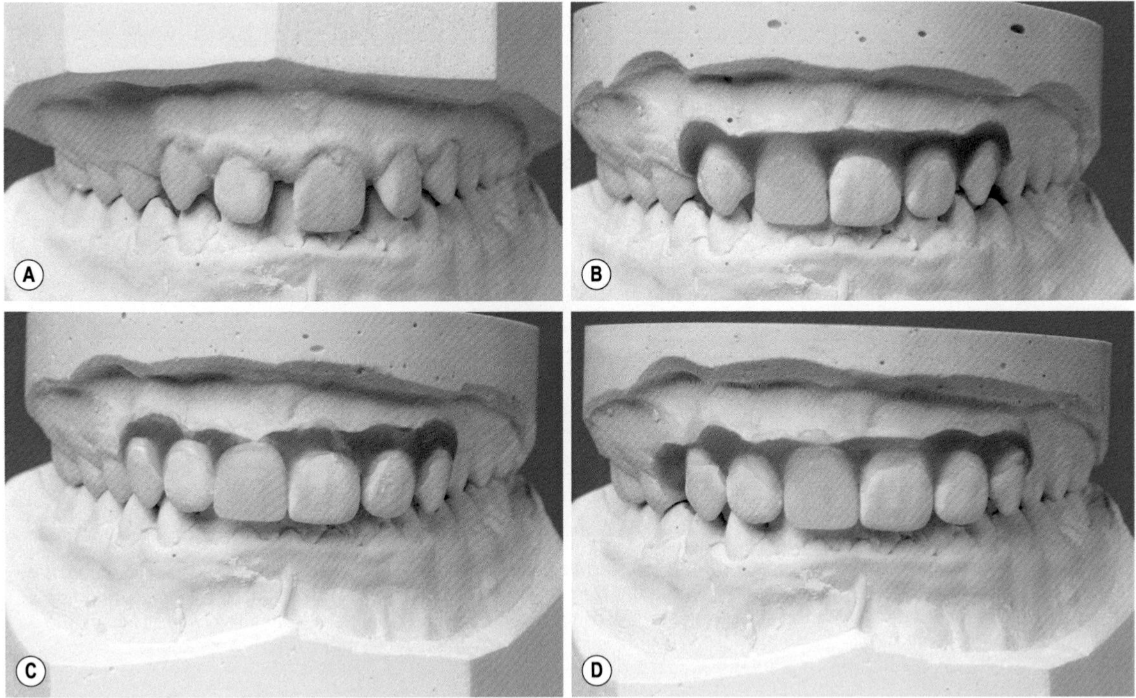

Figure 5.17 Kessling set-ups for a patient with a missing upper right central incisor (A). The treatment options explored are: (1) no orthodontics and build up the upper right lateral incisor with composite (B); (2) create space orthodontically for the upper right central incisor replacement (implant or minimum preparation (resin retained) bridge) without extractions (C) and with upper right premolar extraction (D).

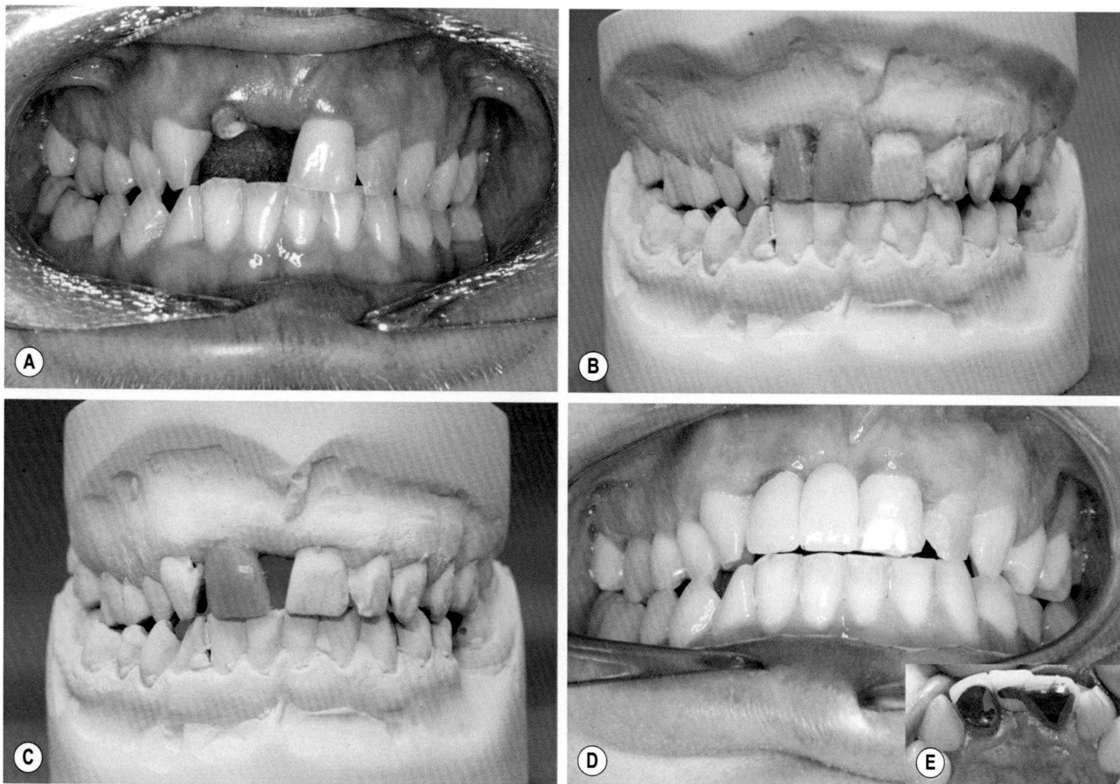

Figure 5.18 This patient has a missing upper right central incisor and retained upper right lateral incisor root. The diagnostic wax-ups show the two possible treatment options and allow the patient to decide on the favoured outcome. A cantilever minimum preparation, resin retained bridge off the upper left central incisor and a post crown on the upper right lateral incisor were provided.

indicated (see Chapters 10 and 11 on metal–ceramic crowns and all-ceramic crowns). Note that if veneers are placed around existing extensive restorations the risk of failure around the margins increases as an inferior bond may result. For those teeth with a problem with shape but not tooth position, a veneer made in either direct composite or porcelain can be the solution. In cases when changes to the tooth position and tooth shape are needed, minimal intervention techniques are often inappropriate and crowns are required. Before embarking upon more extensive restorations, particularly those involved with tooth position, an orthodontic approach must be considered first.

BLEACHING

Vital bleaching

Hydrogen peroxide (H_2O_2) has been used to whiten teeth for over a century. The molecule is minute and able to pass through the enamel to affect the dentine. It is believed that most of the action of bleaching is on the dentine rather than the enamel which is much more translucent. The mode of action is not fully understood but the small size of the molecule penetrates the dentine and removes stains from the tissue. The high reactivity of hydrogen peroxide and the subsequent release of the superoxide ion are understood to be the reason why it is so effective but how the stain is removed is less clear.

The most commonly available form of hydrogen peroxide is carbamide peroxide, otherwise known as urea peroxide, which breaks down to form hydrogen peroxide and urea. The hydrogen peroxide forms the superoxide ion and water whilst the urea breaks down to form ammonia and carbon dioxide. The urea formed as part of the breakdown is too small to have any toxicological consequence. There have been no clinical studies suggesting bleaching has any serious systemic risk other than that normally encountered with restorative materials. The effects on restorative materials themselves is largely transient and reversed within 24 hours but most practitioners recommend a few days between completion of bleaching and any restorative work involving bonding.

The main advantage of bleaching is that it is conservative of tooth tissue. The bleaching product can be delivered at the chairside or at home. Both techniques utilize

Table 5.1 List of stains successfully managed with bleaching. All require either unrestored or minimally restored teeth. Some of the acquired forms may be simply removed by scaling and polishing the teeth

ACQUIRED	DEVELOPMENTAL (MILD FORMS)
• Mild generalized staining • Age-related yellow discoloration • Tobacco staining • Dietary stains, e.g. tea and coffee • Colour change related to pulpal trauma	• Fluorosis • Tetracycline staining • Amelogenesis imperfecta

the same chemistry, namely the use of hydrogen peroxide. Chairside bleaching is particularly suitable for patients without the motivation for home care and who prefer dentists to manage their treatment. It is generally more expensive in surgery time and often more costly to patients but the result from both techniques is likely to be the same. Table 5.1 shows those cases most successfully treated with vital bleaching.

For home care a vacuum-formed splint is made to overlay the teeth. It is generally cut back just below the gingival margins and usually has no palatal coverage. It is loaded with bleaching agent by the patient and worn each night for 2–3 hours (Figure 5.19). In most superficial discolorations the results are seen within a couple of weeks (Figure 5.20). For more intense stains, particularly those associated with tetracycline or fluorosis, the bleaching may need considerably more time. It is worth using a shade guide to determine the colour before treatment and to monitor if and how well the bleaching is working.

The gingival margin area around teeth can be more resistant to bleaching and it is worthwhile warning patients if a particularly darkened area along the cervical margin exists (Figure 5.20C). The colour stability of bleached teeth is also not predictable as people respond differently to bleaching. Generally, teeth that have bleached well can remain stable for 2–3 years, after which further bleaching may be required. Patients should be warned about this potential risk prior to commencing treatment.

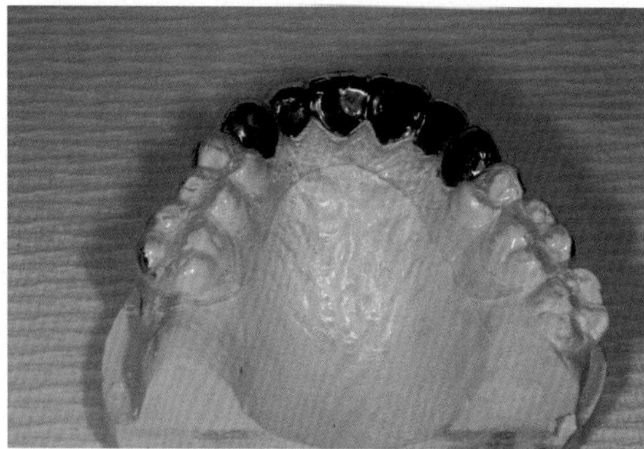

Figure 5.19 The bleaching tray is made over the teeth with a vacuum-formed plastic. Some technicians paint a spacer over the teeth to be bleached but this is not essential.

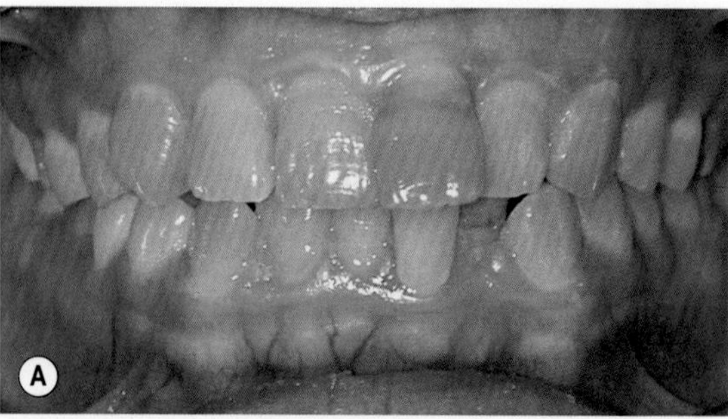

Figure 5.20A Two changes are needed to improve the appearance. Firstly to orthodontically move the teeth to remove the overlap and then bleaching to improve the colour.

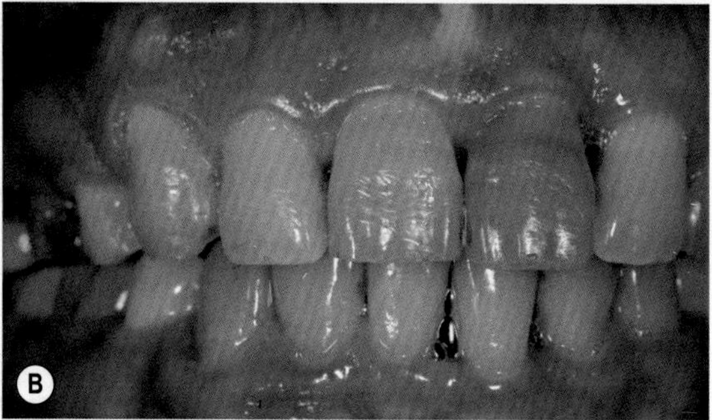

Figure 5.20B Patient seen in Figure 5.20A. Following orthodontics the teeth are better aligned.

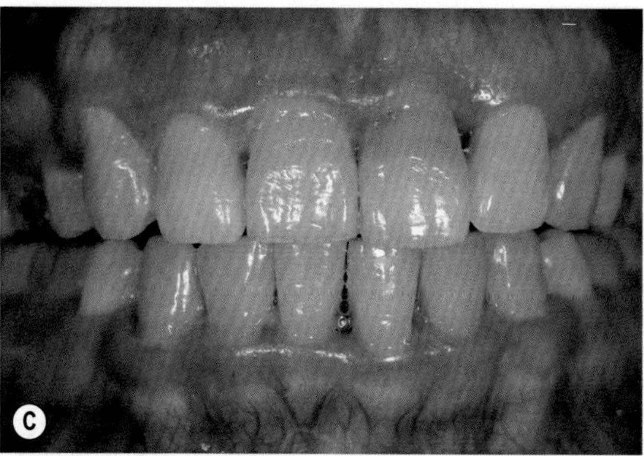

Figure 5.20C Patient seen in Figure 5.20A and 5.20B. Following bleaching the teeth have whitened but the gingival margin on the upper left central incisor has been more resistant.

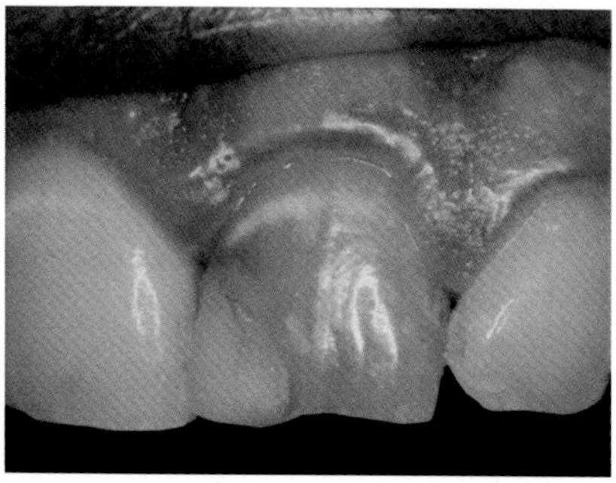

Figure 5.21 An extensively restored and discoloured tooth unsuitable for bleaching. A new restoration (core) and crown would be more appropriate.

The most common side effect of vital bleaching is dentine sensitivity as the bleach has a low pH and opens up dentinal tubules. Generally, the symptoms are transient and do not threaten the pulp. Intermittent use or using desensitizing toothpastes should provide relief from pain for most sufferers, allowing the bleaching to continue, but in some cases the intensity of the pain prevents further bleaching.

The choice between bleaching and other options depends on the restorative status of the teeth and the severity of the discoloration. Extensively restored teeth or severely discoloured teeth (Figure 5.21) are more appropriately treated with crowns, whereas bleaching can be tried in teeth with less severe defects and restorative status.

Non-vital bleaching

Non-vital bleaching following successful endodontic treatment may avoid the need to use a crown to improve the appearance of anterior teeth that are minimally restored (Figure 5.22). Bleaching virtually unrestored root-filled anterior teeth preserves the tooth tissue. However, cases involving extensive restorations (more than a small Class III or IV) and dark discolouration (Figure 5.23) may need crowns and often a post to retain the core (see Chapter 7). Bleaching will generally improve the brown discolouration which occurs once the vitality of teeth is lost. The darker the stain, the more resistant to bleaching the tooth becomes.

Before embarking on non-vital bleaching a periapical radiograph is needed to ensure a good and effective root canal treatment is present. The gutta-percha should be removed from the pulp chamber and root canal to below the gingival margin and sealed with a glass ionomer cement. These two factors ensure that no bleaching products enter into the periradicular tissues. Rubber dam should be placed to ensure protection of the soft tissues. Sodium perborate is commonly used in non-vital bleaching. It is another product of the hydrogen peroxide family which breaks down to form sodium metaborate, hydrogen peroxide and nascent oxygen. This material has been used for over half a century to bleach non-vital teeth using the 'walking technique'.

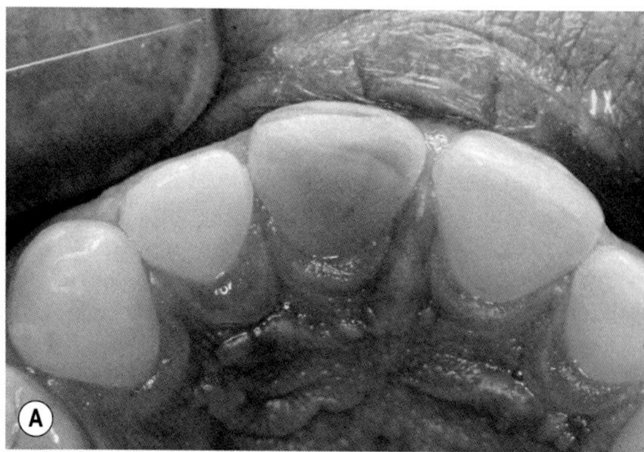

Figure 5.22A Palatal view of a less severely discoloured and fractured upper right central incisor which is more appropriately treated with a bleaching agent and a conservative composite restoration.

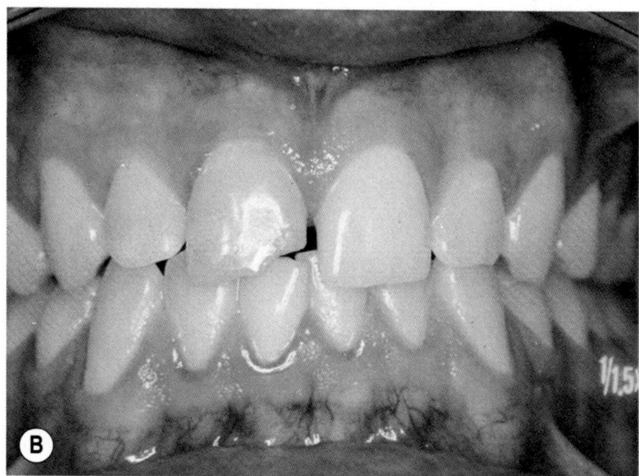

Figure 5.22B Labial view of less severely discoloured and fractured upper right central incisor seen in Figure 5.22A.

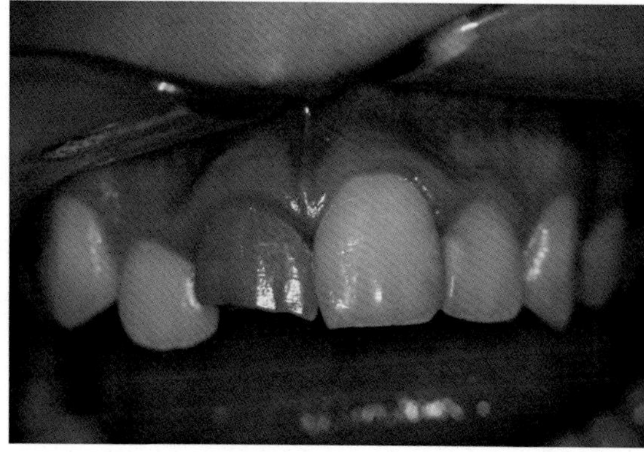

Figure 5.23 Severely discoloured and fractured upper right central incisor requires a crown.

Sodium perborate mixed with hydrogen peroxide is placed in the coronal cavity and packed against the buccal wall and then sealed in with a temporary restorative material for about 2 weeks (Figure 5.24). This may need to be repeated a number of times to achieve the correct shade. Some practitioners acid etch the inside of the pulp chamber to open up the dentinal tubules to ensure better penetration of the active bleach products; however, there is no evidence to support its efficacy. As an alternative to the walking bleach technique, following placement of a well-sealed restoration in the coronal aspect of the root canal, carbamide peroxide delivered in a splint can be used by the patient in a similar way to vital bleaching.

Where non-vital bleaching is concerned some have reported external cervical root resorption, but this is more likely to be a result of the trauma that led to the discolouration in the first instance. The risk of resorption as a result of non-vital bleaching can be reduced with an appropriate technique described above.

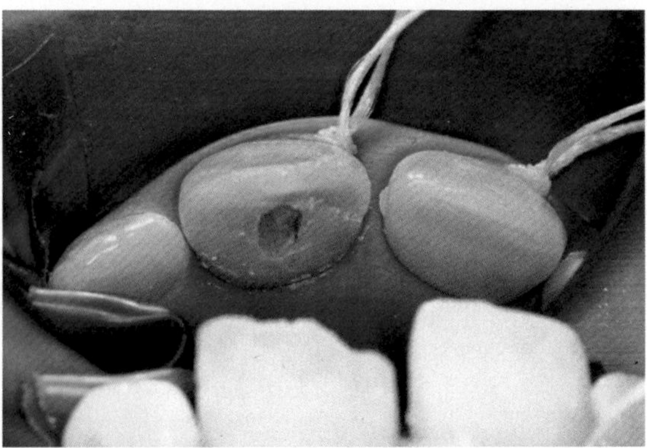

Figure 5.24A Gutta-percha has to be completely removed from the pulp chamber for non-vital bleaching. The gutta-percha should be covered with a layer of glass ionomer to provide a coronal seal. Rubber dam is essential.

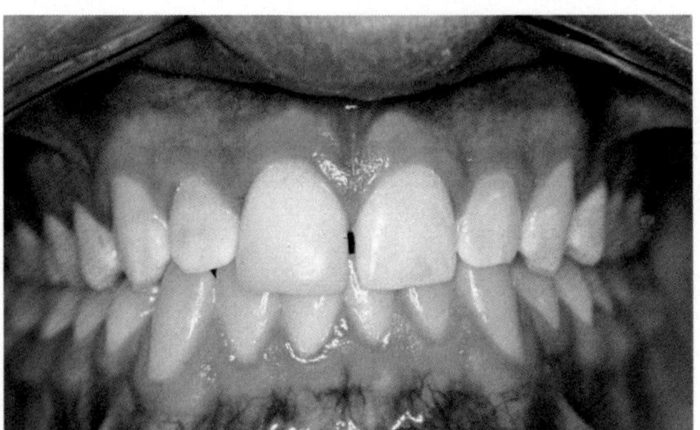

Figure 5.24B Patient seen in Figure 5.22 with upper right central incisor having undergone non-vital bleaching and composite addition. The definitive composite should be placed after bleaching for accurate colour matching. Note the dehydration and whitening of adjacent teeth following rubber dam placement.

Whitening strips and topically applied systems

Over-the-counter products are available outside many parts of Europe and over the internet. Their efficacy is based on the in-surgery techniques and these products have proven to be successful. It should be borne in mind, however, that there are always dangers with patient-applied products that are not prescribed and supervised by a dentist.

ACID MICROABRASION

Acid abrasion or microabrasion is essentially a simultaneous process of erosion and abrasion used to remove superficial defects and discolouration within enamel. Strong acids (e.g. 18% hydrochloric acid) and pumice slurry are applied to the enamel and gently agitating using special rubber agitators similar to a rubber point or a rotating rubber cup in a speed-reducing handpiece (to reduce the risk of acid splatter). The acid dissolves the outer layer of enamel which is then worn away by the agitated pumice. The technique is only suitable for superficial defects in enamel such as mild fluorosis; it should not be used for defects in dentine. The process is essentially a controlled way of removing the surface layer of enamel and when 18% hydrochloric acid and pumice are used in this way for approximately 100 seconds, about 360 ± 130 μm of enamel thickness is lost (Tong et al., 1993). The obvious major issues of using concentrated hydrochloric acid in the mouth are safety should the product be spilt onto the soft tissues; rubber dam is therefore mandatory (Figure 5.25).

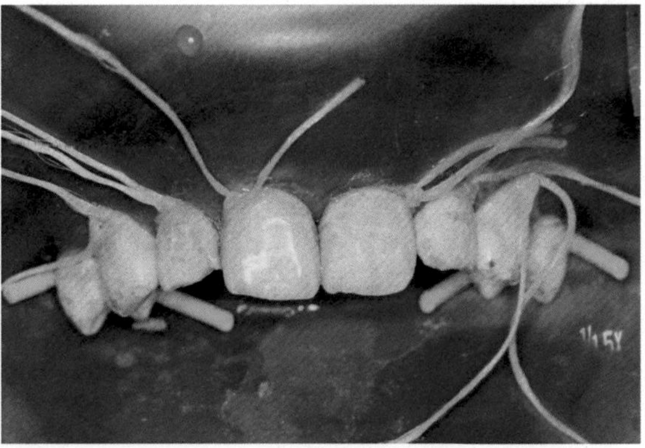

Figure 5.25 Patient seen in Figure 5.7A with fluorosis where microabrasion was planned. Rubber dam isolation is essential when carrying out microabrasion. Note the use of floss ligatures to retract the rubber dam, ensuring complete exposure of the crown. Microabrasion failed to improve the appearance in this case.

SUMMARY

This chapter has detailed the most common causes that patients complain about in relation to the appearance of their teeth. Carefully listening to the patient's issues will direct the dentist to the chief complaint. Planning treatment in patients with a heightened concern about their appearance is often difficult and a combined orthodontic restorative approach is often necessary for more complicated cases. This chapter has also dealt with minimally invasive methods of addressing various aspects of appearance such as bleaching for discolouration and microabrasion for superficial enamel defects. More advanced operative methods of dealing with issues of appearance such as the placement of veneers and crowns are dealt with in the relevant subsequent chapters.

FURTHER READING

Brunton, P.A., Aminian, A., Pretty, I.A., 2006. Vital tooth bleaching in dental practice: 2. Novel bleaching systems. Dent. Update 33, 357–358, 360–362.

Pretty, I.A., Ellwood, R.P., Brunton, P.A., Aminian, A., 2006. Vital tooth bleaching in dental practice: 1. Professional bleaching. Dent. Update 33, 288–290, 293–296, 299–300.

Pretty, I.A., Brunton, P., Aminian, A., Davies, R.M., Ellwood, R.P., 2006. Vital tooth bleaching in dental practice: 3. Biological, dental and legal issues. Dent. Update 33, 422–424, 427–428, 431–432.

Tong, L.S., Pang, M.K., Mok, N.Y., King, N.M., Wei, S.H., 1993. The effects of etching, micro-abrasion, and bleaching on surface enamel. J. Dent. Res. 72, 67–71.

Chapter | 6 |

Occlusion

David Ricketts

CHAPTER CONTENTS

WHAT IS OCCLUSION?

Occlusion is the way in which the maxillary and mandibular teeth come together. This definition conjures up a static relationship; however, in function the teeth move across one another and this articulation or dynamic occlusion is equally important. These tooth contacts cannot be looked at in isolation as the masticatory system also involves the periodontium, the skeletal components (including the temporomandibular joints) and the neuromusculature.

For some the study of occlusion is shrouded in mysticism and for others there is a conviction in philosophy that has seen occlusal adjustments and rehabilitations carried out solely to ensure a patient's occlusion fits the perfect ideology. Such conviction has been based upon subjective workings of various individuals and little sound evidence. Every patient is an individual and their occlusal management should be customized accordingly. However, when extensive rehabilitation of the dentition is required, some of the traditional teachings are useful.

It is important when restorations are placed that they are in functional harmony with the masticatory system to ensure a comfortable functioning apparatus. Failure to do so has been implicated in the aetiology of temporomandibular disorders and bruxism.

BRUXISM

Bruxism is a parafunctional activity which involves the clenching and grinding of teeth. This can occur consciously when awake (awake bruxism) or at night when asleep

(sleep bruxism). Awake bruxing is more common in females, has been linked to anxiety and stress, and is thought to affect 20% of the population. The prevalence of sleep bruxism decreases with age, with it being reported in 14–18% of children, 8% of adults and only 3% of elderly. Sleep bruxism is frequently noisy and reported by partners, and individuals may wake up with stiffness and aching of the jaws. Complaints of headaches are also common. Occlusal interferences were once thought to provoke sleep bruxism, but it is now thought of as a sleep-related movement disorder.

Most bruxism is mild and non-damaging to tooth tissue; as such, no treatment is required. However, for some, tooth wear and fracture may occur or the noise of grinding is unacceptable for partners and treatment is sought. For these patients a correctly adjusted hard acrylic splint can be supplied for night-time or daytime wear to protect the teeth. Such splints are referred to as stabilization splints and can be worn in the maxillary (Michigan splint, Figure 6.1; see also Chapter 4) or mandibular (Tanner appliance) arch.

An alternative splint is the localized occlusal interference splint (LOIS appliance, Figure 6.2). This consists of an acrylic plate retained by suitable clasps and two ball-ended wires which are placed between opposing teeth to interfere with the occlusion. Occlusal loading of the ball interferences leads to stimulation of periodontal mechanoreceptors, afferent feedback and reduction in occlusal loading. When used for bruxing habits, both splints act as a 'habit breaker' and patients can be gradually weaned off them.

If tooth destruction has taken place as a result of bruxism and restorative management is required, damage to any restorations can occur and it is important that the patient is aware of this. Damage to new restorations can be reduced by correct choice of dental materials, namely metal occlusal surfaces where possible and protection of restorations with a stabilization splint which can be worn at night for sleep bruxism and during the day if necessary for awake bruxism.

TEMPOROMANDIBULAR DISORDERS

Within the dental literature there seems to be no agreement as to a definition for temporomandibular disorders (TMD). What is clear is that TMD covers a number of

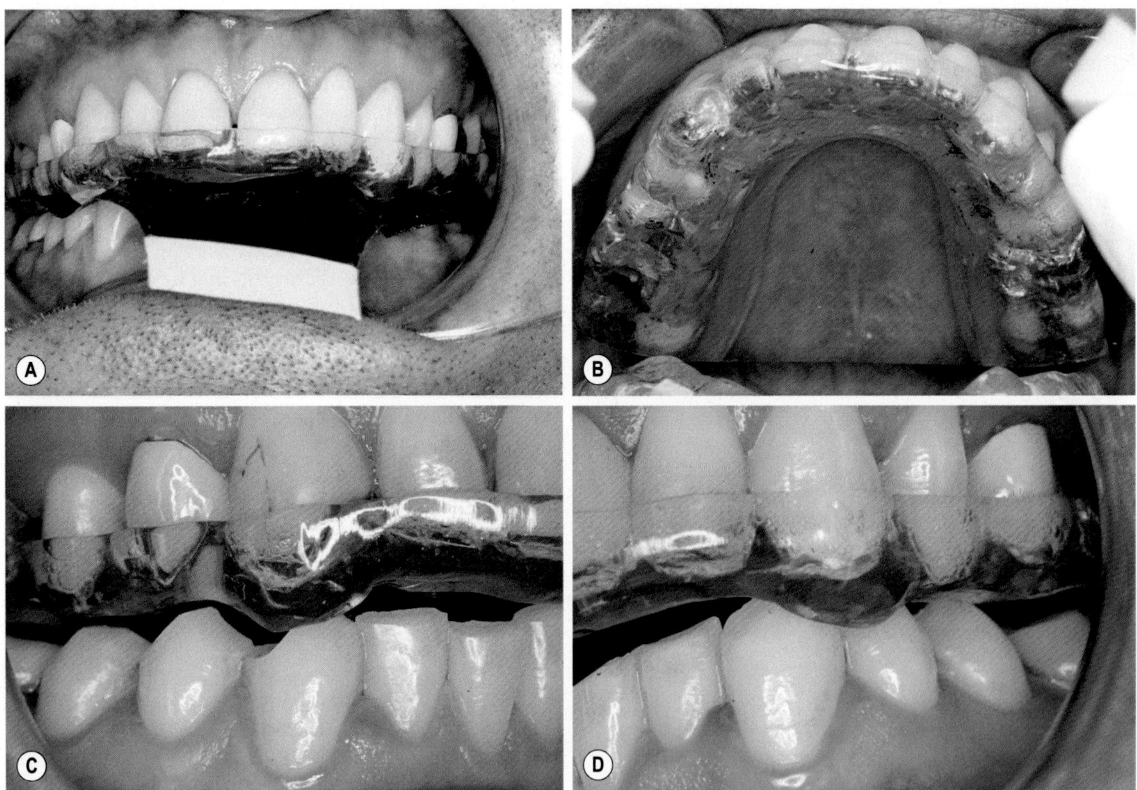

Figure 6.1 A Michigan splint being fitted and occlusion being checked to ensure all lower teeth occlude with the splint (A, B). Manufacture using casts mounted on an articulator reduce the amount of adjustment. The splint should have a canine rise in lateral excursions (C, D).

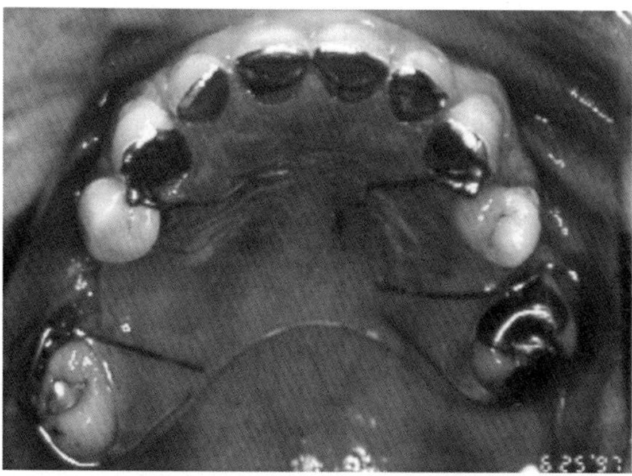

Figure 6.2 Localized occlusal interference splint (LOIS appliance). The ball-ended wires on the occlusal surface of the canine–premolar teeth interfere with the occlusion and are aimed at breaking a bruxism habit.
(Courtesy of Dr John Radford)

complex conditions with common signs and symptoms. The conditions are defined in the glossary of prosthodontics terms as those producing 'abnormal, incomplete or impaired function of the temporomandibular joint(s)'. The most common conditions making up these disorders, together with their signs and symptoms, can be seen in Figure 6.3. A number of terms have been given to the signs and symptoms allotted to pain dysfunction syndrome, some of which include myofascial pain, craniomandibular dysfunction and mandibular dysfunction. Rarer causes of TMD are rheumatoid arthritis, psoriatic arthritis, developmental defects, infection, neoplasia and ankylosis.

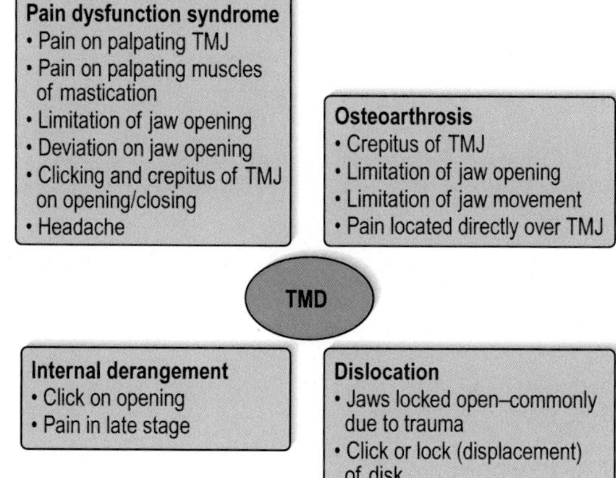

Figure 6.3 The most common conditions with their signs and symptoms which make up the temporomandibular disorders (TMD).

Epidemiological data indicate that signs and symptoms of TMD are relatively common (50–75% and 20–25%, respectively) and are evenly distributed between men and women; however, only 3–4% of the population actually seek treatment and these are more likely to be women, hence it is frequently and incorrectly cited that women are affected more than men.

Many theories on the aetiology of TMD have been put forward and, to a degree, management has been dictated by these thoughts. Whilst bruxism is a separate entity, it has been linked with TMD, possibly as one of the aetiological or exacerbating factors. Historically the occlusion (malocclusions, interferences and non-working side contacts) was also incriminated in causing TMD but as more is known about the condition it is realized that it has a complex and multifactorial origin and that occlusion plays a relatively minor role. Occlusal adjustments have been shown in numerous studies neither to prevent nor treat TMD and should therefore not be considered. TMD patients have been shown to have higher levels of stress, anxiety, depression and aggressive behaviour and as such it is thought that psychological factors may be more important.

TMD can be treated in a number of ways. Simple advice and reassurance that the condition is relatively common and not sinister may be sufficient. A simple change to a soft diet for a period of time, jaw rest and a hot pack over the tender areas can be advised. Medical management can include non-steroidal anti-inflammatory drugs which can be used topically (Mentholatum Deep Relief gel containing ibuprofen) or systemically if not contraindicated by any other medical condition such as asthma or gastritis. For the restorative dentist, the most common, time-honoured and least invasive form of treatment is to provide the patient with a stabilization splint. This treatment is often successful but why it is, is less clear. It may be: (1) a simple placebo effect; (2) the splint may disengage the occlusion, so eliminating any occlusal interferences and a reflex reduction in muscle activity; (3) the splint's repositioning effect may allow recapture of an anteriorly displaced disc; or (4) the increased occlusal vertical dimension alone may lead to relief. It has been shown that the greater the splint thickness, the more rapid the relief of symptoms. If these simple non-invasive treatments are not successful, thought should be given to referral to a specialist where other modalities of treatment such as prescription of muscle relaxants or antidepressants can be considered.

It is advisable to avoid complex and advanced restorative work in patients who are or have suffered from TMD. Their adaptation to the smallest changes in occlusion may be poorly tolerated and signs and symptoms of TMD may be exacerbated. Such patients can also be very focused on their 'bite' and have unrealistic expectations. If restorative treatment is unavoidable, treatment of the TMD needs to be carried out first and great care needs to be taken to ensure that any changes to the occlusion are gradual and staged.

PATIENT EXAMINATION

To enable the correct management of the occlusion, an understanding of its components and their function is important; this unfortunately is frequently overlooked in a clinical examination. This section details what should be examined and recorded.

Extraoral examination

Facial appearance

The facial appearance can firstly be assessed for facial asymmetries and skeletal relationship. With the patient's teeth in contact, the lower face height should be assessed in proportion to the total face height, especially in patients complaining of missing teeth and tooth wear. Loss of teeth and occlusal stops could result in an overclosed appearance but a reduction in lower face height is unusual in patients with tooth wear. This is because of dento-alveolar development or compensation which counterbalances the loss in coronal tooth tissue height. In fact it has been suggested that dento-alveolar development takes place in the absence of tooth wear and some researchers have shown an increase in face height with age. This is the mechanism which leads to overeruption of teeth when taken out of occlusion – for example, by loss of an opposing tooth (Figure 6.4).

Temporomandibular joints (TMJ)

The patient should be asked to open and close their mouth. The extent to which they can open should be measured between the incisal edges of the upper and lower incisor teeth. At maximum opening this should be more than 35 mm for women and 40 mm for men. Any limitation to opening should be recorded. Any deviation of the mandible on opening and closing from a normal vertical straight line should be observed and described. Gentle pressure over the head of the condyle should be applied when the patient opens and closes. This should be repeated with a finger in the external auditory meatus. Any tenderness, clicking or crepitus (grating sensation) should be noted and when they occur in the opening–closing cycle.

Intraoral examination – examination of the occlusion

Intercuspal position (ICP)

Intercuspal position can be defined as the position of the jaws when the maxillary and mandibular teeth are in maximum intercuspation. This has also been referred to as centric occlusion. Patients usually close from a rest position immediately into this position due to a conditioned path of closure. It is important to establish whether the occlusion in ICP is stable; that is, an occlusion where there is no possibility of tooth movement, namely overeruption, drifting or tilting of teeth (Figure 6.5). If teeth are extracted or lost due to other causes, or if they lose their contour (a carious lesion cavitating, tooth fracture, tooth wear), occlusal contacts and interdental contacts, teeth can move, often complicating any subsequent restorative work (Figures 6.4 and 6.6).

When teeth overerupt in the absence of periodontal disease, the alveolar process remodels and the gingival margin moves with the tooth (see Figure 5.3, Chapter 5). This dento-alveolar compensation can happen quickly in some patients and is a reason why temporary crowns

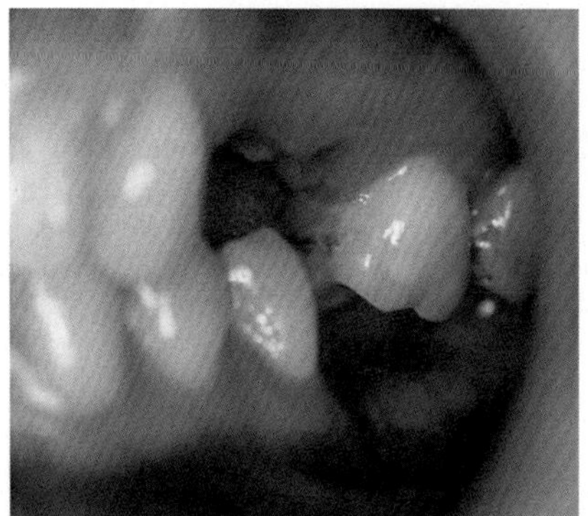

Figure 6.4 Loss of the lower left first and second molar teeth and upper left first and second premolar teeth has allowed overeruption of the opposing teeth. This now complicates their replacement as there is reduced height above the edentulous ridges.

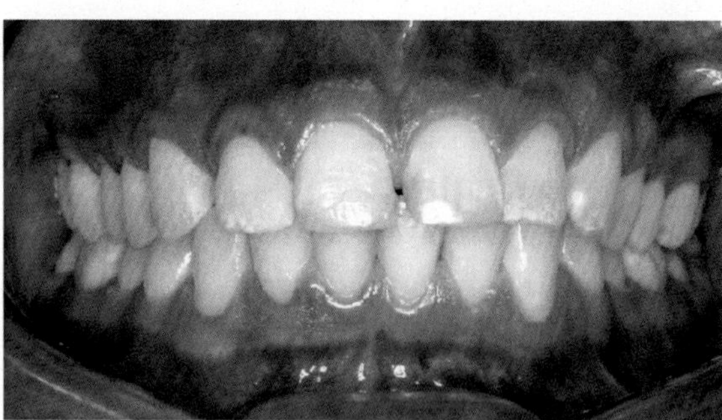

Figure 6.5 Patient with a stable intercuspal position (ICP): all interdental and occlusal contacts are intact preventing any tooth movement.

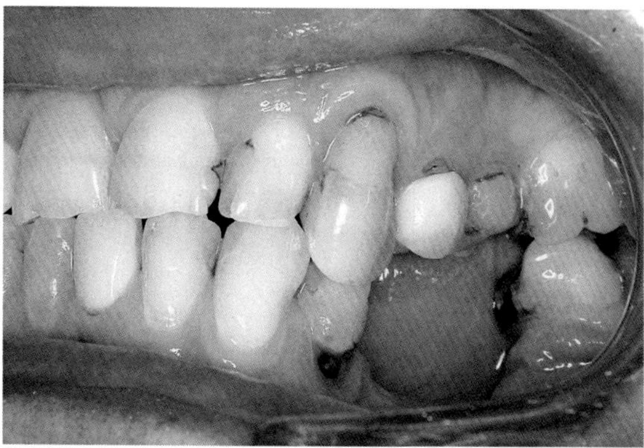

Figure 6.6 Patient with a heavily restored dentition. Repeated loss of the restoration in the lower left first premolar tooth has allowed overeruption of the upper left canine.
(Courtesy of Suzanne Blacker)

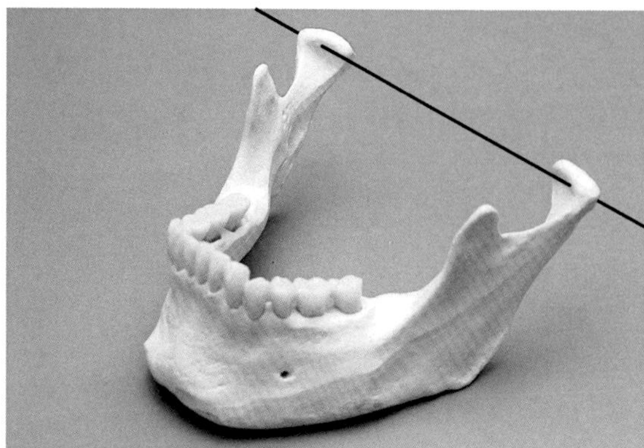

Figure 6.7 When the mandible is bilaterally in the most comfortable posterior location in the glenoid fossa, the mandible opens and closes around an arc of curvature through an imaginary axis drawn through the centre of the head of both condyles. This imaginary axis is termed the terminal hinge axis.

should be placed following tooth preparation for crowns or bridges; the occlusal and proximal reduction will result in an unstable occlusion and if no temporary is placed, overeruption and drifting of teeth could occur. This would result in a prosthesis that does not seat fully and appear to be occluding prematurely or appear 'high' in ICP.

Centric relation, terminal hinge axis position and retruded contact position (RCP)

Centric relation describes the jaw relationship between the maxilla and mandible when the mandible is in a retruded position. Differing definitions of centric relation have focused on slightly different positions of the condyle in the glenoid fossa and some on the relationship of the head of the condyle to the interarticular disc. These are rather academic arguments as clinically the position of the condyle cannot be visualized or confirmed without complex equipment. A more pragmatic and practical definition was proposed by Christensen in 2004 which conforms to most dentists' clinical practice. He described centric relation as the 'most comfortable posterior location of the mandible when it is bilaterally manipulated gently backward and upward into a retrusive position'. When this is done the mandible opens and closes on an arc of curvature around an imaginary axis drawn through the centre of the head of both condyles; this imaginary axis is termed the *terminal hinge axis* (Figure 6.7). Measured in the incisor region the arc of opening around the terminal hinge axis position takes place for about 20 mm before the condyles start to translate down onto the articular eminence (Figure 6.8). When the mandible closes in the terminal hinge axis position the first tooth contact is called the *retruded contact position* (*RCP*). The terminal hinge axis position is said to be the most reproducible jaw relationship; however, small variations from day to day and at different times during the day may occur. For most dentate patients there is a slide of the teeth and mandible from RCP into ICP of about 1–2 mm in an anterior and upwards direction. It is important to identify the RCP contact and record the direction and smoothness of the slide.

Excursive movements of the mandible

Retruded contact position is the most posterior tooth contact. All movements of the mandible occur anterior to this and can be guided by either the teeth when in contact and limited by the musculoskeletal system when the teeth are together or on jaw opening. With the teeth together the mandible can move forwards (protrusion), directly to the left or right (left or right lateral excursions) or in a pathway between these extremes. Some texts refer to anterior and posterior guidance, where the anterior guidance is provided by the tooth contacts and posterior guidance by the temporomandibular joints and associated ligaments, disc and musculature. In this terminology, the anterior guidance does not necessarily have to be on the anterior teeth; it can be on posterior teeth.

Posterior guidance

If the TMJ is viewed in three dimensions, its movements can be described when the mandible is moved into protrusion and lateral excursion.

Protrusion

When the mandible moves into protrusion, the condyles move from the glenoid fossa in a forward and downward movement onto the articular eminence. The angle this path makes with the horizontal when the individual is sitting upright is termed the *condylar inclination* (Figure 6.9).

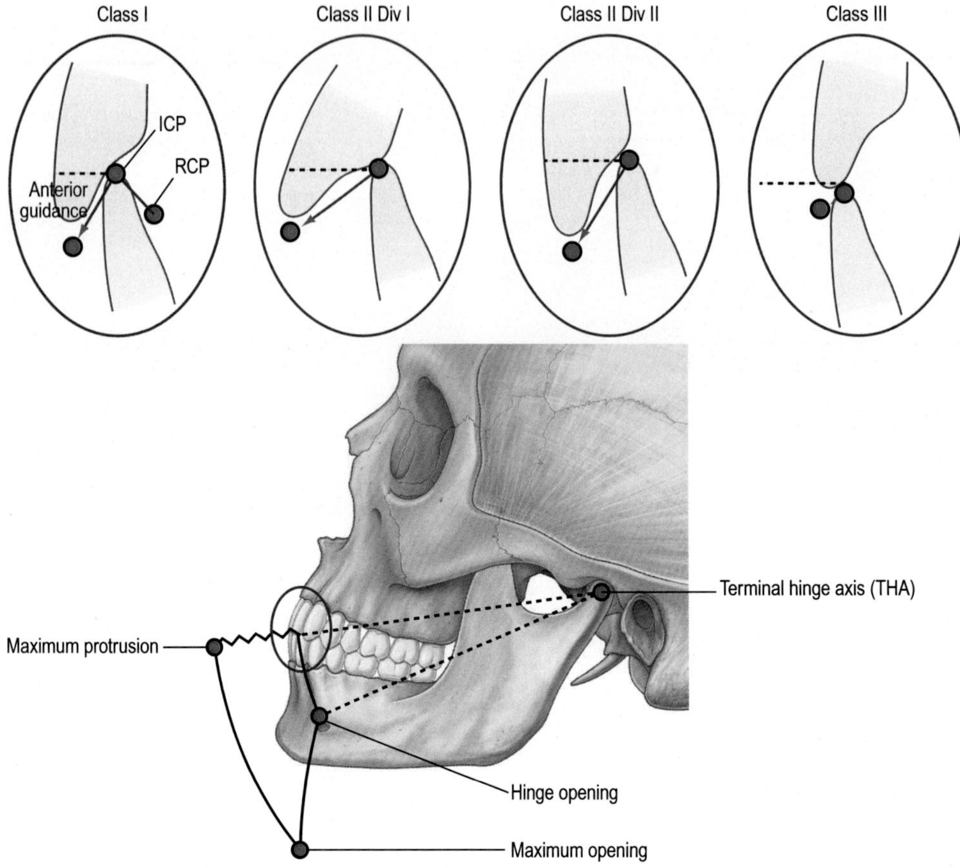

Figure 6.8 Main picture depicts Posselt's envelope of movement – a tracing made by an imaginary point between the lower incisor teeth in the sagittal plane. The inset images show how the incisor relationship can affect the amount of anterior guidance. ICP, intercuspal position; RCP, retruded contact position.

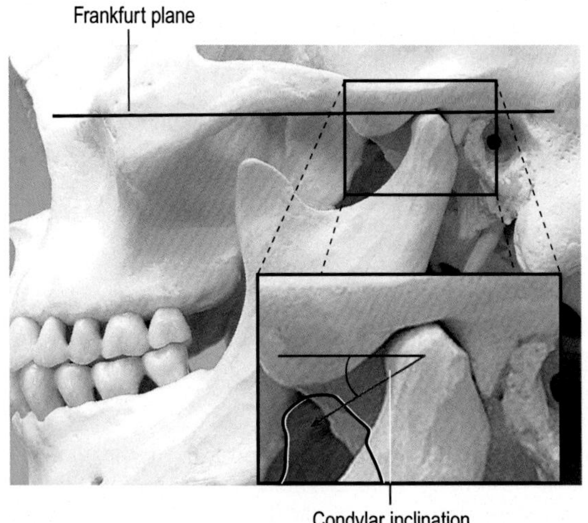

Figure 6.9 In protrusion the condyle moves down and forward onto the articular eminence. The angle this makes with the horizontal is the condylar guidance.

Lateral excursion

In lateral excursion, the side to which the mandible moves is called the working side and the opposite side from which the mandible moves is the non-working side. In Figure 6.10 the inferior surface of the skull can be seen with the outline of the mandible superimposed; the mandible is moving to the right and hence the right-hand side is the working side and the left-hand side the non-working side.

When the mandible moves into lateral excursion the non-working condyle moves forward and medially; the angle this makes with the parasagittal plane is termed Bennett angle (Figure 6.10) and is viewed in the horizontal plane. The working side condyle also moves laterally and this is called Bennett movement.

Anterior guidance

Protrusion

In protrusion the posterior teeth or anterior teeth may contact and this is governed by the incisor relationship

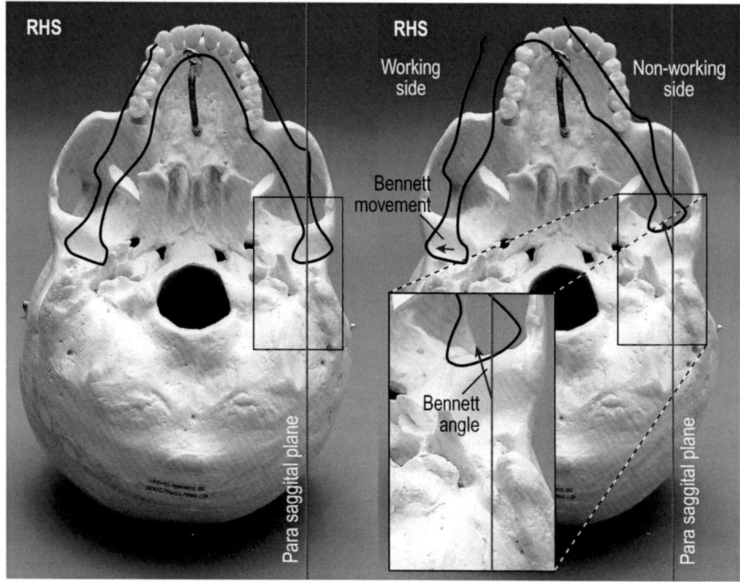

Figure 6.10 View of base of skull with outline of mandible in intercuspal position superimposed (left). In right lateral excursion (right) Bennett movement and Bennett angle can be seen.

and incisal guidance. There are four classifications describing the incisor relationships based upon their inclination, and horizontal (overjet) and vertical (overbite) overlap (see Figure 6.8):

- *Class I.* The lower incisors occlude within the middle third of the palatal surface of the upper incisors (Figure 6.11). In Class I incisor relationships the overjet is normally 2–3 mm and the overbite 2–4 mm. As the mandible moves forwards the mandible drops and the posterior teeth usually separate or disclude.
- *Class II.* In a Class II incisor relationship the lower incisors occlude or potentially occlude with the gingival third of the palatal surface of the upper incisors or palatal gingivae. This classification is divided into two subdivisions depending on the inclination of the upper incisors:
  - Class II Division I. The upper incisors are proclined and the overjet is increased. Depending on the severity of the incisor relationship, the incisal guidance is reduced and the likelihood of posterior teeth contacting in protrusion is increased.
  - Class II Division II. The upper incisors are upright or retroclined and the overbite is increased. In protrusion the incisal guidance is marked and the posterior teeth separate or disclude immediately (Figure 6.12). Posterior tooth contacts are therefore unlikely.
- *Class III.* In Class III incisor relationships the lower incisors occlude with the incisal third of the upper incisor teeth, the teeth may have an edge-to-edge relationship or the lower incisors may occlude in front of the upper incisors (Figure 6.13), a so-called reverse overjet. In this incisor relationship the incisal guidance is reduced and the posterior teeth are likely to contact in all excursive movements.

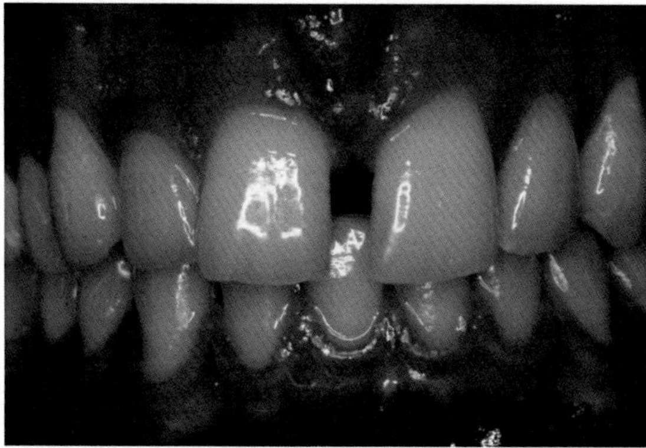

Figure 6.11 Patient with a Class I incisor relationship.

In addition to these incisor relationships, there may be an anterior open bite (Figure 6.14), where there is no anterior tooth-to-tooth contact or there is bimaxillary proclination where both upper and lower anterior teeth are proclined. In both these situations incisal guidance is non-existent or reduced, respectively.

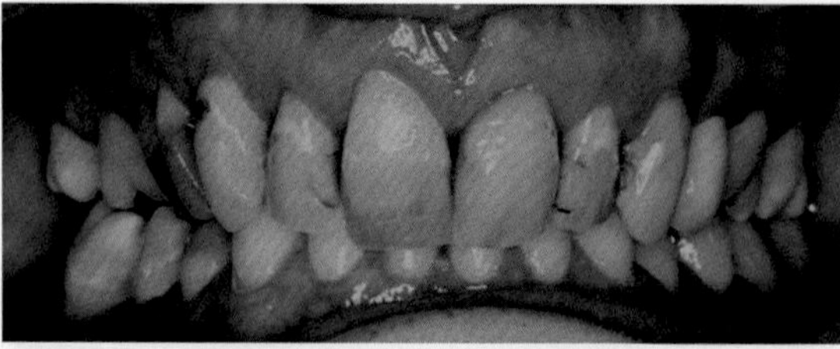

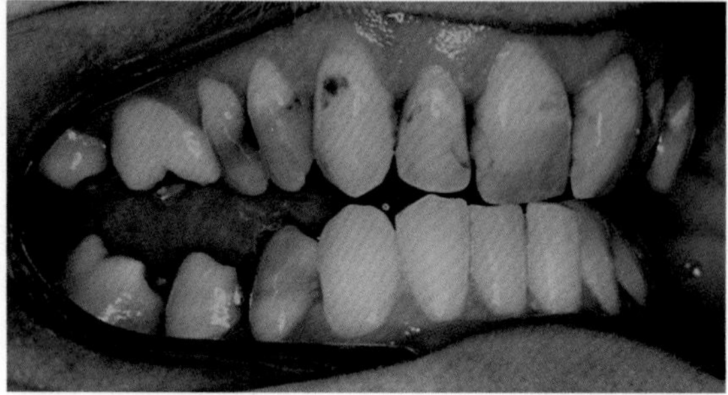

Figure 6.12 Patient with a Class II Division II incisor relationship. The deep overbite means that in protrusion the posterior teeth immediately disclude, making the placement of posterior restorations much easier and anterior restorations much more difficult.

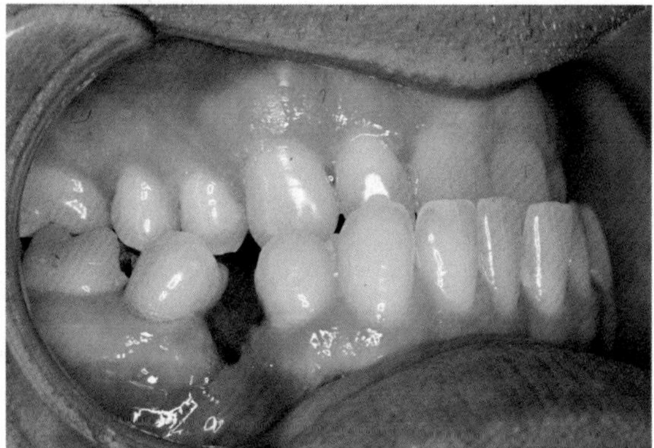

Figure 6.13 Severe Class III incisor relationship with reverse overjet. In protrusion there is no guidance on the anterior teeth and posterior teeth will remain in contact, making the occlusion on posterior restorations more difficult to achieve.

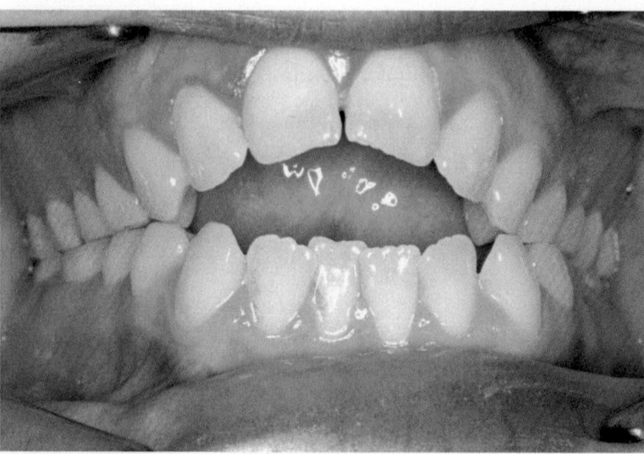

Figure 6.14 Patient with a severe Class II Division I incisor relationship and an anterior open bite. In all excursive movements the posterior teeth are in contact and making posterior restorations will be more difficult.

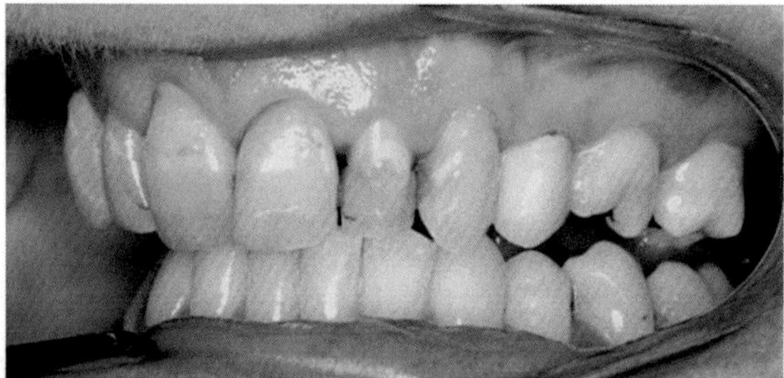

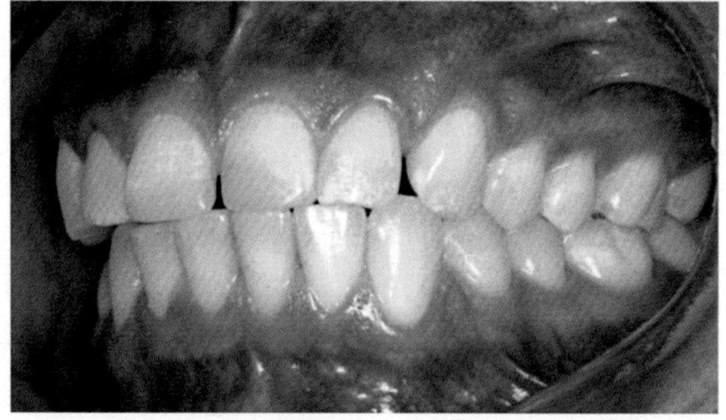

Figure 6.15 In lateral excursion the guidance on the working side can either be canine guided (top) or group function (bottom).

Lateral excursion

In lateral excursion tooth contacts on the working side can be either between the canine teeth, termed canine guidance, or between one or more posterior teeth, termed group function (Figure 6.15).

Whilst guidance in lateral excursion is usually provided by the teeth on the working side, non-working side contacts can occur (Figure 6.16). This is more likely if the condylar inclination is shallow or if the tooth guidance on the working side is shallow. Both will mean that the body of the mandible moves more horizontally into lateral excursion with the non-working side teeth not dropping downwards and hence more likely to make contact.

TWO APPROACHES TO MANAGING THE OCCLUSION

Current management of the occlusion in operative dentistry is very much based on what is regarded as good clinical practice and will depend upon whether single

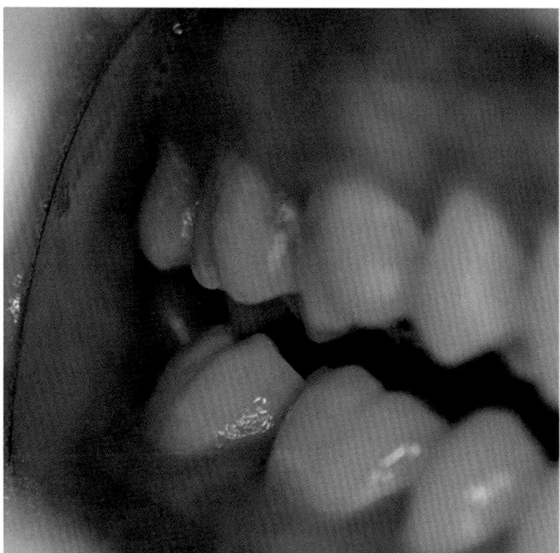

Figure 6.16 This patient is moving into left lateral excursion. There is an obvious non-working side contact between the molar teeth.

individual restorations are placed or whether extensive work means that all or most of the occlusal surfaces are being restored. In the former situation when individual or small numbers of restorations are being placed a *conformative approach* to the occlusion is adopted whereby the restoration(s) is made to fit in harmoniously with the existing occlusion and articulation. This does not mean that the occlusion is adjusted until no 'high spots' are detected, but rather simultaneous, even occlusal contacts need to be achieved with both the restoration placed and the adjacent teeth. When most or all of the teeth are to be restored with fixed prosthodontics or a combination of fixed and removable prostheses, it is usual to adopt a *reorganized approach* to the management of the occlusion. Here the occlusion is reorganized so that the RCP and ICP coincide at a predetermined vertical dimension.

ARTICULATORS

To assist in the detailed examination of the occlusion, aid treatment planning and facilitate the laboratory in making indirect restorations, study casts are often mounted on an articulator. An articulator is a hinged device connecting maxillary and mandibular members, onto which corresponding casts can be attached, enabling the relationship between opposing teeth to be reproduced as accurately as possible. Articulators vary in their complexity and hence in their ability and accuracy to reproduce jaw movements.

Probably the most commonly used method to locate opposing casts is to hand-hold them. This simple but effective method is only suitable for individual crowns in a Class I incisor relationship. In accepting hand-held models the dentist should appreciate that some intraoral occlusal adjustment will be needed at the chairside. If the occlusion is group function or the tooth involved with guidance, the time needed for occlusal adjustment can be excessive. Articulators attempt to mimic the relationship between the upper and lower jaws and should reduce the time needed to adjust an indirect restoration to fit the existing occlusion.

Simple hinge articulator

In its simplest form there is a simple hinge articulator (Figure 6.17), which is often used for simple fixed prosthodontics as only opening and closing of the jaws is possible. The arc of opening on the simple hinge articulator is different from that of a patient as the hinge is closer to the teeth on the model than the TMJ would be to the teeth in the mouth. Lateral excursive and protrusive movements are also not possible.

Average value articulators

Average value articulators allow for some degree of protrusive and lateral excursive movements (Figure 6.17). The condylar inclination is set at a single predetermined angle by the manufacturer which is usually 30° and not adjustable. The Bennett angle and Bennett movement are not reproduced and the maxillary cast is usually mounted in an arbitrary position. Whilst average value articulators allow some movement of the casts, this is not precise and therefore their use is limited to the reproduction of intercuspal position. They are not commonly used as they are neither semi-adjustable articulators which give more precision, nor do have they any significant advantage over hand-held models or simple hinge articulators.

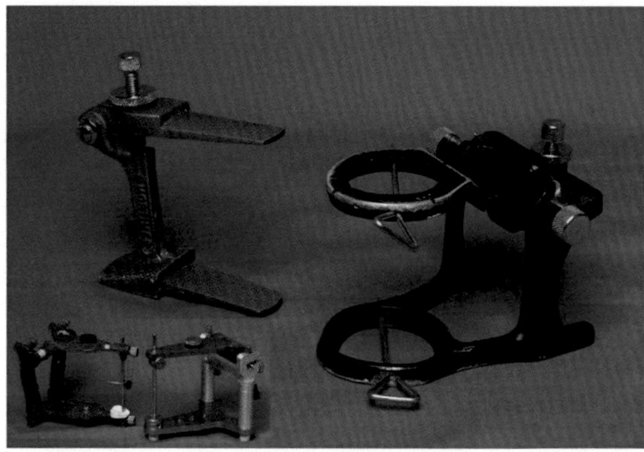

Figure 6.17 A simple hinge articulator (left) and an average value articulator (right). Two further average value articulators are seen inset.

Semi-adjustable articulators

When planning and executing more advanced restorative dentistry, the semi-adjustable articulator is invaluable (Figure 6.18). The design of articulators varies with manufacturers but most allow adjustment of condylar inclination, Bennett movement and Bennett angle. In relation to articulators, the Bennett movement is often referred to as immediate side shift and the Bennett angle as progressive side shift. The height of the incisal pin can also be altered and the incisal table can usually be adjusted or modified/customized. The intercondylar width cannot be altered and is usually set at 11 cm.

Arcon vs non-arcon articulators

Semi-adjustable articulators can be either arcon (*ar*ticulating *con*dyle) or non-arcon in design. An arcon articulator is one in which the condylar component or sphere is attached to the mandibular member of the articulator and the glenoid fossa component to the maxillary member; it is therefore anatomically correct and thus easier to conceptualize. A non-arcon articulator is one in which the condylar component or sphere is attached to the maxillary member and sits in a track connected to the mandibular member.

Fully adjustable articulators

Fully adjustable articulators are more complex devices allowing the clinical scenario to be most closely reproduced. Instead of flat tracks and planes that reproduce the condylar movements on semi-adjustable articulators, fully adjustable articulators have further components that can be adjusted and use curved condylar inserts that can more accurately reproduce the three-dimensional nature of the glenoid fossa anatomy. These articulators require more complex information and time to program them, and pantographic (see Cadiax system) and stereographic recordings are needed. As these articulators are only as accurate as the recordings used to program them and are usually reserved for the most complex of restorative procedures, the semi-adjustable articulator is the articulator of choice for the vast majority of clinical situations.

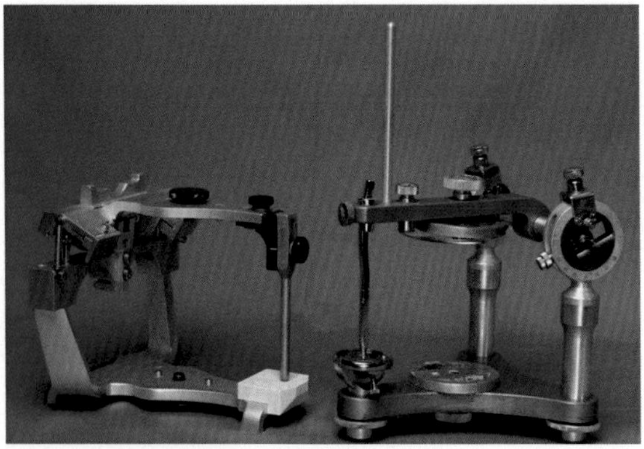

Mounting models on a semi-adjustable articulator

A facebow and interocclusal record are required to mount maxillary and mandibular casts onto an articulator.

Facebows

Facebows are calliper-like devices that record the relationship of the maxillary teeth to the position of the condyle when it is in the terminal hinge axis position and allows this information to be transferred to the articulator when mounting dental casts. To use a facebow, firstly the position of the condyle needs to be identified and this can only be done accurately with a kinematic facebow (Figure 6.19). This consists of a clutch, which is essentially an impression tray that is fitted to the mandibular teeth, and a rigidly attached facebow which has condylar pointers on arms which can be extended or retracted and an adjustable angulation mechanism. The patient is then guided into the terminal hinge axis position and asked to open and close slightly. The adjustable components on the facebow arms are then altered until the condylar pointers no longer arc and pure rotation occurs: the condylar pointers are then directly over the terminal hinge axis.

Identifying the hinge axis position using a kinematic facebow is time consuming and most clinicians use arbitrary positions. The use of an earbow is convenient and

Figure 6.18 An arcon (Denar, Whip Mix Co.) semi-adjustable articulator (left) and a non-arcon (Dentatus, Dentatus Company) semi-adjustable articulator (right).

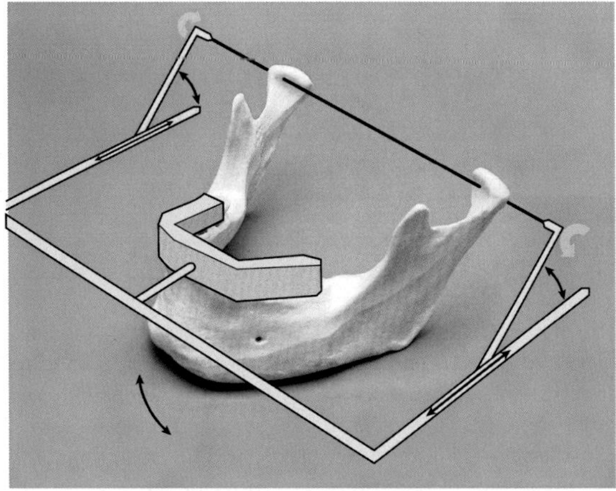

Figure 6.19 Diagrammatic representation of a kinematic facebow.

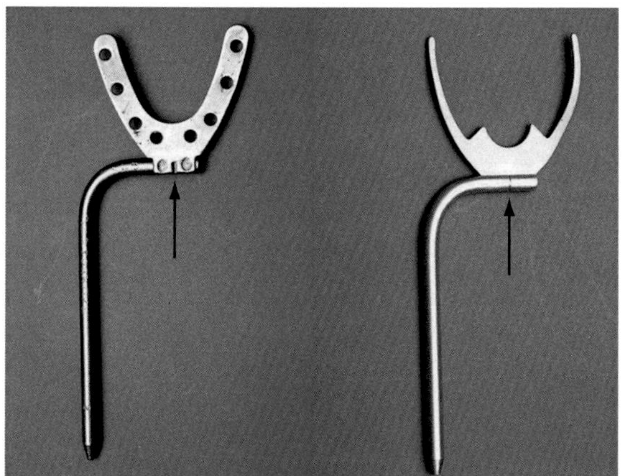

Figure 6.20 Bite fork for Denar and Dentatus facebows. Note both have a notch on the upper surface (arrowed) to allow alignment with the patient's centre line. The bite fork can be covered with either wax or an addition cured silicone bite registration paste.

in nearly 90% of patients the earbow axis will be within 6 mm of the true terminal hinge axis. The other most commonly used arbitrary hinge axis position is 13 mm along an imaginary line from the tip of the tragus of the ear to the outer canthus of the eye.

Once the positions of the condyles have been located, an imprint of the cusp tips and incisal edges of the teeth in the maxillary arch need to be recorded on a bite fork (Figure 6.20). Dental wax such as Beauty Pink wax or a silicone bite registration paste is an ideal material for this. It is important that the bite fork is seated firmly on the teeth and not rocked in an attempt to get an imprint of all teeth whilst the wax is cooling or when the silicone is setting. This ensures that the dental cast made in the laboratory seats precisely into the imprint without rocking during its mounting on an articulator. The bite fork is then linked to the facebow via a jig. The bite fork is then reseated on the maxillary teeth and held firmly in place, ideally by the patient. The condylar locators are then placed into position either in the external auditory meatus in the case of the earbow, or over the marked arbitrary or kinematically determined hinge axis position. The facebow needs to be centralized around the patient's head, which in the Denar Slidematic earbow is automatic and in the Dentatus facebow is achieved by ensuring the measurements on two rulers attached to each condylar pointer are equal.

To allow the occlusal plane of the maxillary cast to be set on the articulator to the correct angulation to the horizontal or Frankfurt plane (plane between the inferior border of the orbit or *orbitale* and the superior margin of the corresponding external auditory meatus or *porion*) in a patient standing upright, a third reference point is needed. The third reference point chosen will depend upon the facebow and articulator system being used; for example, the Denar MK II (Whip Mix Co.) uses a point on the face which is 43 mm above the incisal edge of the lateral incisor and the Dentatus (Dentatus Company) uses the *orbitale*. Finally, a pointer is aligned with the third reference point and all components tightened together.

The entire facebow (Dentatus) or jig and bite fork (Denar) can then be released from the patient's head, disinfected and sent to the laboratory for mounting of the maxillary cast. Figures 6.21 and 6.22 show how the Denar facebow is recorded and transferred to the laboratory for mounting of maxillary casts on the Denar MK II articulator, and Figures 6.23 and 6.24 show how this is done for the Dentatus facebow and articulator.

Interocclusal record

To enable the technician to mount the mandibular cast on the articulator in the correct relationship to the maxillary cast, an occlusal record is required. If all movements of the mandible are to be reproduced, including the RCP–ICP slide, a terminal hinge axis record should be taken; however, if the articulated casts are to be used to aid the manufacture of simple restorations, an ICP record is frequently sufficient.

Taking a terminal hinge axis record can be difficult in some patients due to preconditioned paths of closure as a result of feedback from periodontal mechanoreceptors and proprioceptors during repeated tooth contacts. Muscle tension or muscle splinting may also make it difficult to guide the mandible back into a posterior position. Even once an RCP contact has been made, for many patients the tooth contact leads them to readily slide into ICP. In these patients a Lucia jig or deprogramming appliance can be constructed at the chairside (Figure 6.25A). This is essentially a cold cure acrylic anterior bite platform which covers the upper central incisors. It is designed so that the lower incisors occlude at 90° to the platform with all posterior teeth separated. Repeated contact on the splint breaks down the programmed paths of closure and allows the operator to guide the mandible into its posterior position. The terminal hinge axis interocclusal record can be taken with the Lucia jig in situ (Figure 6.25B), thus preventing any sliding into ICP. Once mounted on the articulator, the incisal pin can be moved until RCP contact is made; this is possible due to the pure rotational closure of the mandible in the terminal hinge axis position. Other methods for deprogramming have been described in order to make a terminal hinge axis record and these include the use of cotton wool rolls between the teeth and a hard occlusal splint.

If sufficient teeth contact, an ICP record or terminal hinge axis interocclusal record can be taken in either

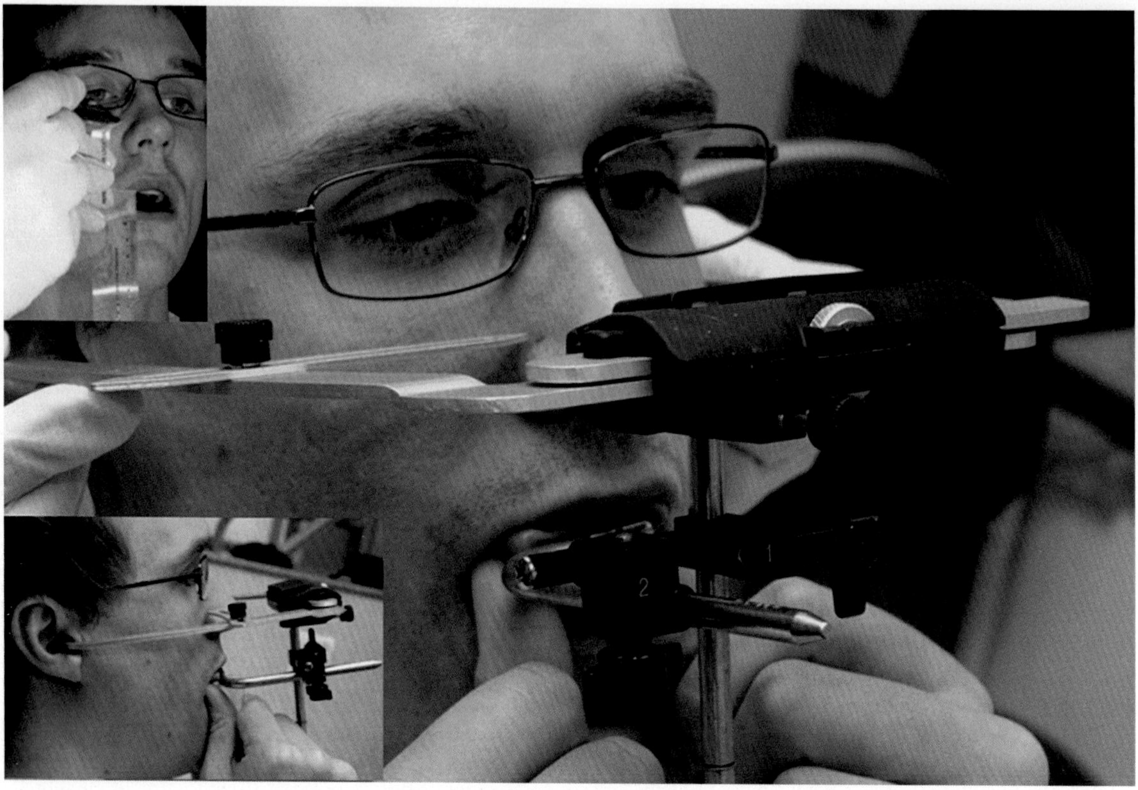

Figure 6.21 Denar Slidematic facebow (earbow) being recorded. The third reference point is recorded first and marked on the side of the nose with a pen (inset, top left). The condylar locators are placed in the external auditory meatus (inset, bottom left) by sliding the bow together. The bite fork and the slidematic earbow are then linked together with the jig making sure the numbers 1 and 2 on the jig face forwards. Once the jig has been adjusted so that the third reference pointer is aligned with the marked third reference point, the screws on the jig can be tightened.

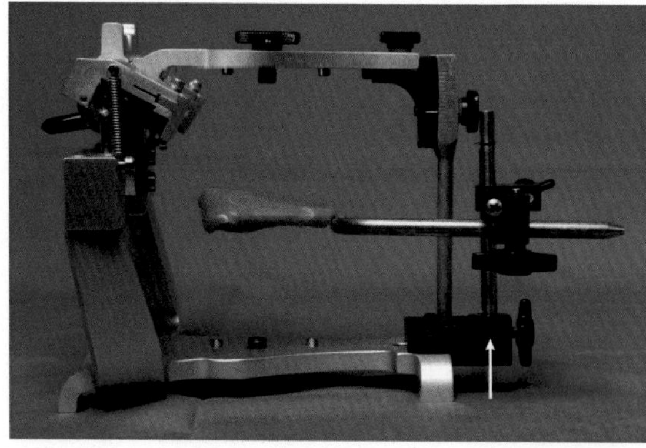

Figure 6.22 Denar bite fork and jig transferred to the Denar articulator. The pillar of the jig sits in a special mounting block (arrowed). The maxillary study cast can now be seated into the wax imprint on the upper surface of the fork and attached to the maxillary arm of the articulator with anti-expansion plaster.

wax or a silicone bite registration paste. If wax is used it is important not to use a 'horseshoe'-shaped record as this can easily distort in transit to the laboratory, and as it is not elastomeric, its original shape is not reformed. Instead the wax should be at least double thickness and extend across the arch. Once the patient has closed down into the warmed and softened wax, it can be removed and the excess cut away with scissors so that the technician can confirm that the study casts are fully seated into the record. This will obviously distort the wax and so it has to be reseated in the same position in the patient's mouth and the record re-established. Once removed from the mouth it is chilled in cold water and disinfected ready to send to the laboratory (Figure 6.26).

Silicone bite registration pastes are presented in double cartridges containing the base and catalyst pastes. These are inserted into a gun and syringed around the occlusal plane of the lower teeth through a double helix mixer tip which ensures a bubble-free, perfectly mixed paste

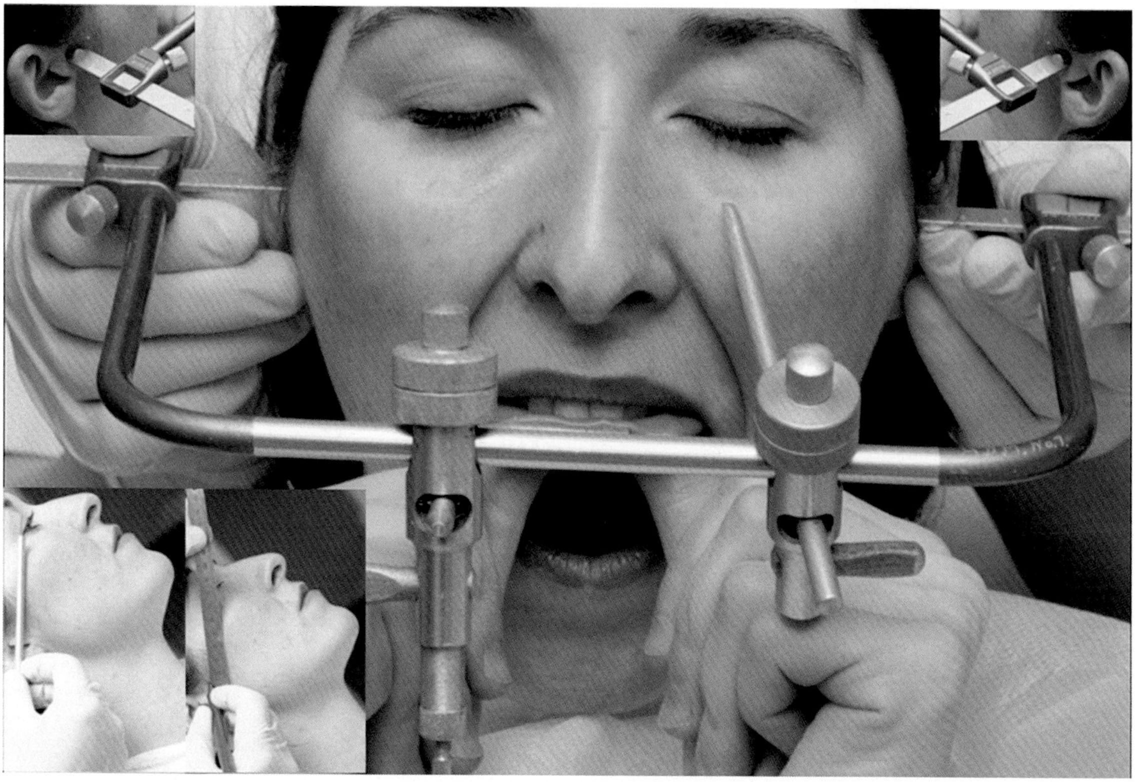

Figure 6.23 Dentatus facebow being recorded. The condylar pointers are placed over the marked arbitrary hinge axis position (inset, bottom left). The facebow is centralized by ensuring that the condylar rulers read the same on left and right hand side (inset, top). The orbital pointer is placed in position and the screws tightened.

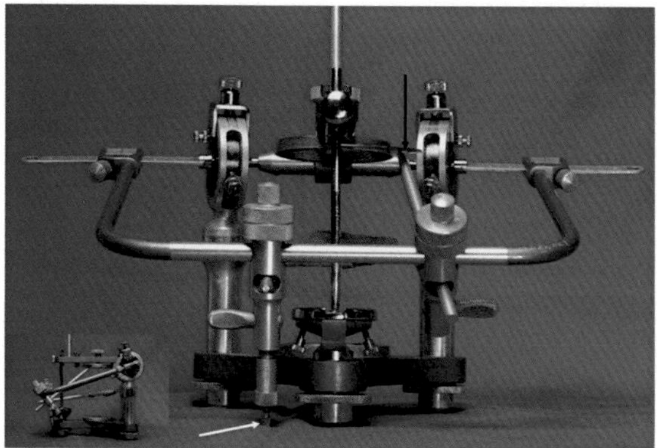

Figure 6.24 The entire Dentatus facebow recording is then transferred to the Dentatus articulator. The pin at the foot of the bite fork jig (arrowed white) is adjusted until the orbital pointer touches the orbital plane on the articulator (arrowed black). The maxillary study cast is then placed on the bite fork imprint and the cast attached to the maxillary arm of the articulator using anti-expansion plaster.

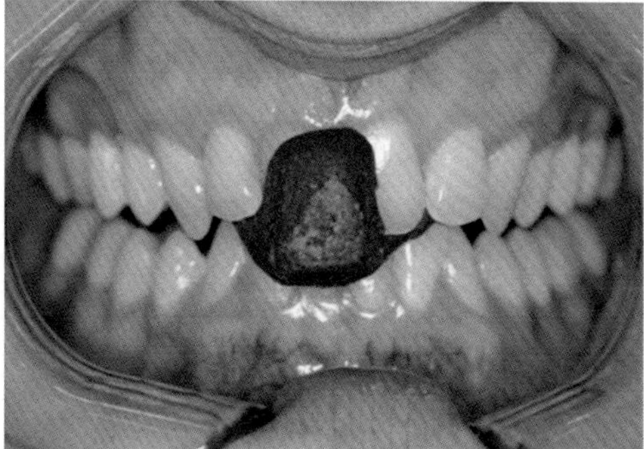

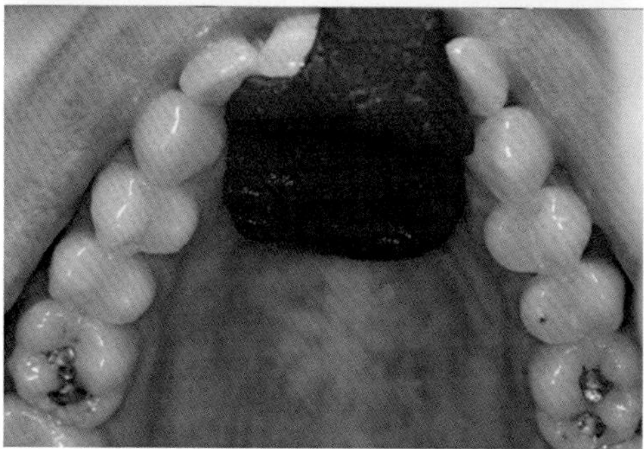

Figure 6.25A Anterior and palatal view of Lucia jig made from cold cure acrylic.

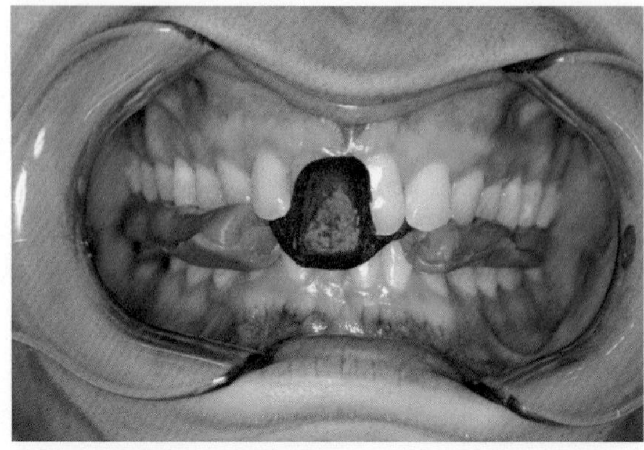

Figure 6.25B Wax terminal hinge axis interocclusal record being taken with the Lucia jig in situ.

(Figure 6.27). Bite registration pastes have a rapid set, avoiding patient fatigue when keeping the jaw in the same position and errors due to jaw movement.

Placing any material between the teeth and then the casts in the laboratory always has the potential to introduce errors; therefore, if the occlusion is obvious, the casts can be manually placed together using marked index teeth (Figure 6.28). If insufficient teeth are present, wax occlusal record blocks may be required and used as for recording the occlusion for removable prostheses.

Programming the semi-adjustable articulator

The adjustable components on a semi-adjustable articulator are commonly set at average values: condylar inclination 25–35°, progressive side shift (Bennett angle) at 7–15° and immediate side shift (Bennett movement) 1–2 mm.

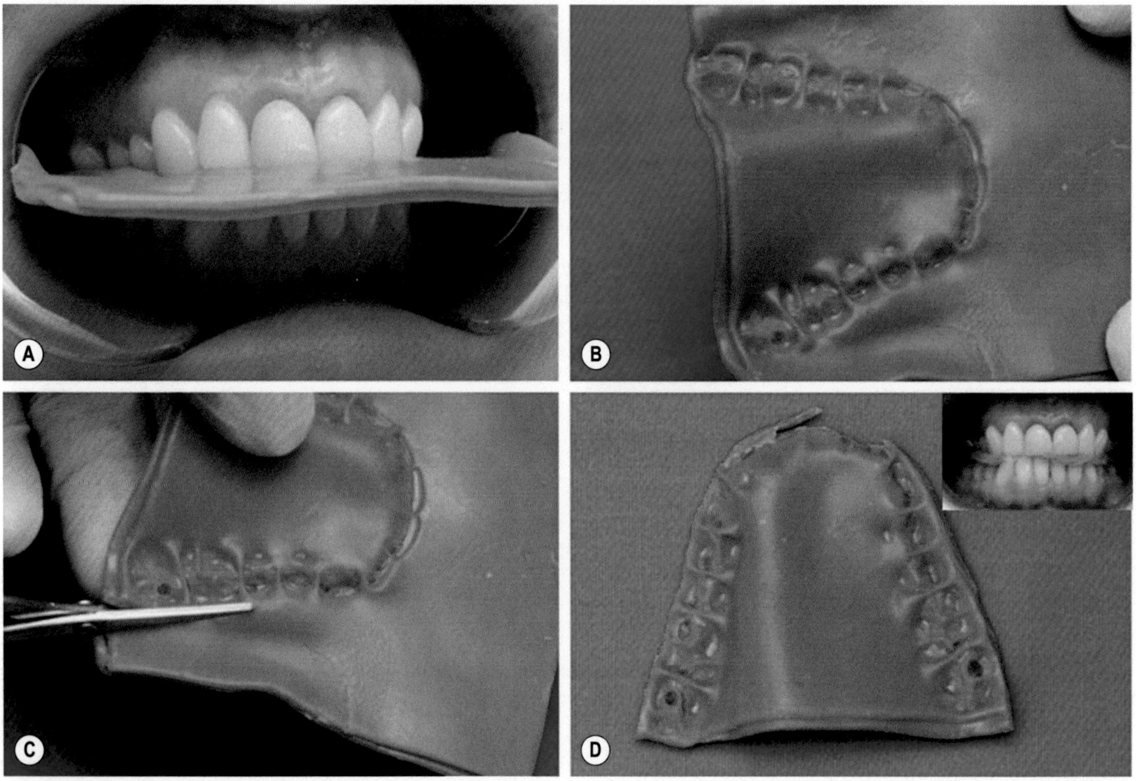

Figure 6.26 Steps for taking a wax interocclusal record. The patient bites into at least a double layer of warmed and softened wax, ideally wax such as Beauty Pink wax (Moyco Union Broach, York, PA) which is hard and brittle when cold (A). When removed (B) and still warm and soft, the excess wax is removed using a scissors (C). As this distorts the wax it is reseated in the mouth, removed again and chilled, disinfected and sent to the laboratory (D).

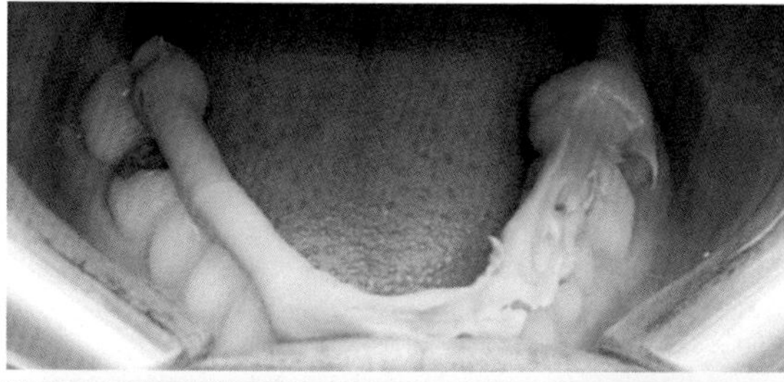

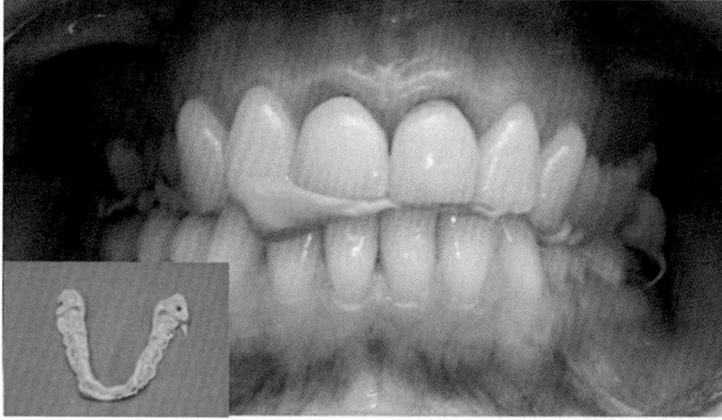

Figure 6.27 Silicone bite registration paste syringed over the occlusal surfaces of mandibular teeth (top). The patient bites through the paste (bottom) and once set is removed, disinfected and sent to the laboratory (inset).

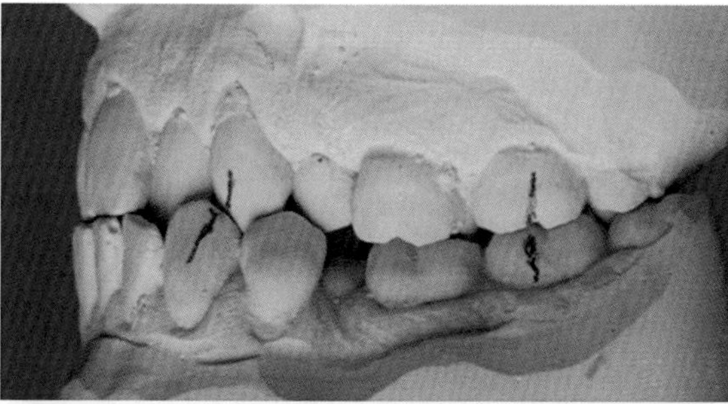

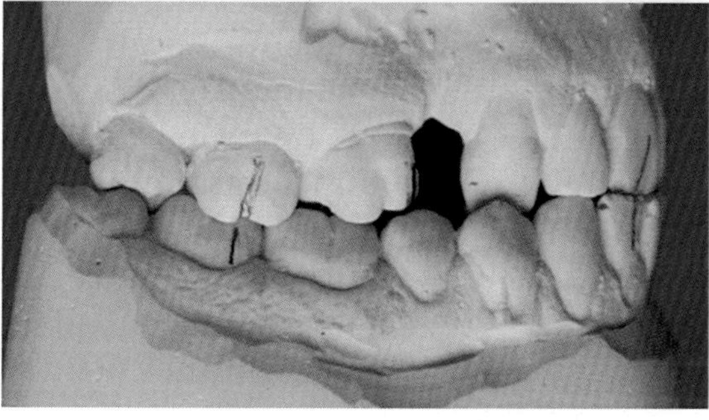

Figure 6.28 Study casts with index teeth marked. The patient's occlusion is obvious and no interocclusal record is needed.

To customize the settings for each patient, excursive occlusal records are required or a pantographic tracing. This is described here using the Denar MK II articulator as an example. The operator should start with all settings on the Denar MK II articulator set at zero. To set the condylar inclination a protrusive wax record is required. Protrusion of the mandible brings the condyles down onto the articular eminence and the posterior teeth will usually separate. This will also depend on the amount of incisal guidance. A protrusive wax record will record this amount of separation. The maxillary and mandibular arms of the articulator should be separated and the protrusive record placed between the casts until they are fully seated. This will bring the condylar spheres downward and forward as in the patient. The condylar inclination element is then released and tilted down until it contacts the condylar sphere and secured; this is the condylar inclination.

To set the Bennett angle and Bennett movement, left and right lateral excursive records are required. In left lateral excursion the left condyle moves laterally and the immediate side shift adjustment is made on the left glenoid fossa component of the articulator until the medial wall contacts the condylar sphere. On the non-working side (right-hand side) the condyle would have moved forward and medially and the Bennett angle component is again adjusted until the condylar sphere seats into the fossa and against the medial wall. The same is repeated with a right lateral excursive record. Figure 6.29 shows the adjustable components on the Denar MK II articulator. Some dentists simply use protrusive records only to set condylar inclination and then set Bennett angle and movement to average settings, and some take lateral records only to set all components.

Alternatively, pantographic tracings or readings can be used. A pantograph is a set of tracing devices similar to facebows which are attached to the mandible and maxilla which records mandibular movements in three planes. A simplified version of such a device is the Denar Cadiax (Whip Mix Co.) (Figure 6.30). The Denar Cadiax consists of a maxillary bow which is strapped to the head. The nasal support is adjusted until the condylar component of the bow sits at the terminal hinge axis position (Figure 6.30, left). The mandibular bow is then attached to the mandibular clutch which is essentially an impression tray, loaded with impression material to keep it securely in place, and an anterior rod to which the bow is attached. A sensor plate is then attached to the maxillary bow and a stylus to the mandibular bow (Figure 6.30, right). Left and right lateral excursive movements are then made by the patient and the Denar Cadiax records these movements both graphically and numerically (Figure 6.31). These readings can then be set on the articulator.

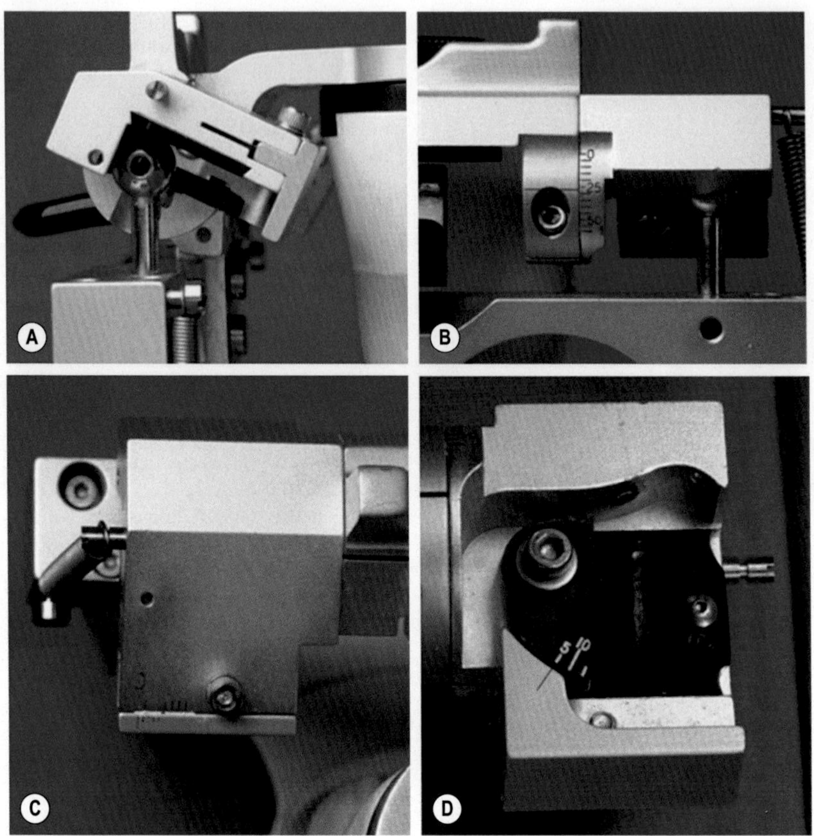

Figure 6.29 Adjustable components on the Denar MK II articulator. Top shows how condylar inclination is adjusted and below how Bennett movement (left) and Bennett angle (right) are adjusted.

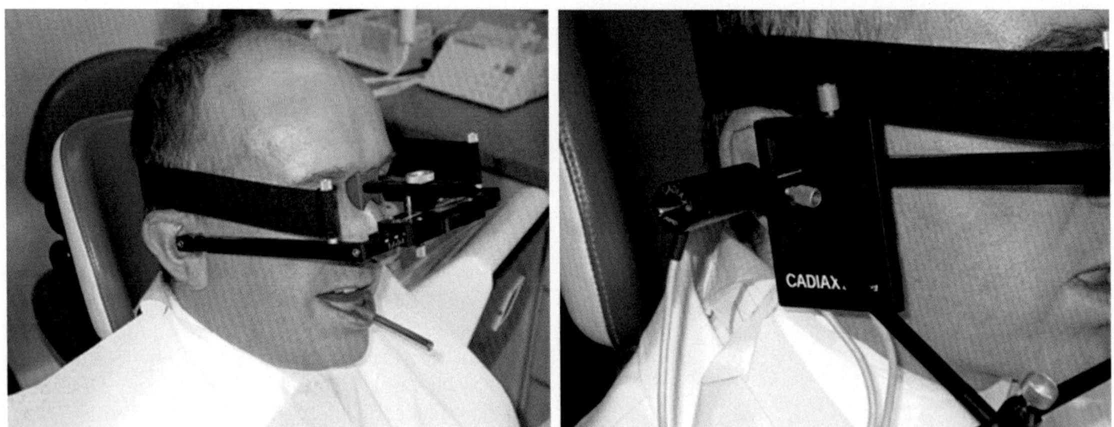

Figure 6.30 The Denar Cadiax consists of a maxillary component strapped to the head and a nasal support adjusted until the condylar component of the bow sits at the terminal hinge axis position. The mandibular component is attached to a clutch which is placed over the teeth with a loaded impression tray.

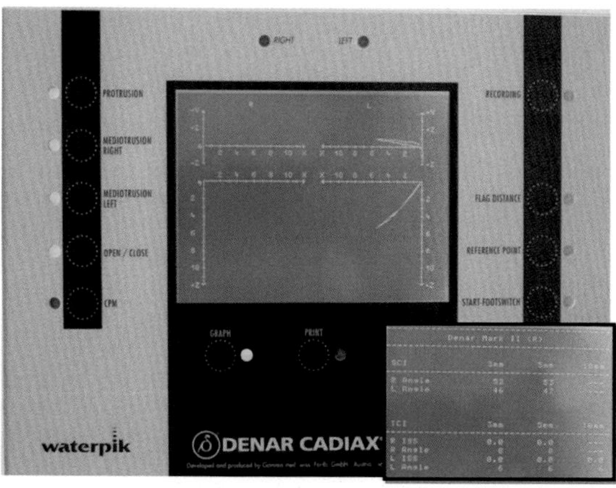

Figure 6.31 The Denar Cadiax gives a graphic recording of the condyle movements seen here for the left condyle. Progressive side shift (Bennett angle) and condylar inclination are illustrated. Numerical values for these angles and immediate side shift (Bennett movement) are also given (inset).

SUMMARY

This chapter has addressed why occlusion is important in restorative dentistry and has attempted to diffuse some of the mystique that has surrounded the subject. Examination of a patient's occlusion is an essential part of any clinical examination and the aspects that should be looked for and recorded in the patient's clinical notes are described, together with the relevance to making restorations whether or not they are direct or indirect. The use of articulators plays an important role in this examination, particularly when the restorative procedures become more complex. Their use is also important for the construction of indirect restorations and, as such, their use has been described in detail. When indirect restorations are fitted the occlusion will need to be checked and adjusted. How this is done is described in Chapter 9. There are also special considerations to managing the occlusion – for example, in reproducing guidance, management of short clinical crowns and reorganizing the occlusion. These are addressed in Chapters 14 and 16.

FURTHER READING

Al-Ani, Z., Gray, R., 2007. TMD current concepts: 1. An update. Dent. Update 34, 278–288.

Christensen, G.J., 2004. Is occlusion becoming more confusing? A plea for simplicity. J. Am. Dent. Assoc. 135, 767–770.

Davies, S.J., Gray, R.M.J., Smith, P.W., 2001. Good occlusal practice in simple restorative dentistry. Br. Dent. J. 191, 365–381.

Davies, S., Gray, R.M.J., 2001a. What is occlusion? Br. Dent. J. 191, 235–245.

Davies, S., Gray, R.M.J., 2001b. The examination and recording of the occlusion: why and how. Br. Dent. J. 191, 291–302.

Gray, R.J.M., Davies, S.J., 2001. Occlusal splints and temporomandibular disorders: why, when, how? Dent. Update 28, 194–199.

Lavigne, G.J., Khoury, S., Abe, S., Yamaguchi, T., Raphael, K., 2008. Bruxism physiology and pathology: an overview for clinicians. J. Oral Rehabil. 35, 476–494.

Palik, J.F., Nelson, D.R., White, J.T., 1985. Accuracy of an earpiece face-bow. J. Prosthet. Dent. 53, 800–804.

Türp, J.C., Greene, C.S., Strub, J.R., 2008. Dental occlusion: a critical reflection on past, present and future concepts. J. Oral Rehabil. 35, 446–453.

Chapter | 7 |

Cores

Carol Tait, David Ricketts

CHAPTER CONTENTS

INTRODUCTION

A core material replaces missing coronal tooth structure prior to restoration with an indirect extracoronal restoration and helps to stabilize weakened parts of the tooth. It is generally recommended that a core should be considered when more than 50% of the coronal part of the tooth is missing. Existing restorations should be investigated radiographically to diagnose residual caries or caries adjacent to the restoration and evaluated clinically to determine if the existing restoration needs replacing. An assessment of the depth of the cervical margins should highlight potential challenges with preparation and impression taking. Some clinicians recommend the routine removal of existing directly placed restorations to confirm these criteria and replacement with a new core to ensure that the newly placed core is adequately retained (see Chapters 3 and 8 for further discussion). But this is not always necessary, particularly if the restoration was placed recently or there are no clinical or radiographic reasons to do so.

MATERIALS

Several dental materials can be used for core build-ups; each has different properties and therefore advantages and disadvantages. Enamel–dentine bonding using adhesive materials, such as composite resins or glass ionomer-based materials, allows a more conservative technique compared to amalgam which often requires additional tooth preparation to achieve adequate retention. Crown preparation can be carried out immediately following core build-up if the material used is command set by light curing. If the core is placed as a transitional restoration at an appointment prior to preparation then it should be sufficiently contoured to give occlusal stability, cause no food packing and maintain gingival health.

There are many materials on the market that are suitable for core build-up, but those based upon composite resin are increasing in use and many may say they are the most appropriate to use in contemporary practice. The use of amalgam has decreased in popularity, mainly because of health and environmental issues over its mercury content, its inability to bond to tooth structure and its colour. In a number of countries the use of dental amalgam has already been banned and this is only likely to extend to other countries in the future. However, it is still in use in sufficient countries and sufficient quantities to warrant its description in this textbook.

Composite resin (Figure 7.1)

Composites consist of a resin, normally an aromatic dimethacrylate such as BisGMA, and filler particles such as quartz, silica and other types of glass. The type, particle size and content of the filler particles control the properties of the material. Barium- or strontium-containing glasses are also added to make the material radio-opaque. Many composites have a variation in particle size. So-called hybrid composites contain large filler particles (15–20 μm) and smaller colloidal silica (0.01–0.05 μm) particles. Microfilled composites (average filler particle size = 0.02 μm) can be highly polished, but this is a property obviously not necessary for a core material. The most effective core materials are hybrid composites and more recently the newly developed low-shrink composites (e.g. Filtek LS Low Shrink Composite (3M ESPE) based on silorane chemistry) might prove to be effective. Composites have a compressive strength similar to dentine and higher tensile and flexural strengths. They can be bonded to tooth structure when used with a dentine-bonding agent; however, placement is technique sensitive.

When using composites it is important to prevent moisture contamination with saliva or blood and, therefore, where possible, rubber dam isolation is recommended. Visible light cured composites should be placed in increments to reduce problems with shrinkage on setting. Polymerization contraction may increase the risk of marginal leakage and post-treatment sensitivity. The lower shrink composites that are being introduced may overcome this problem in the future but will need assessing as the materials develop. Water sorption occurs with composites and can lead to expansion of the material. This, however, takes some time to occur and is unlikely to have an impact on the provision of indirect restorations. Any dimensional

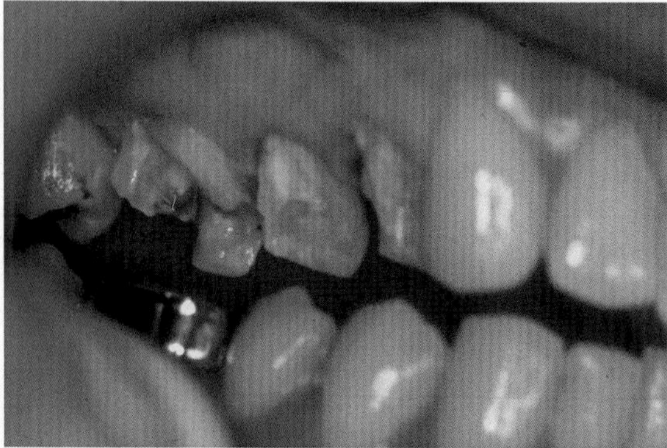

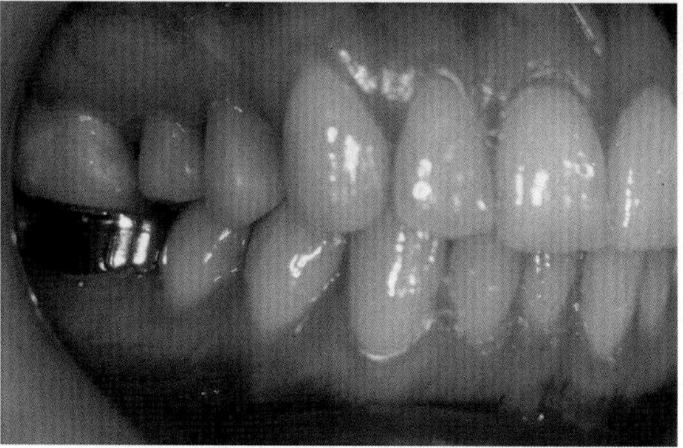

Figure 7.1 Composite resin cores placed in root-filled teeth in the upper right sextant in preparation for all ceramic dentine-bonded crowns. See Chapter 11 for preparations and cemented restorations.

change that does occur will be easily compensated for by the placement of die relief on the master die in the laboratory. Composite is the material of choice for a core when an all-ceramic crown is planned (Figure 7.1).

Newer hybrid composite core materials are available with various additives such as fibres, ceramic fillers, titanium and lanthanide, that claim to improve the mechanical properties of the material. Examples of these are Paracore (Coltène Whaledent), Ti-core (Essential Dental Systems, Inc.), Light-Core (Bisco, Inc.), Coradent (Vivadent) and Core Paste XP (Den-Mat). Composite core materials are available with a blue pigment to allow the clinician to distinguish between tooth structure and material during preparation (e.g. MultiCore Flow Blue, Ivoclar). Some composites are also packable, facilitating contact point formation and reducing the risk of voids.

Advantages of composite resin as a core material

- Strong and can therefore be placed in thinner sections compared to amalgam
- Immediate setting with light-cured composites
- Can be bonded to tooth structure
- No mercury
- Tooth coloured, hence ideal under all ceramic crowns

Disadvantages of composite resin as a core material

- Technique sensitive – moisture contamination and polymerization shrinkage should be avoided
- Can be difficult to distinguish between composite and tooth structure when preparing crown margins

Glass ionomer cement (GIC)

The original cements contain a fluoroaluminosilicate glass, which reacts with a polyalkenoic acid to form a cement. Many studies have shown that glass ionomer is not sufficiently strong to be used as a core build-up material unless there are two intact walls remaining. There should also be at least 1–2 mm of remaining sound tooth structure coronally that can be prepared as a ferrule. This is an important distinction when compared to composite materials that have greater strength and are more suitable for extensive restorations. Glass ionomer can also be useful as a filler to block out undercuts (e.g. when preparing a tooth for an inlay) and to make good any defects or irregularities in a tooth preparation for an indirect restoration (e.g. when a filling or piece of tooth is lost during tooth preparation; see Chapter 12). Variations of glass ionomer cements have been developed in the past in an attempt to improve the physical properties of the material and these have included the addition of metal particles by a fusion process resulting in a cermet, or addition of amalgam alloy particles resulting in an admix.

Resin-modified glass ionomers (RMGIs)

In the early 1990s a water-soluble resin (hydroxyethyl methacrylate, HEMA) was added to conventional GIC to improve the physical properties, as such the material cures by an acid–base reaction (the glass ionomer component) and a resin polymerization, which is either chemical or light activated or both (dual cured). Some RMGIs are specifically advocated as core materials such as Vitremer core build-up material (3M ESPE). Whilst most of these materials are tooth coloured, their use beneath all-ceramic restorations should be avoided as they undergo hygroscopic expansion which could lead to ceramic fracture. Resin-modified glass ionomer is an ideal core material for metal or metal–ceramic crowns, inlays, onlays or bridges, or reinforced core ceramics; however, like chemically cured glass ionomers, it needs significant remaining tooth structure to be effective.

Advantages of GIC and RMGIs as core materials

- Sets quickly, allowing immediate preparation
- Adhesive
- Fluoride release – The clinical significance of this is controversial and there appears to be no conclusive evidence in the literature for or against the anti-cariogenic properties of fluoride release from GICs or RMGIs in clinical trials (Randall & Wilson, 1999)
- Low thermal expansion coefficient

Disadvantages of GIC and RMGIs as core materials

- Low compressive and tensile strengths
- Weak material only suitable when significant proportion of the tooth remains
- Deterioration at low pH
- Sensitivity to moisture during setting

Amalgam (Figure 7.2)

Dental amalgam consists of mercury combined with a powdered silver–tin alloy with the addition of copper, palladium and other elements. High copper amalgam

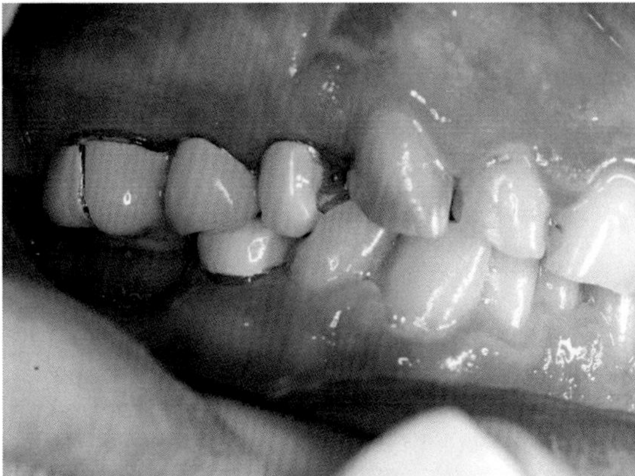

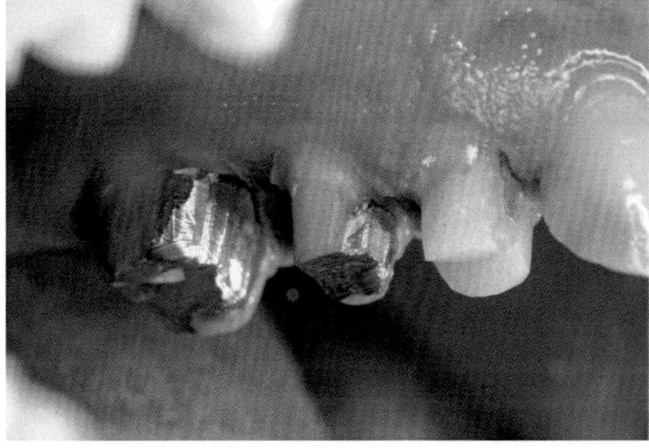

Figure 7.2 Failed metal–ceramic crowns in the upper right sextant being removed (top) and the amalgam cores beneath (bottom).

alloys have a copper content of 30% and on setting have a smaller concentration of the gamma-2 phase, which means they are less easily deformed, stronger in compression, and have reduced potential for corrosion. The alloy particles can be spherical, lathe cut or admixed. Amalgam can be the material of choice for core build-ups on posterior teeth and is still used by some practitioners. Its use is, however, on the decline and is only likely to decline further in the future. Unfortunately, as the material takes 24 hours to reach maximum compressive strength, crown preparation has to be carried out at a second appointment. The spherical, high copper alloys reach their maximum strength faster and can be prepared 10–15 minutes following placement rather than the normal 24 hours; however, even this is a long time to wait in a busy practice. As amalgam does not adhere to tooth structure it has to be mechanically retained or chemically bonded. It performs well if properly condensed and is not contaminated by large amounts of blood or saliva during placement.

Advantages of amalgam as a core material

- Not particularly technique sensitive
- Strong if placed in sufficient bulk
- Can be used as a bonded amalgam
- Easy to distinguish between amalgam and tooth structure
- Packable – if condensed well voids are avoided

Disadvantages of amalgam as a core material

- Long setting time
- Low initial tensile/compressive strength
- Weak in thin section
- Mercury may be of concern to some patients
- Potential for electrolytic galvanic action between amalgam and other metals in crowns for example
- Not adhesive and so needs mechanical retention derived from the cavity

VITAL TEETH

Preoperative assessment (see also Chapter 3 on endodontology)

It is important prior to planning an indirect restoration that the tooth and any existing restoration are carefully assessed to ensure long-term success. The tooth should be symptom free, ideally provide a positive sensitivity test and a periapical radiographic examination made to ensure an absence of periradicular pathology. If needed, endodontic treatment should be carried out. The existing restoration needs careful examination and if doubt exists it should be removed to ensure that the core is placed on sound tooth structure and that no previous carious exposure exists.

Methods of core retention for vital teeth

There are no absolute guidelines, but if more than 50% of tooth structure has been lost or removed, additional methods of retention are usually required. Retention can be either mechanical, when using amalgam, or adhesive. The latter is the most common as composite is the preferred material for a core.

Adhesive retention

Composite resins and dentine bonding

Bonding of composite to etched enamel has made a huge advance in operative dentistry, allowing aesthetic restorations to be placed and clinical techniques such as minimum preparation (resin retained) bridges. Bonding of hydrophobic composite resins to physiologically wet dentine has also made a massive leap forward over the last two decades. Generally the dentine surface is chemically treated with an acid to allow the mechanical interlocking of resin around the dentinal collagen, producing a layer known as the hybrid layer. The bonding agent, which is normally an unfilled resin, is then applied to the dentine surface and light cured. It copolymerizes with the resin already present in the collagen matrix, locking it onto the dentine and providing a more suitable surface for bonding with resin composite materials.

The steps involved in dentine bonding have changed over the years. Initially a separate etch, primer and bond were used. With this technique there was a risk that during drying the collagen may collapse and ruin formation of the hybrid layer. Two-step systems have either a separate etch with the prime and bond combined in one bottle or the etch and prime combined with a separate bond. The latter has the advantage that the self-etching priming agent does not have to be washed off the dentine. One-step bonding systems are similar to self-etching priming materials but have the bonding agent added also. They have been shown not to etch the enamel as effectively as phosphoric acid.

Adhesive retention for amalgam restorations – amalgam bonding

Whilst dentine bonding was developed for use with composite, its use has also been applied to the more traditionally used amalgam. Amalgam-bonded restorations are thought to improve restoration retention, reinforce remaining tooth tissue and enhance the marginal seal against bacterial leakage. This philosophy is not new; in 1897, Baldwin suggested placing a thin, wet layer of zinc phosphate cement on the cavity walls prior to condensing the amalgam in an attempt to improve the bond and marginal seal; the acidity of the unset zinc phosphate cement probably etched the tooth, creating micromechanical retention. Today, the technique has been modified using modern dental materials including self- or dual-curing metal adhesive resins or glass ionomer cements. Specific products such as All-Bond 2 (Bisco), Amalgambond Plus (Parkell), Optibond 2 (Kerr), RelyX ARC (3M ESPE) and Panavia EX, Panavia 21 (Kuraray) have been studied regarding bond strengths and prevention of microleakage.

Amalgam bonding – technique

- Gain as much mechanical retention as possible using conventional means, such as undercuts, occlusal key ways and grooves.
- Isolate the tooth using rubber dam or cotton wool rolls and saliva ejector.
- Consider if a lining is needed in a deep cavity, keeping this to a minimum, bearing in mind this might interfere with the subsequent bonding technique.
- Check the fit of matrix band, remove and lightly coat its inner surface with petroleum jelly.
- Isolate the cavity but do not over-dry as this may result in postoperative sensitivity. Place the matrix band using wedges to maintain a tight fit gingivally.
- Either use a total etch technique in the cavity, rinse thoroughly, dry and apply a compatible dentine-bonding agent according to the manufacturer's instructions (e.g. Scotchbond for use with RelyX ARC) or use a compatible self-etching bonding agent.
- Using a microbrush, apply a thin coat of freshly mixed resin (e.g. RelyX ARC) over the entire cavity surface.
- Condense the amalgam onto the unset resin, beginning in the deepest areas such as grooves and boxes first. The wet cement will be extruded towards the occlusal surface.
- Once the cavity has been completely packed, remove the top layer of amalgam/cement with a cotton pellet and replace with a final layer of amalgam. Complete initial carving before removal of the matrix band.

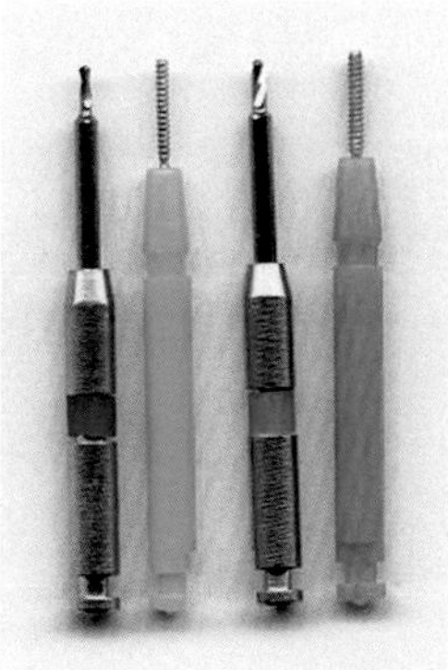

Figure 7.3 Self-threading intradental pins. The pin drills cut a hole in the dentine slightly narrower in diameter to the thread on the pins. The pins shear off once they have penetrated the full depth of the pin hole.

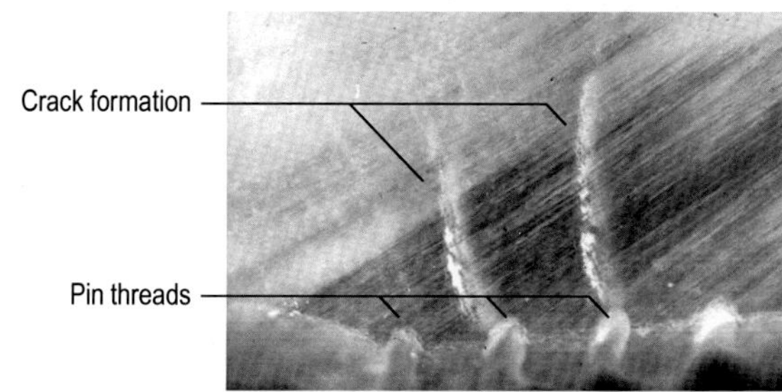

Figure 7.4 Micrograph showing crack formation in dentine radiating out from the pin threads cut into the pin hole seen at the bottom of the image.
(Courtesy of Professor A Grieve)

Mechanical retention for amalgam restorations

Intradental pins

The use of dentine pins has decreased as the use of amalgam has declined (and hence its need). Pin placement is also fraught with problems, but, like amalgam, some practitioners continue pin use so it is sufficient to warrant description in this text. Most intradental pins are self-threading; a pin hole is cut within dentine which is slightly narrower in diameter than the thread on the corresponding pin (Figure 7.3). Therefore, as the pin is inserted into the hole, it cuts its own counter-thread on the walls of the pin hole, causing stresses within the dentine (Figure 7.4). As the pin is inserted deeper into the hole, the frictional forces increase and often the pins shear off before they reach the base of the pin hole (Figure 7.5). This leaves a void at the base of the pin hole, an unretentive and potentially loose pin in dentine, and a pin too long coronally which is likely to interfere with the occlusion. Any attempt at shortening the pin with a high speed bur will cause vibration of the pin, shattering the dentine counter-threads, and will lead to loss of the pin. Clamping the pin with a self-locking tweezers will dampen down the vibration and will reduce the risk of loosening the pin. Alternatively, the pins can be bent slightly to avoid the occlusion and to ensure that they are surrounded by sufficient core material (Figure 7.6).

The use of pins to aid retention should only be employed as a last resort due to their complications. In addition, if placed in the wrong direction, they can completely or partially perforate into the pulp or the

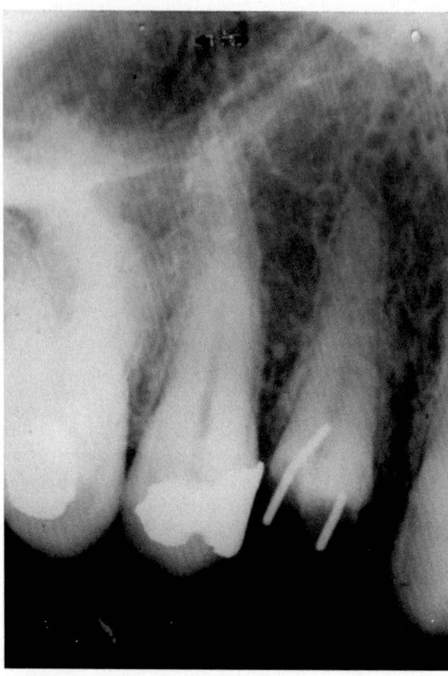

Figure 7.5 Radiograph of two pins in the upper right first premolar tooth. The mesial pin has not completely entered the dentine and the distal appears to be perforating into the pulp (note this is a two-dimensional image and the pin may be buccal or lingual to the pulp).

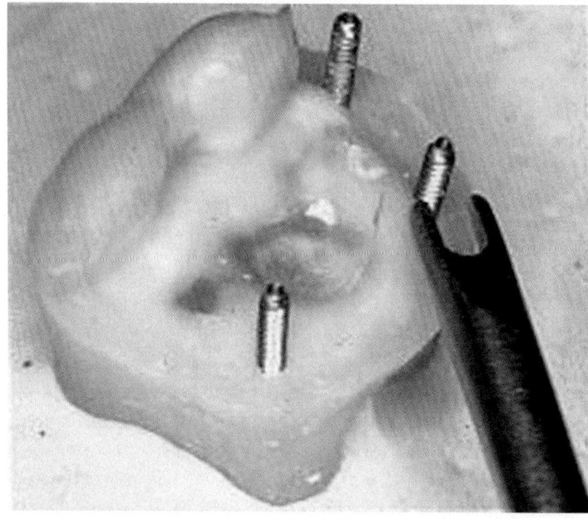

Figure 7.6 Three pins placed in an extracted molar tooth. The pins are tilted and need to be bent to ensure sufficient core material surrounds them.

periodontal ligament (Figures 7.5 and 7.7, respectively). On the few occasions where pins are thought to be necessary the following guidelines should be considered:

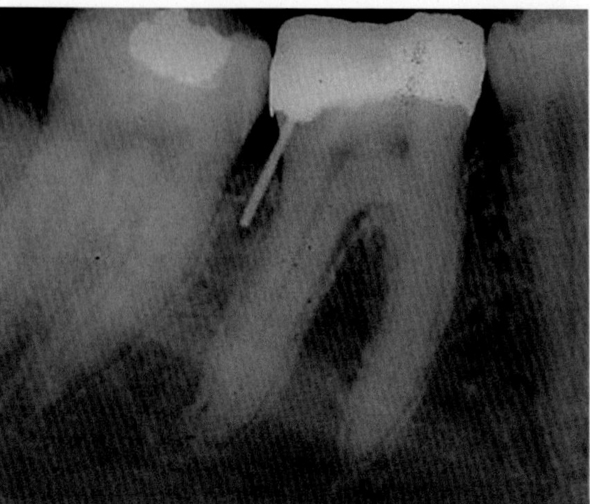

Figure 7.7 The pin placed in this molar tooth has perforated into the periodontium and will be extremely difficult to remove – this may need to be done surgically.

- As pins weaken the amalgam restoration use the minimum number. As a guide, use one pin for every missing cusp or marginal ridge up to a maximum of four. The stresses formed in pin-retained cores can be reduced by coating the pin with an adhesive such as Panavia and 4-META (4-methacryloxyethyl trimellitate anhydride).
- The pin should be placed 2 mm into dentine and 1 mm away from the enamel–dentine junction.
- Pins should be placed parallel to the external tooth surface and away from furcation areas and proximal boxes.

It is important to check the pin channel carefully for any perforations prior to inserting the pin; failure to do so can lead to the need for complicated endodontic treatment or periodontal surgery to remove the pin (Figure 7.7). If preparation of the pin channel causes perforation into the pulp chamber the channel should be filled with mineral trioxide aggregate (MTA). If the perforation is into the gingival sulcus this should be included within the margin of the preparation; however, if below the epithelial attachment the channel may again be filled with MTA.

Circumferential slots and grooves

Introduced by Outhwaite and colleagues (1979), these were originally prepared in dentine using a very small inverted cone bur (a small round bur could also be used) and were found to be equally retentive as the placement of four dentine pins. The core, however, is more easily displaced during removal of the matrix band when amalgam is used. If amalgam is used, consideration should be given to the placement of an orthodontic band (Figure 7.8) or a correctly contoured and polished copper band, which can be left in place whilst the amalgam sets.

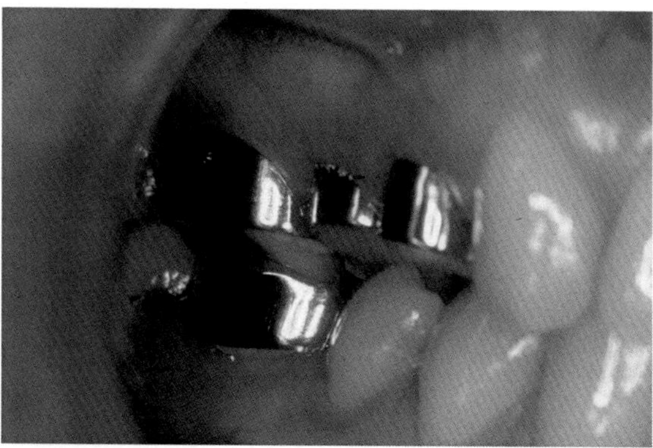

Figure 7.8 Orthodontic bands placed on heavily broken-down teeth to stabilize the core and aid their retention to allow endodontic treatment. Such bands can be used when placing amalgam cores and removed once the amalgam has set.

Elective root canal treatment

Teeth with a doubtful pulpal status can be considered for elective root canal treatment prior to provision of an indirect restoration. The success rate of endodontic treatment carried out when teeth are vital with minimally infected pulp tissue is higher than when the pulp has become necrotic and heavily infected, and when pathology of the periradicular tissues has become involved.

Elective endodontic treatment may also be necessary in teeth that have lost substantial coronal structure because of caries, tooth wear, trauma or fracture of weakened tooth tissue around restorations. These teeth may have so little remaining tooth structure that there is insufficient retention for a core and an elective endodontic treatment is required to allow placement of a post (usually in single rooted teeth) or utilization of the pulp chamber (in molar teeth) to help retain the core.

Vital teeth that have overerupted into an opposing edentulous space or where there is an inadequate opposing restoration may require occlusal correction to bring the tooth/teeth back into an acceptable occlusal plane. This may necessitate endodontic treatment as decreasing the occlusal height can expose significant amounts of dentine, causing intractable sensitivity or in some cases may itself expose the pulp (Figure 7.9). In these situations it is important to re-establish a stable occlusion to prevent further overeruption.

Occasionally tooth preparation may result in irreversible pulpitis; this can occur because of a history of repeated restorations, overzealous tooth preparation or insufficient water spray during preparation (see Chapter 3 on the stressed pulp). Patients should be warned of this complication in advance. Often the symptoms do not present until after the final restoration has been fitted, presenting the dentist with the embarrassing dilemma of either carrying out root canal treatment through the newly placed restoration (which is technically much more difficult) or removing the restoration and replacing it following root canal treatment.

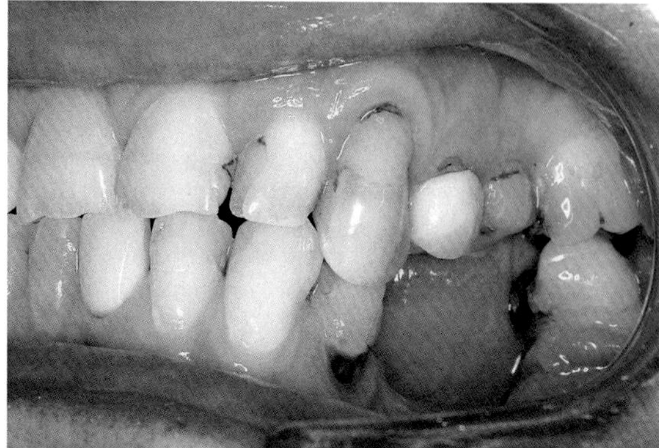

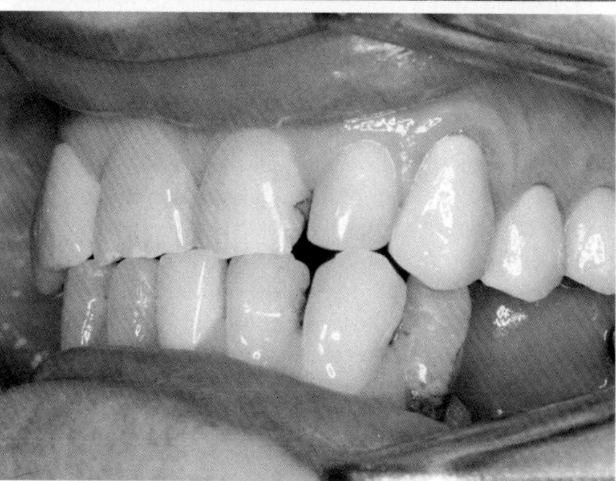

Figure 7.9 Patient with an overerupted upper canine (top). To align this tooth it has had to be root treated to enable sufficient reduction in height for alignment and further reduction to allow for crown coverage (bottom). Note the lower premolar tooth has been built up into occlusion to prevent further overeruption.
(Courtesy of Suzanne Blacker)

ENDODONTICALLY TREATED TEETH

It was a traditional belief that endodontic treatment caused teeth to become more brittle and therefore prone to fracture. This was thought to be because of loss of moisture content and changes in collagen cross-linking in dentine. This has, however, been disputed by recent research, which has found that the brittleness occurs as a result of the combination of loss of coronal tooth structure and structural integrity caused by the access preparation. Since tooth fractures are more common in endodontically treated teeth, the design and prompt placement of the definitive restoration is of huge importance to increase the longevity of the tooth. The type of restoration will depend on the following:

- *The amount of remaining tooth structure.* The loss of tooth structure is one of the most important factors that determine the type of definitive restoration. Whilst endodontically treated teeth with only minimal access cavities can be restored conservatively, those weakened by considerable damage, including loss of one or both marginal ridges, will require more extensive restoration, sometimes involving post placement for core retention and a crown. In all situations, preservation of as much coronal tooth tissue as possible is important as it affords the crown a ferrule effect, protecting the tooth from an increased risk of root fracture.
- *The position of the tooth.* Anterior teeth that are intact other than the endodontic access cavity are at little risk of fracture and generally do not require a crown. An endodontically treated tooth that has lost substantial tooth structure will require a crown and possibly a post if there is insufficient tooth structure to retain a core. Posterior teeth are subjected to greater occlusal loads and must therefore be protected against fracture. Cuspal coverage restorations are generally indicated. Wherever possible the core should be mechanically or adhesively retained and posts avoided if possible.

When to place a post?

Anterior teeth with minimal palatal access cavities require restoration only with a simple composite filling. All traces of gutta-percha and sealer should be removed from the pulp chamber to the level of the amelo-dentinal junction and sealed with a layer of resin-modified glass ionomer to form a coronal seal. A lighter shade of composite is used to maximize the aesthetics of the tooth and for obvious reasons anterior teeth should not be restored with amalgam.

A palatal access cavity often weakens teeth with existing extensive mesial and distal restorations to the point where a crown should be placed as the definitive restoration. If there is sufficient coronal tooth structure to retain a composite core once the tooth has been prepared for a crown, then a post is not essential or required as generally this does not strengthen the tooth/root (Figure 7.10); a post is only indicated when there is insufficient remaining coronal tooth structure to retain a core.

Placing posts in posterior teeth provides more challenges, partly because of the difficulty of access but also because the root canals tend to be narrower. A post is only needed in posterior teeth if there is insufficient coronal tooth tissue remaining to support a core. In most cases a Nayyar core can overcome the need for a post. This core utilizes the shape of the access cavity to retain the restoration (see later in the chapter). If there is little pulp chamber present as a result of extensive tooth tissue loss, a Nayyar core is unsuitable and in this case a post is appropriate. When situations like this arise the overall prognosis for the tooth is generally poor.

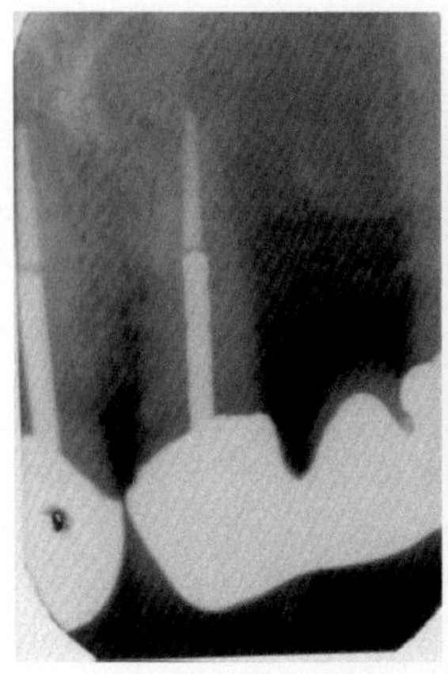
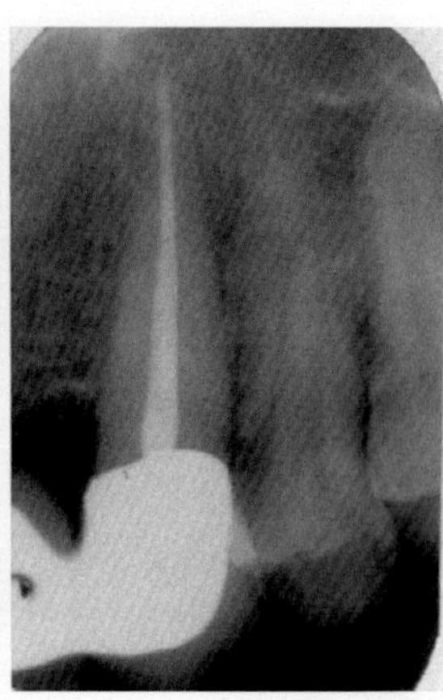

Figure 7.10 Periapical radiographs of upper left central incisor and upper left canine. The teeth are bridge abutments. The central has a serrated ParaPost and ~5 mm of apical gutta-percha. The canine did not require a post as there was an adequate amount of coronal tooth tissue remaining.

The most important determinant to the successful restoration of a root-filled tooth is the presence of a ferrule. This is the name for a rim of supragingival tooth tissue which is used to assist retention of the restoration and is explained in more detail later in the chapter.

ANTERIOR AND SINGLE-ROOTED TEETH

Post space preparation

Post space preparation should be carried out with care so as not to disrupt the apical seal or cause a lateral perforation. At least 4–5 mm of gutta-percha should be left to provide an adequate apical seal (Figure 7.10). If this leaves insufficient length of root canal for retention of a post, then the root should be extracted as the restoration will be compromised because of lack of retention. Root canals that have been obturated using a heated carrier technique such as Thermafil make it more difficult to remove only the coronal portion without disrupting the apical part; therefore, if it is obvious that a tooth will require a post, this type of obturation technique should not be used.

Removal of root canal filling prior to preparation of post space

Chemical

Historically, solvents such as oil of turpentine or chloroform have been used to soften gutta-percha, making it easier to remove by instrumentation with, for example, Hedstrom files. This technique is not advisable for removal of gutta-percha prior to post space preparation as there is no control over the depth of softening, which could disrupt the apical seal and allow leakage of the solvents into the periradicular tissues.

Thermal

This is a very easy way to remove a predetermined length of gutta-percha from a root canal. Using a preoperative radiograph, a correct size of System B tip (SybronEndo), chosen to bind at the desired post length, is marked with a rubber stop. The System B is set at 100°C and the tip inserted into the gutta-percha for 3 seconds. The heat is removed and apical pressure maintained for a further 10 seconds. A short burst of heat is then applied, and the tip rotated and removed, bringing the coronal mass of gutta-percha with it. A plugger is then applied vertically to compact the residual gutta-percha. The canals walls can be examined under magnification to ensure all traces of material have been removed from the root canal walls.

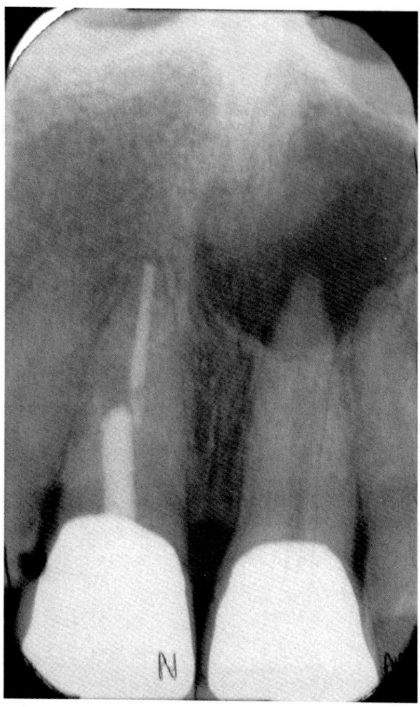

Figure 7.11 Inappropriate post space preparation in the upper right central incisor has nearly led to a distal perforation.

Mechanical

This technique is popular but if not carried out with care can weaken or result in perforation of the root (Figure 7.11). It is advisable therefore to use a non-end cutting bur such as Gates Glidden (Figure 7.12) or a Peeso reamer. Modern rotary nickel titanium retreatment instruments such as the ProTaper D series (Dentsply, Surrey, UK; Figure 7.12) make gutta-percha removal very easy. As with heat removal, the apical gutta-percha should be vertically compacted to ensure a good seal.

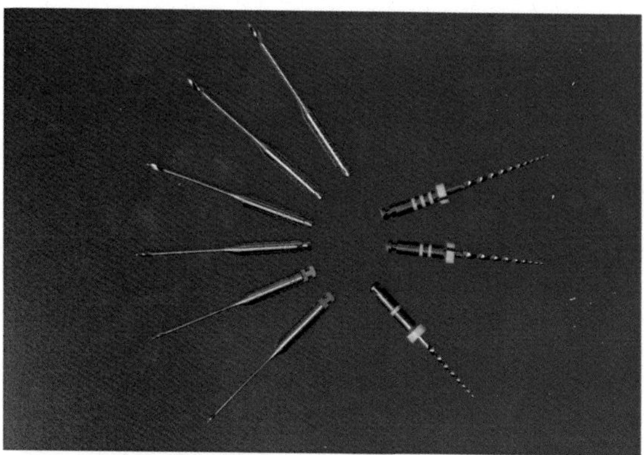

Figure 7.12 Gates Glidden burs (left) and ProTaper D series (right) used to remove gutta-percha prior to post space preparation. Note a rubber stop should be placed on the instrument at the desired post length.

Creating the post space

The longer the post, the better the retention; however, as mentioned previously, at least 4–5 mm of gutta-percha must be present apical to the post. A space between the end of the post and the root canal filling should be avoided as this will compromise the seal and may predispose to leakage and possible failure of the root canal filling. An adequate width of post is required for strength and resistance to post fracture and this will vary with each post system; however, broad posts should be avoided as there is a high risk of lateral perforation and a greater chance of root fracture. It has been suggested that the ideal post diameter at its apical end should be no more than one-third of the root width at this level.

When using the twist drills to create the post space it is important to start with the smallest size, gradually increasing to the optimum size to minimize heat build-up, reducing potential for damage to cells within the periodontal ligament. This technique will also keep dentine removal centred along the root canal and reduce the risk of lateral perforation.

Types of post

Metal posts

Metal posts are available in a variety of metals including stainless steel, titanium and titanium alloys, gold alloys, non-precious metals and gold plated brass. Stainless steel and brass posts can form corrosion products within the post space that can lead to discolouration of the root and compromise the aesthetics. Titanium posts do not corrode but fracture more easily and have a similar radio-opacity to gutta-percha, often making them difficult to differentiate on a radiograph. This can, on occasion, lead to a surprise finding when a decision is made to carry out root canal retreatment.

Posts are either parallel or tapered in design. Although parallel posts are more retentive, there is a greater risk of perforation of the apical root during preparation if a wide post is placed in a narrow canal.

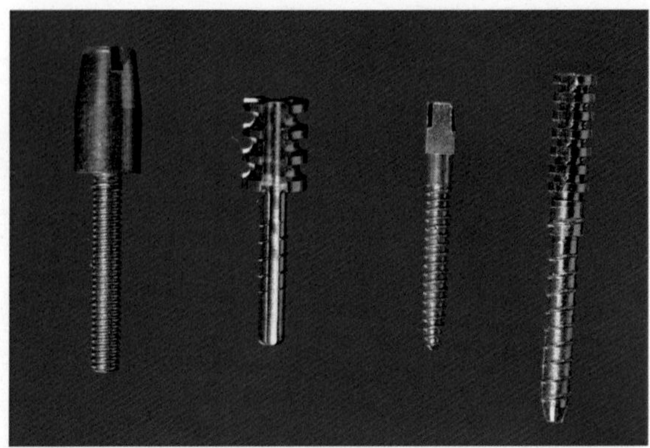

Figure 7.13 Examples of active (threaded) posts. Starting left with two parallel sided posts the Kurer K4 and Radix Anchor, then two tapered posts, the Dentatus screw and FlexiPost. The last has a split down its centre which allows the post to collapse when screwed into place.

Active posts

These involve cutting threads in the root canal dentine prior to placement and therefore tend to be more retentive than passive posts of a similar design. They are either self-threading or pre-tapped.

Self-threading posts have a shank that is slightly narrower than the prepared post space and a thread that is slightly wider. As the post is rotated into place it cuts its own counter-thread into the dentine. The procedure is quite unlike using a wood screw since dentine is hard and brittle. Careful placement is needed, using concepts more similar to metal working than wood, as there is potential to introduce stresses in the root dentine. Once the post hole has been prepared, it is tempting to coat the self-threading post with luting cement and rotate it into place in one stage; however, this introduces stresses into the dentine. Instead, the threaded post should be tried-in, cutting its own counter-thread in the dentine, and if retentive it is removed and reinserted into place coated with a cement lute. Used in this way the amount of stress introduced into the dentine can be reduced.

Self-threading posts can be either tapered or parallel in design. An example of a tapered, threaded post is the Dentatus screw (Dentatus) (Figure 7.13). This post can cause high stresses within the root as it is inserted, causing a wedging effect and possible root fracture. The Radix Anchor (Dentsply) is an example of a parallel, self-threading post. The threads are located at the coronal portion of the post only (Figure 7.13). Again the post should be placed initially without cement to cut the counter-thread. When it is reinserted to the full length of the prepared post space it should be derotated by a quarter turn to minimize stresses within the root dentine.

Pre-tapped posts have a higher frequency of threads around a parallel-sided shank. The post space is prepared and then the counter-thread is cut into the dentinal walls by using a thread cutter or pre-tapping device (Figure 7.14). This is designed to reduce the stresses created compared to that induced when self-threading posts are used in a one-stage technique. The higher frequency of threads and the lack of a vent to provide an escape route for excess cement can cause excessive stresses within the dentine. An example of this type of post is the Kurer K4 anchor system (Sabre Dental; Figure 7.13).

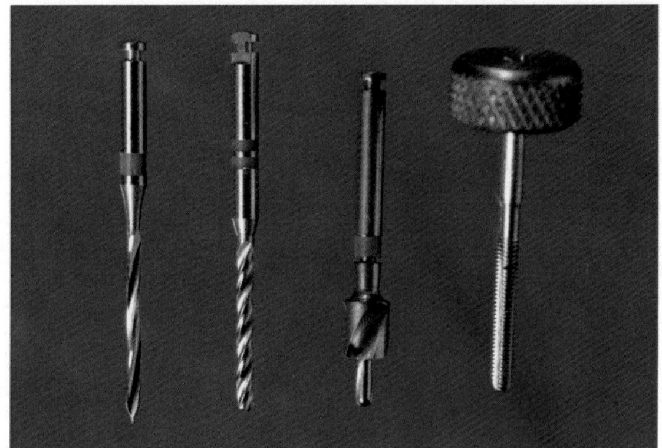

Figure 7.14 Kurer K4 post drills and tapping device (right). From left to right: reamer to remove gutta-percha, post space drill, root facer (to produce a flat surface to seat the post down to) and the tapping device to cut the counter threads on the post hole wall. The actual post is seen in Figure 7.13.

Although active posts allow for greater retention, the stresses they produce on the root dentine are not favourable, even when the pre-tapped varieties are used, and may result in root fracture. It would be sensible to reserve these posts for cases where retention is compromised such as short or curved roots.

Passive posts

These are either custom-made cast posts or prefabricated posts. Custom-made cast posts and cores can be made from type III, type IV gold alloy or base metal alloys. The latter are harder and may predispose the tooth to root fracture. The impression technique produces a smooth-sided, tapered post that matches the original taper of the root canal preparation. This is an ideal choice for an irregular canal such as that seen in an upper second premolar tooth, which is wide and oval bucco-palatally at its entrance and much narrower apically (Figure 7.15). To take an impression of an irregular post hole the wash material is syringed around the entrance to the post hole and the plastic impression post is pushed through the unset wash, dragging it into the post hole. Before the wash sets the loaded impression tray is seated (see Chapter 13).

Although the use of cast tapered posts decreases the risk of root perforation apically, the retention of the post is compromised. Parallel-sided posts give better retention than tapered posts and can be used provided the rules set out under post space preparation are adhered to. Serrated posts have negative recesses in them and give more retention than smooth-sided posts. It is possible to custom-make a parallel-sided serrated post by using a system such as the ParaPost XP (Coltène Whaledent, UK; Figure 7.16). For each size post there is a smooth plastic impression post (the blue one can be seen in Figure 7.15). A retentive 'mushroom' shape can be created in the impression post at the end which is embedded into the impression by melting it with a hot metal instrument such as a flat plastic. The serrated burn out plastic post is then sent with the impression to the laboratory for the technician to wax a core around and cast using the lost wax technique (see Chapter 9). The final post type within the parapost XP kit is the metal temporary post which can be used in conjunction with temporary crown materials and techniques (see Chapter 14).

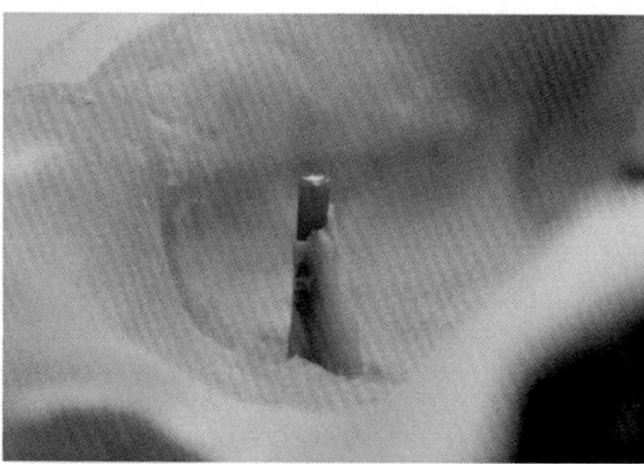

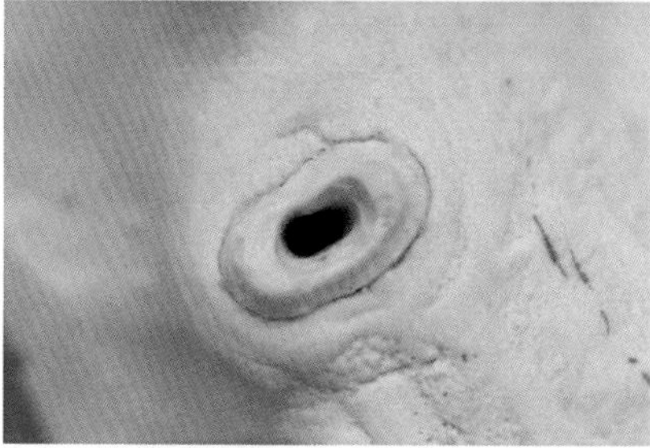

Figure 7.15 Impression taken for a cast post and core (top). A blue plastic impression post has been used with an addition cured silicone putty and wash impression material. The resultant die stone model can be seen below.

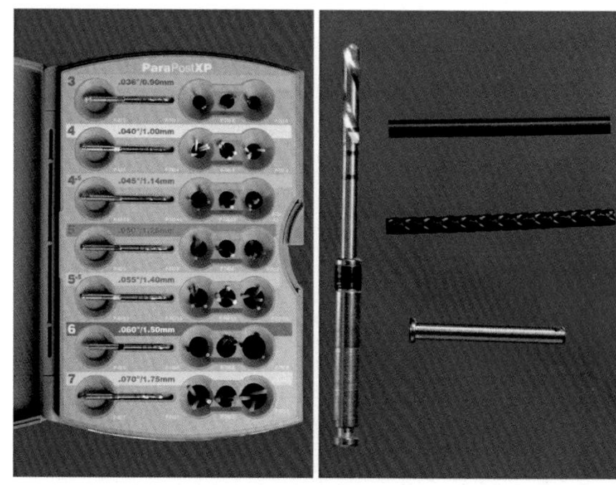

Figure 7.16 ParaPost XP system for making custom-made cast post and cores. On the right magnified image, from top to bottom is the plastic impression post, the serrated burnout post and the metal temporary post.

The use of custom-made cast posts and cores is more time consuming as additional clinical time and laboratory costs are incurred. It is preferable to fit the cast post and core and then take a further impression for the crown to reduce the chance of a compromised marginal fit (Figure 7.17). However, cast posts are preferred by many practitioners and so continue to have a use in operative dentistry.

Prefabricated passive posts

These can be either tapered or parallel in design. They have a vent that allows the escape of excess luting cement. Examples of posts from the ParaPost series (Coltène Whaledent, UK) have parallel sides and a diamond-shaped retentive feature (serrations) along part of (ParaPost XT) or along the entire length of (ParaPost XH) the post. The diamond-shaped serrations interconnect, effectively acting as a vent for excess luting cement (Figure 7.18). Once cemented into the post hole, the core is built up directly in the mouth with the chosen core material.

Non-metal aesthetic posts

These were introduced to improve aesthetics as metal posts can be visible through all-ceramic restorations and can cause the marginal gingival tissues to appear dark. Aesthetic clear, white or tooth-coloured posts can be made from quartz fibre, ceramic and zirconia.

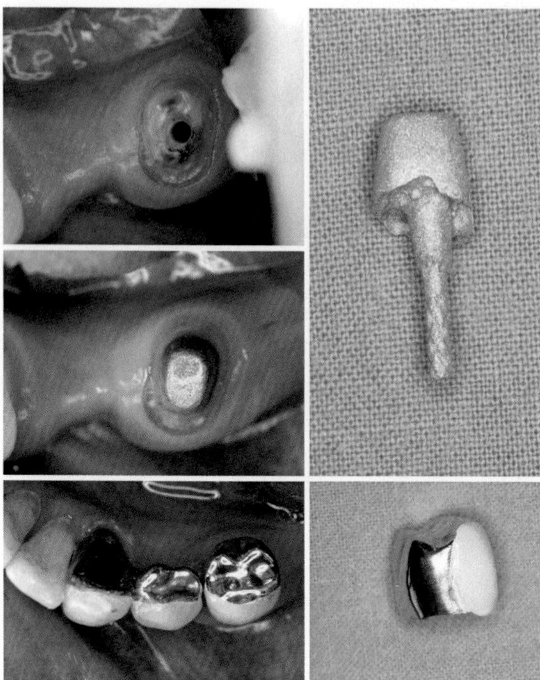

Figure 7.17 Preparation for cast post and core and metal–ceramic crown (top left). The cast post and core (top right) is cemented (middle left) and a second impression taken for the metal–ceramic crown (bottom). A minimum preparation (resin retained) bridge was made at the same time to replace the lower left first premolar tooth.

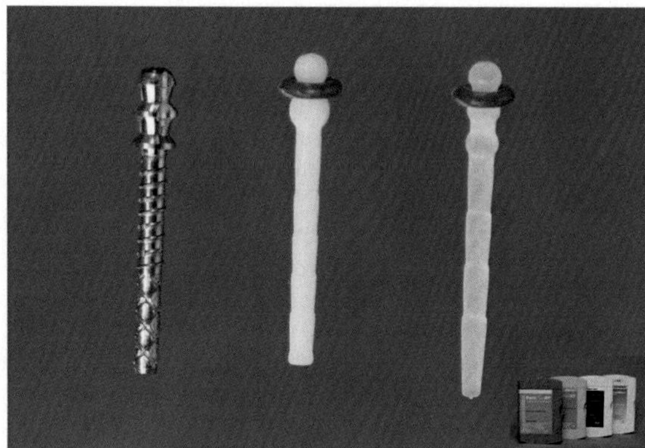

Figure 7.18 Examples of prefabricated posts which are taken from the ParaPost series (Coltène Whaledent, UK). Left is the ParaPost XT which has an apical serrated pattern and a coronal 7 mm of threaded post. The ParaPost XH has the same serrated design along its entire length (not shown). The two quartz fibre posts are the Fiber White (middle) and Taper Lux (right). The red ring is for colour coding only and should be removed before the core is built up.

Fibre posts

Carbon fibre posts were introduced in the 1990s in an attempt to overcome the complication of root fracture that existed with metal posts. They were more flexible, having a similar stiffness to dentine, and were bonded to the post space using adhesive resin cements. These have since been replaced by tooth-coloured quartz, silica and glass fibre posts, which give superior aesthetics. The typical composition by weight is 42% fibre, 29% filler and 18% resin. The quartz fibres run longitudinally along the length of the post embedded in an epoxy resin (Figure 7.19). There are tapered and parallel designs available that are compatible with placement of a composite core; some even have retentive head designs to improve core retention (Figure 7.18).

Whilst the microflexure of these posts reduces the risk of failure due to vertical root fracture, in the authors' opinion they are best used when a ferrule can be achieved. If there is no coronal tooth tissue, the composite core can debond from the root face and the microflexure can lead to either post fracture or delamination of the post due to leakage of moisture (Figure 7.20).

When preparing the post space for a quartz fibre post it should be meticulously cleaned of traces of gutta-percha and sealer, especially sealer containing eugenol which could interfere with the resin luting cements advised for cementing these posts. The post space should be carefully dried prior to cementation using a paper point. Self-etching, resin luting cements are ideal for cementing quartz fibre posts as the reliable application of acid etch, rinsing, drying and application of primer and bond is difficult in the narrow confines of a post hole.

Should endodontic retreatment be required, quartz fibre posts can be removed by cutting along the post.

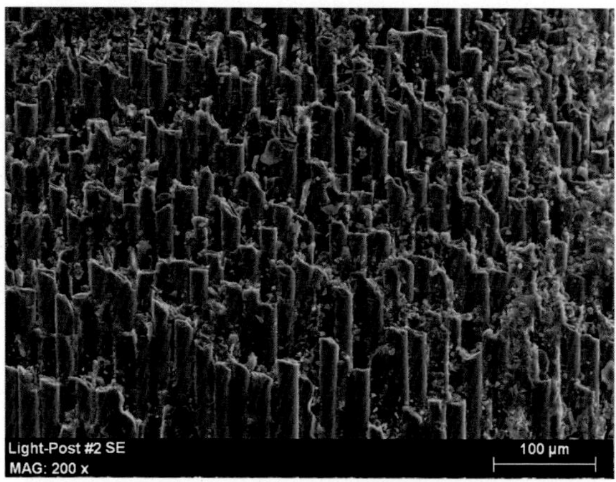

Figure 7.19 Micrograph of a quartz fibre post – Light-Post. The fibres can be seen running longitudinally along the length of the post embedded in an epoxy resin.
(Courtesy of RTD, France)

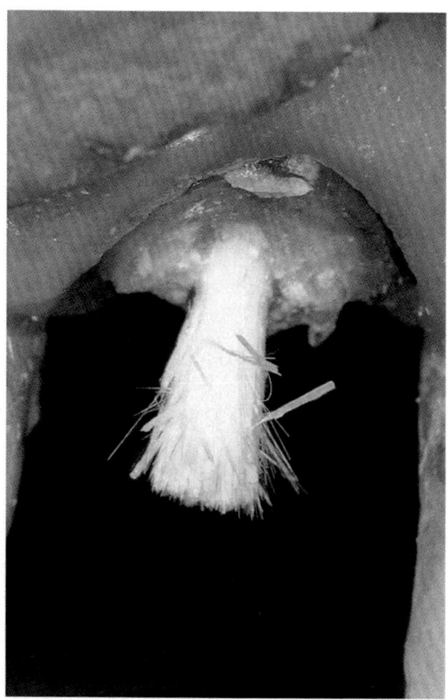

Figure 7.20 This tooth has no coronal tooth tissue present for a ferrule. The composite core has debonded and fluid microleakage has led to delamination of the post and loss of the crown. The make of post is unknown.

A pilot hole is cut using a pin drill followed by a non-end cutting rotary instrument such as a Peeso drill (Figure 7.21). Removing quartz fibre posts can be difficult because they are tooth coloured and in the depths of a post hole it is almost impossible to determine what is post and what is tooth tissue. Recherches Techniques Dentaires (RTD) has overcome this problem with their new post system, D.T. Light-Post Illusion. These posts have a colour added to them which is temperature sensitive; at body temperature they are clear/tooth coloured but when cooled with a three-in-one syringe, for example, the colour reappears, assisting in their removal if required (Figure 7.22).

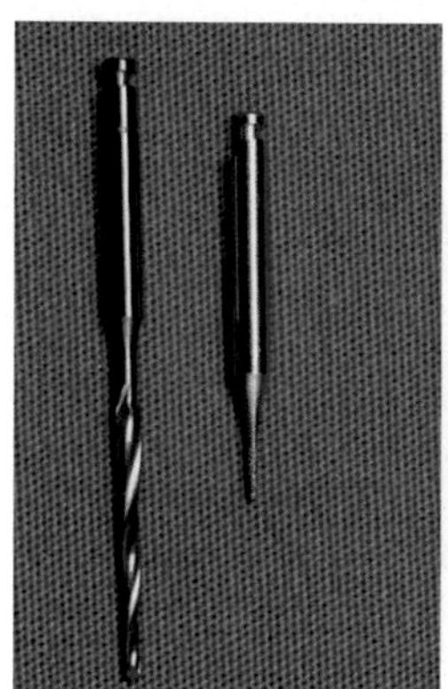

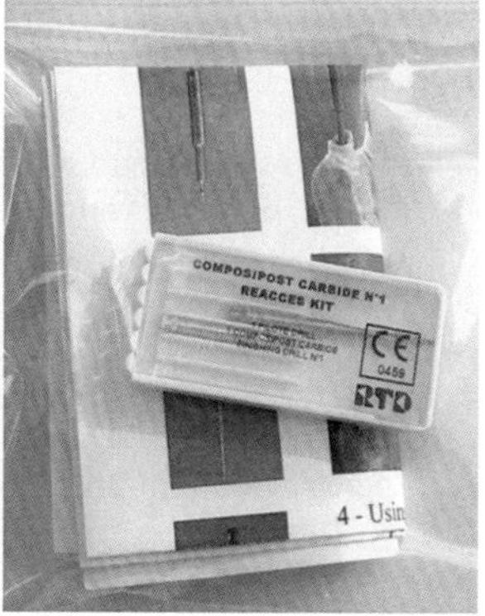

Figure 7.21 Quartz fibre post retrieval kit provided by RTD. *(Courtesy of RTD, France)*

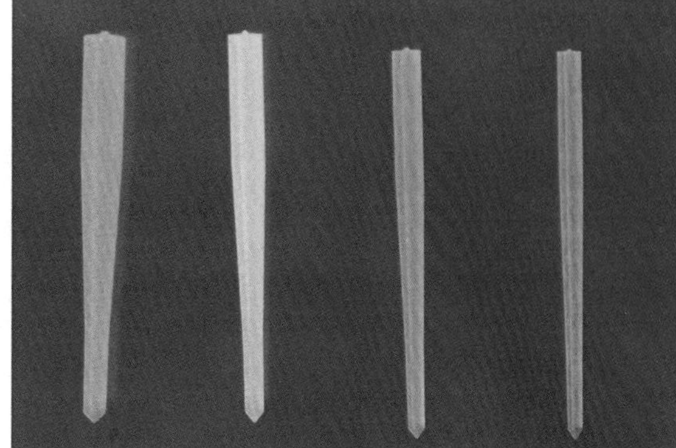

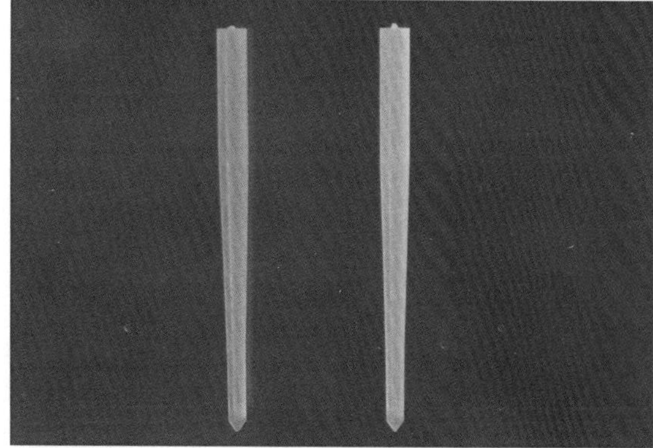

Figure 7.22 D.T. Light-Post Illusion. The colour-coded posts have double tapered configuration (top). When warmed to body temperature the colour disappears (bottom post on right).

Fibre posts and weakened roots

In cases of weaken roots such as immature teeth or those compromised by caries or operative procedure, the internal surface of the root can be strengthened using composite bonded to the root dentine, prior to placement of a quartz fibre post. In order to ensure the composite material is cured along its length, a clear plastic sprue (Luminex, Dentatus) is placed through the middle of the composite and then removed following curing. This leaves a ready-made channel that just requires refinement before bonding the post (Figure 7.23).

Ceramic and zirconium posts

Although these posts are tooth coloured they have several disadvantages in that they are weaker than metal posts and therefore have to be made broader, resulting in a wider post-space preparation that may result in perforation. Zirconium posts cannot be etched, making retention of a composite core very difficult. Both are extremely

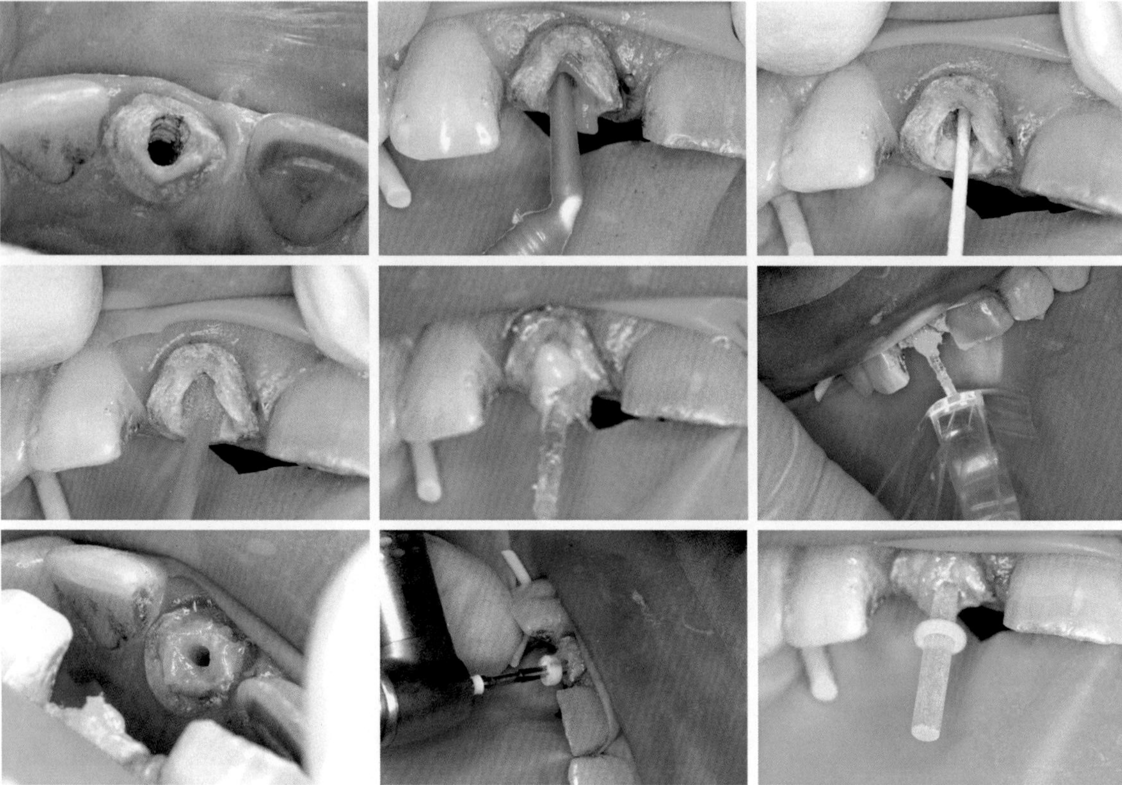

Figure 7.23 From left to right and top to bottom. Severely compromised root due to poor post hole preparation and near perforation. Acid etch applied and agitated in post hole with microbrush for 10 seconds. After rinsing thoroughly the post hole is dried with a large paper point. Bond is then applied with a microbrush. The post hole is filled with composite and the petroleum jelly-covered Luminex post inserted through the composite and light cured. The post is removed, post hole modified with a suitable twist drill and the chosen quartz fibre post cemented with a resin luting cement. The post length can now be reduced if required and a composite core built up.

difficult to remove and often this can only be done using a diamond high speed bur; however, this is very tedious and carries with it a high risk of the bur skating off the post into the dentine and perforating. It is best to avoid this type of post.

POSTERIOR TEETH

Endondontically treated posterior teeth should be restored with a cuspal coverage restoration to protect the remaining tooth structure and prevent failure due to fracture or coronal leakage. The type of restoration depends on the amount of remaining tooth structure and the occlusal forces on the tooth. Placing posts in premolar and molar teeth can cause complications such as a strip or lateral perforation and can weaken the root, predisposing to root fracture. As retention can be gained from the undercut shape of the pulp chamber in combination with mechanical and adhesive retention, posts are generally not required to retain the core material and are therefore unnecessary.

Nayyar described a core that used the pulp chamber and the coronal 2–4 mm of the root canals for retention. The roots of posterior teeth usually diverge from the pulp chamber and removing 2–4 mm of root filling material and packing core material into the space provided affords excellent retention. This technique therefore prevented the need for the placement of pins and posts in posterior teeth. More recent research has shown that removing gutta-percha at the entrance to the root canals is no longer necessary. If the access cavity for the endodontic treatment has been cut correctly, the pulp chamber itself should be undercut. The cross-sectional area of core material within the pulp chamber is also adequate for acceptable strength

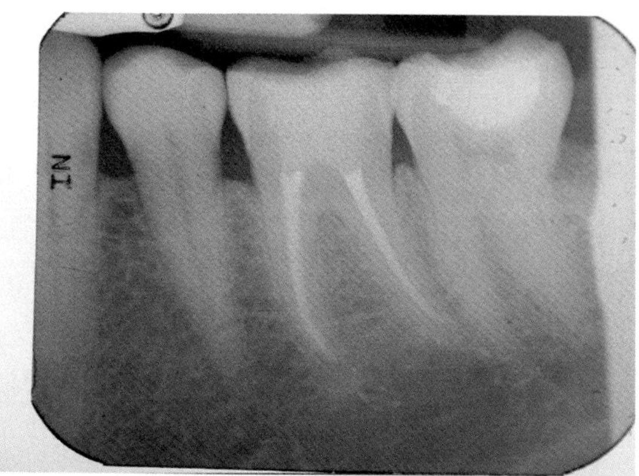

Figure 7.24 Modification of a Nayyar core. The pulp chamber is utilized for retention; however, no gutta-percha has been removed from the entrance to the root canal. The core has been built up in composite.

of any of the core materials in use. If amalgam is used it can be bonded to the tooth structure for added retention and to improve the coronal seal; however, the evidence for this is weak. Composite can also be used as a core material but should not be placed into the root canals as this would be difficult to remove, in that it would be difficult to differentiate it from tooth tissue, should root canal retreatment be required (Figure 7.24).

SUMMARY FOR PLACEMENT OF POST AND CORE MATERIALS

Retention and resistance

Retention is the ability to resist vertical displacement and is influenced by the post's length, diameter, taper, whether active or passive, and the type of luting cement used. Parallel posts are more retentive than tapered posts but have a higher risk of perforation with increasing diameter. Active posts are more retentive than passive posts but if placed with too much torque can result in root fracture. The post should be as long as possible but maintain an apical seal of 4–5 mm gutta-percha. For success, the length of the post should be equal to if not greater than the clinical crown height.

Resistance is the ability of a post to withstand lateral and rotational forces. This is determined by the amount of remaining coronal tooth structure, the length of post, the presence of a ferrule, and whether or not an anti-rotational key has been cut in the root surface. The last is only required with cylindrical posts when there is no coronal tooth tissue for a ferrule and should be cut on the palatal/lingual aspect of the post hole to a depth of about 2–3 mm.

Ferrule effect

The length of the post and creation of a ferrule are the two most important determinants for a successful post crown. The presence of a ferrule is an important feature that will increase the longevity of the restoration. It refers to the presence of the coronal tooth structure that the crown will encompass and should be at least 2 mm in height. This will improve the fracture resistance of the tooth and reduce the risk of vertical root fracture, especially when metal posts are used. The band of extracoronal material that covers this tooth structure is the ferrule and is usually provided by the crown that is placed over the core (Figure 7.25).

Posterior teeth

Avoid the placement of posts in posterior teeth whenever possible as preparation for these can easily result in a strip perforation. Rely instead on retention from placement of the core material within the pulp chamber, together with the aid of bonding.

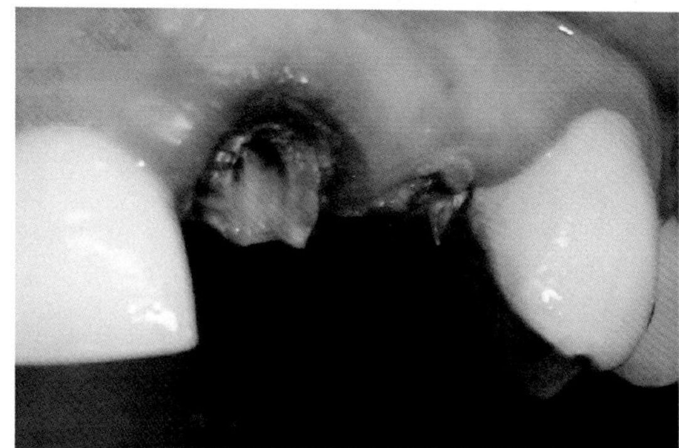

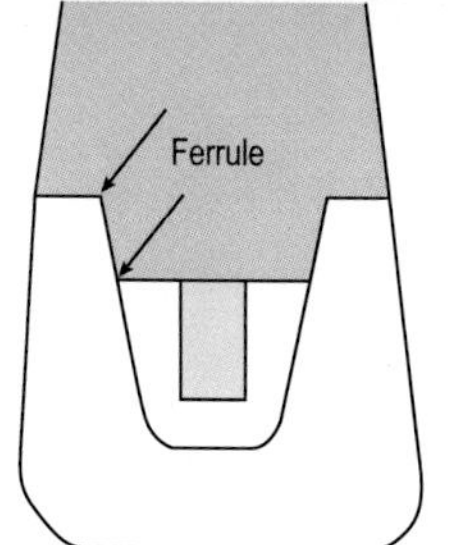

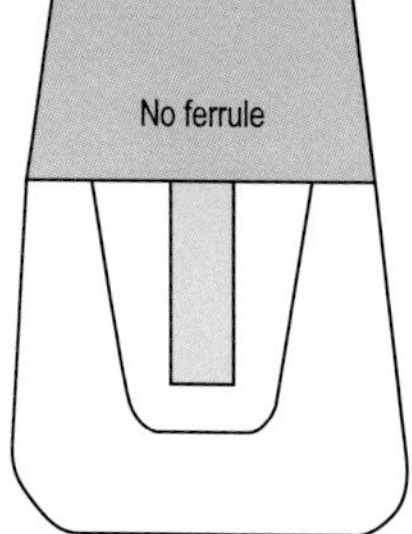

Figure 7.25 Two examples of teeth that require posts to retain cores, the left with a 2–3 mm ferrule mesio-distally and the right with no coronal tooth tissue and no ferrule. The tooth with the ferrule has a much better prognosis than the one without.

FURTHER READING

Bateman, G., Ricketts, D.N., Saunders, W.P., 2003. Fibre-based post systems: a review. Br. Dent. J. 195, 43–48.

Fedorowicz, Z., Nasser, M., Wilson, N., 2009. Adhesively bonded versus non-bonded amalgam restorations for dental caries. Cochrane Database Syst. Rev. 4, CD007517.

Outhwaite,, W.C., Garman,, T.A., Pashley,, D.H., 1979. Pin vs. slot retention in extensive amalgam restorations. J. Prosthet. Dent. 41, 396–400.

Randall, R.C., Wilson, N.H., 1999. Glass–ionomer restoratives: a systematic review of a secondary caries treatment effect. J. Dent. Res. 78, 628–637.

Ricketts, D.N., Tait, C.M., Higgins, A.J., 2005a. Tooth preparation for post-retained restorations. Br. Dent. J. 198, 463–471.

Ricketts, D.N., Tait, C.M., Higgins, A.J., 2005b. Post and core systems, refinements to tooth preparation and cementation. Br. Dent. J. 198, 533–541.

Setcos, J.C., Staninec, M., Wilson, N.H., 2000. Bonding of amalgam restorations: existing knowledge and future prospects. Oper. Dent. 25, 121–129.

Tait, C.M., Ricketts, D.N., Higgins, A.J., 2005a. Restoration of the root-filled tooth: pre-operative assessment. Br. Dent. J. 198, 395–404.

Tait, C.M., Ricketts, D.N., Higgins, A.J., 2005b. Weakened anterior roots – intraradicular rehabilitation. Br. Dent. J. 198, 609–617.

Chapter | 8 |

Gold crowns

John Radford, Brian Stevenson

CHAPTER CONTENTS

INTRODUCTION

Are gold castings the Cinderella of advanced restorative dentistry? Anecdote would suggest they are excellent restorations; dentists often think that they are the restoration of choice but patients frequently state that the dental aesthetic associated with them is unacceptable. It should be borne in mind that the outcome for gold crowns may appear more favourable because dentists provide such restorations for patients they consider would benefit most; that is, patients are highly selected.

So why should dentists be competent in providing castings, particularly as the provision of densely sintered ceramic restorations are continually being refined? As health care professionals there is an imperative to discuss with the patient the advantages and disadvantages of all restorative options. Indeed, not doing so may result in consent being invalid. A carer's role is to empower the patient such that they can decide how they wish their dental treatment to be advanced.

It is traditional to consider full gold crowns, three-quarter crowns or variations of such, and overlays separately. However, there is commonality between the provisions of such restorations. Such shared characteristics will be stated, but when there are differences, these will be identified. This chapter will exclude gold inlays and onlays which are discussed in Chapter 12.

GENERAL CONSIDERATIONS

Targeted history and examination

These are central to offering the patient what is considered in their best interest. A history should identify the pertinent and ignore the trivial.

Sharing of information (for real consent)

Common to all aspects of treatment, it is important to discuss with the patient their history and examination findings, and to offer different treatment options. The patient should be given time to make an informed choice and contemporaneous clinical notes must be made of this process. If the treatment is of high impact, as is often the case with advanced operative procedures, the decision-making process and the agreed treatment approach should be confirmed in writing.

Indications for full coverage gold crowns

These are listed in order, the first being the most common:

- When a plastic restoration has a history of repeated failure within a short defined time interval (Figure 8.1A). This would include failed adhesive restorations used in the management of tooth wear.
- When difficulty has been experienced in placing a large direct restoration with an adequate contour, contact point and occlusal contacts.
- As a retainer for a fixed prosthesis (see Chapter 19).
- To minimize the *real* risk of tooth fracture, for example after endodontic treatment (Figure 8.1B). Many authorities consider that an overlay/onlay may be the most appropriate restoration for a tooth that has been root-treated.
- To include design characteristics to accommodate a metal-based removable prosthesis (Figure 8.2). Such an indication *per se* may be difficult to justify and the decision to crown the tooth will take other factors into consideration, such as its restorative status. The patient must be made aware that any oral health gain must outweigh the removal of tooth tissue and resources required to provide such restorations.

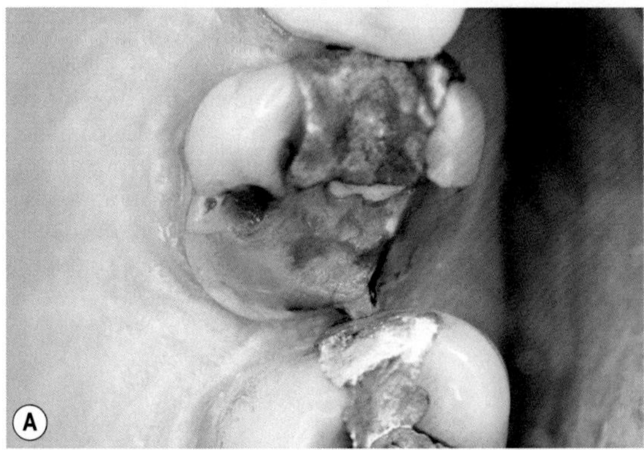

Figure 8.1A The large restoration in the upper left first molar tooth has undergone repeated fracture. To place a direct restoration in this tooth with adequate contour and contact areas, would be clinically demanding.

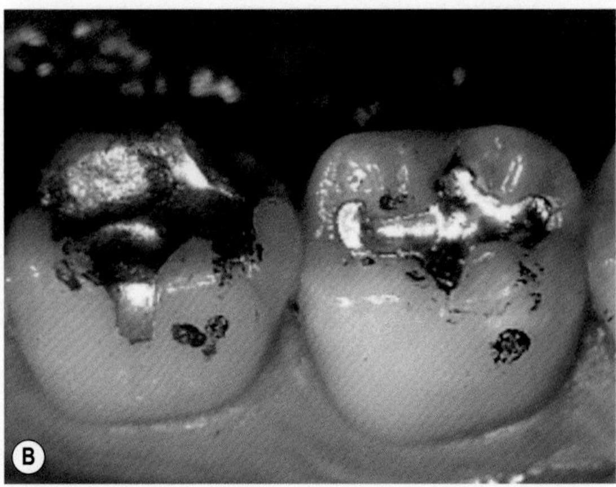

Figure 8.1B The lower left first molar tooth has reduced structural integrity and, as a consequence, the disto-lingual cusp has fractured. A full gold crown is indicated in order to preserve the remaining core and coronal tooth tissue.

Contraindications to full coverage castings

Contraindications to providing such restorations include a lifestyle which adversely influences oral health; these are relative and can usually be overcome should the patient so wish. This must be supported by evidence of change such as quitting smoking, modifying the use of erosive drinks, dietary changes to reduce the frequency of sugar consumption or improved home care. Other 'dental' contraindications such as 'active' caries, 'active' periodontal and periradicular disease have been discussed in Chapters 1–3.

A targeted preventative and preparatory phase is at the heart of a treatment plan which includes the provision of successful laboratory fabricated restorations. If this has not been carried out as part of the treatment plan, apart from the dentist not discharging their moral and statutory covenant/contract, a prosecuting barrister may claim, for example: 'My client would not have consented to this crown if they had been informed beforehand of the subsequent necessity for endodontic therapy…or regenerative periodontal procedures etc.'

Partial coverage castings may be the restoration of choice in certain circumstances. For example, if full coverage preparation removes the bulk of the remaining tooth structure.

Absolute contraindications

These are few. Systemic sclerosis could be such an example as the patient may not be able to open their mouth sufficiently to receive such treatment. Profound xerostomia would also be considered by some to be another absolute

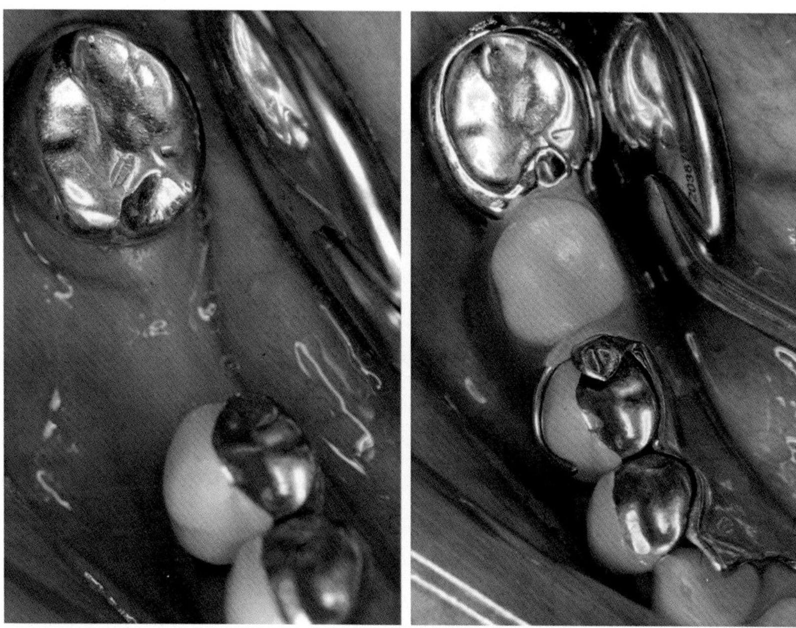

Figure 8.2 Full coverage gold crown on lower right second molar. A rest seat, mesial guide plane and mesio-lingual undercut have been created to optimize the success of the removable cobalt chromium prosthesis.

contraindication but this has to be balanced against the alternative treatment of repeat restorations and loss of function. Another would be if the patient was fearful (dental anxiety). However, supportive therapy may facilitate them receiving such treatment.

Funding and access to health care should never be a contraindication.

STEPS IN TOOTH PREPARATION FOR A GOLD CROWN

General considerations

Occlusal design

- *Conformative or reorganized occlusion*. The dentist can elect to adopt a conformative approach or to reorganize the occlusion. A conformative approach is when the patient is given the same occlusal configuration after the fitting of the restoration as when they attended for the preparation; the occlusion remains unchanged. A reorganized approach is when the relationship between the maxilla and mandible is changed by the gold crown/prosthesis. This approach is usually adopted when most or all of the occluding teeth are to be restored in complex full mouth rehabilitations. In this section, only a conformative approach will be described.
- *Incisal/canine/anterior guidance*. It may be considered more useful to tease this subject apart by considering disclusion of teeth in excursive movements as opposed to occlusion. If the patient has incisal/anterior guidance, the focus will be on establishing a maximum number of bilateral occlusal contacts in maximum intercuspation (ICP). In excursive movements the posterior teeth will disclude and occlusal contacts between posterior teeth will not pose a problem (see Chapter 6). Some authorities suggest that if the patient has incisal/canine/anterior guidance, bodily side shift of the mandible (Bennett movement) is minimized.
- *Group function*. If the patient demonstrates group function, all excursions must be accommodated by the gold crown. Some consider that refinement of the occlusion will be necessary when fitting the casting. This is because Bennett movement (bodily movement of the mandible) is difficult to accurately transfer to an articulator (see below).
- *The occlusal table*. Traditionally, the occlusal table of the restoration is punctuated by fissures and is highly polished. There is no evidence that creation of an intricate fissure pattern has any beneficial effect on function. This is not, however, to denigrate the gnathological approach that had its zenith with full mouth rehabilitations placed on natural teeth (these are beyond the scope of this chapter). The most logical approach is one based around function. A sandblasted

occlusal surface will pick up articulating paper marks more readily than a polished surface and it is often useful to prescribe this to the dental technician. If the patient prefers a polished surface, however, the casting can be polished once the occlusion has been checked and adjusted if necessary.

Whether or not to remove previous restorations before preparation for the casting?

This will depend to a degree as to why the casting is being prescribed and the predicted future integrity of the restoration. Some would assert it is good practice to remove all previous restorations and bases and then replace them with an adhesive core before preparation for a casting. This would avoid embarrassing loss of the restoration during preparation. Others would consider resources could be more productively spent giving oral health messages and a more pragmatic approach would be to carry out the preparation incorporating the existing restoration(s) as the core. If these remain intact and the dentist's intuition is that they can support an indirect restoration, then refrain from placing another core. Advocates of this approach highlight the fact that trauma to the pulp is cumulative and that each time a restoration is replaced more tooth tissue is lost. The final decision as to whether to replace the existing restoration and place a new core will need to be made on an individual basis in consultation with the patient.

Where to finish the gold crown preparation with respect to the gingival margin?

There is an enduring tension between engaging as much tooth structure as possible and encroaching on the gingival domain. In the former case this is performed for reasons of retention and resistance; however, the disadvantage of encroaching on the gingival tissues is that an environment is created in an important area that is unfavourable for the patient to maintain plaque free.

Unequivocally, all restorations should be finished on tooth tissue. The reasons for finishing on tooth tissue are to remove any ledges created by the core and to restrict potential leakage to only that between the casting and tooth.

Burs and instruments

In this subsection, only selected areas will be discussed. In the UK it is conventional to prepare teeth for crowns and bridges using medium-grit diamond burs (Figure 8.3). This is in contrast to other countries where tungsten carbide burs are more commonly used. There is no clinical evidence to show that preparations cut with one or another type of bur result in restorations with a superior outcome.

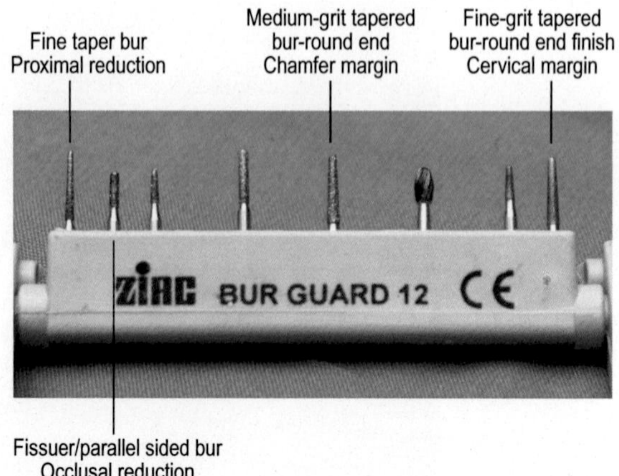

Figure 8.3 Typical crown preparation bur kit. Finer-grit diamond burs (right two) are used to finish the preparation.

Some dentists use fine-grit diamond burs to finish the preparation (Figure 8.3) and argue that the reason for this is to reduce the very small undercuts created by the diamond grit. It has been suggested that these could distort the wax pattern when it is removed from the working die. The routine use of die-spacer on stone dies 'blocks-out' any small undercuts and this should not be an issue (see Chapter 9). In fact the surface roughness of the preparation may improve micromechanical retention when the crown is cemented.

Photographic mirrors are also useful in assessing the axial reduction and taper of the crown preparation. This allows the whole preparation to be examined for possible undercuts without having to change the angle of the mirror or moving the head (Figure 8.4). In addition, a photographic mirror reflects light more effectively.

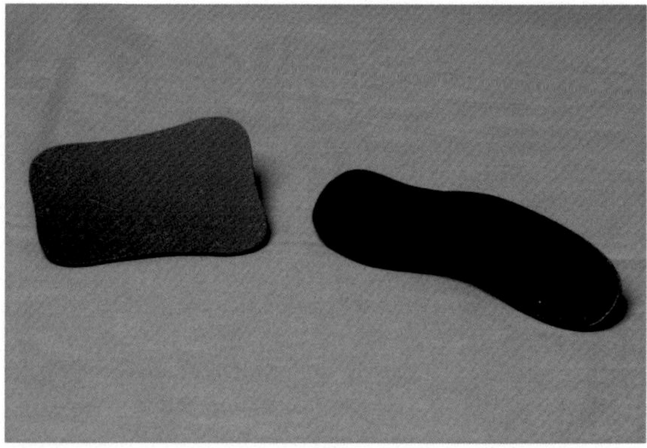

Figure 8.4 Photographic mirrors are useful in assessing the axial reduction for crown preparations and in assessing the alignment of bridge preparations.

Allocation of time between performing basic preparation outline and refining the preparation

The basic preparation of a tooth can be carried out effectively and safely in a relatively short time. However, a disproportionate amount of time should be spent refining the preparation. It is always important to remember to keep the initial preparation as conservative as possible because more tooth tissue and core can be removed in refinement, but it is not always easy or possible to replace it once it is gone. When carrying out multiple preparations, final refinement may be carried out at a second visit with reference to a stone model. This model is poured from a silicone impression of the preparations after the process of initial preparation has been carried out at the first visit. The most difficult area to prepare and refine is the disto-lingual/palatal angle.

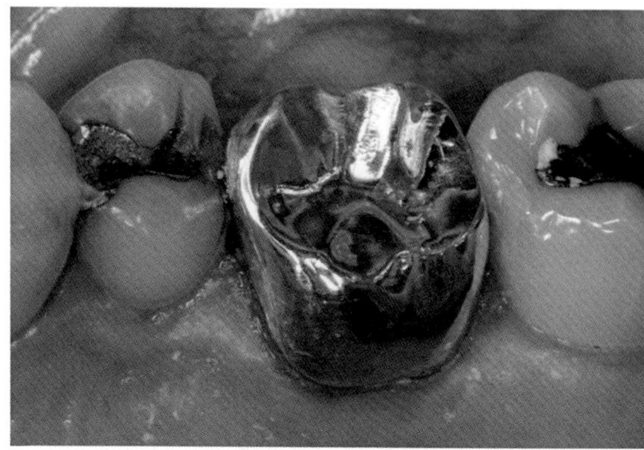

Figure 8.6 The tooth seen in Figure 8.5 restored with an adhesively luted three-quarter gold casting. Note the satisfactory emergence angle of the restoration achieved by thinning the casting with stones before cementation.

Has the use of adhesive cements relegated many of the traditional design characteristics to the archive?

Some may argue that the slavish following of traditional design characteristics in order to achieve retention and resistance is now not so important. Adhesive cements compensate when traditional characteristics cannot be achieved (Figures 8.5 and 8.6). However, others argue that adhesive cements should only be used when absolutely necessary as the removal of crowns cemented with these can be problematic and time consuming. It is a moot point, but possibly the dentist should not entertain retrievability as these restorations should be there for life. The truth of the matter is that many are not (for a number of reasons) and conventions of crown preparation and cementation should be followed. This also keeps preparations as conservative as possible and in a time when the price of gold is at a high premium the amount of gold used is kept to a minimum; some have referred to gold crowns as gold shell crowns as the crown should consist of a thin even thickness of gold in all aspects.

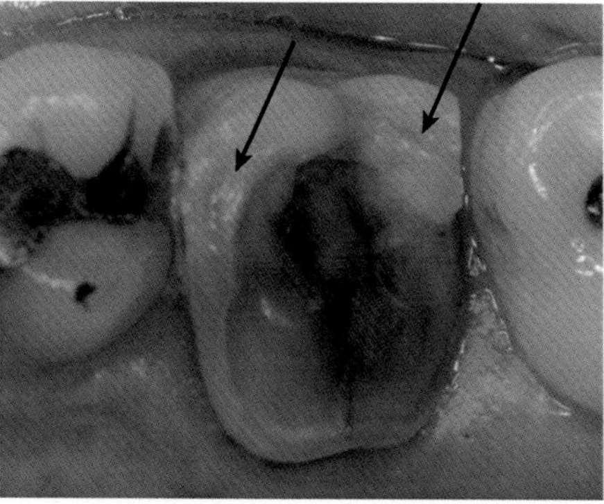

Figure 8.5 The upper left first molar tooth has been prepared for an adhesively luted three-quarter gold crown. Note the occlusal off-set prepared on the buccal cusps (arrowed) in order to aid location of the restoration during cementation. Apart from this, no occlusal preparation was carried out as 'tooth reduction' had occurred through a combination of a lost restoration and tooth wear.

Tooth preparation for gold crowns

Occlusal reduction

Before carrying out occlusal reduction, occlusal contacts when the patient is in intercuspal position (centric stops) and if group function, excursive contacts should be identified using articulating paper. The tooth of the patient illustrated in Figure 8.1B has group function; centric stops and contacts in lateral excursion are identified and differentiated from one another by using different coloured articulating paper.

The occlusal reduction should mirror the anticipated normal morphology of the occlusal table of a tooth. This is best carried out using fissure burs angled according to the cuspal slope (Figure 8.7); this ensures even reduction of the occlusal surface. If the diameter of the bur chosen is consistent with the amount of occlusal reduction needed, the bur can be sunk to its full diameter. If rounded burs are used then there is a potential for insufficient reduction at the centric stops. Not only should sufficient occlusal reduction be carried out to accommodate the gold crown in intercuspal position (~0.5–1 mm) but the dentist should also remove tooth tissue such that there will be no occlusal interferences in all excursive movements including the retruded contact position–intercuspal position (RCP–ICP) slide.

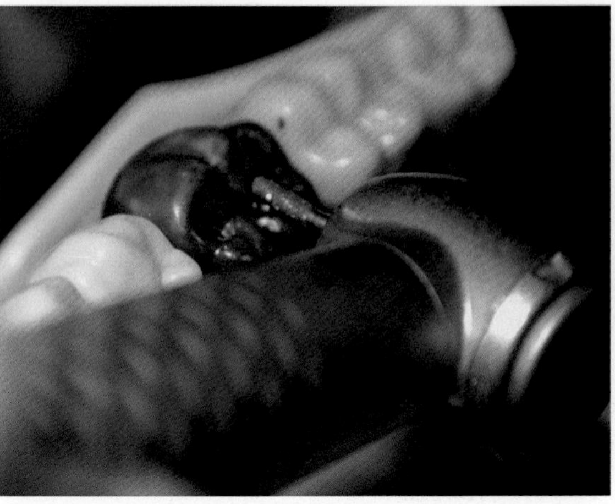

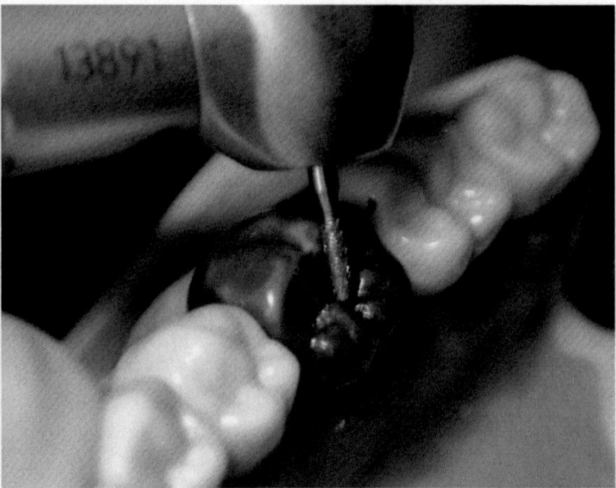

Figure 8.7 To create an occlusal reduction that conforms to the original morphology of the tooth a fissure bur should be used and inclined according to the cuspal slopes. Depth cuts are optional.

When should depth cuts been used?

Some suggest these should always be used as they ensure consistently sufficient and uniform reduction. However, the depth cuts can sometimes be difficult to remove without leaving the preparation with a rippled effect. Figure 8.8 shows a plastic tooth in which depth cuts have been prepared. When removing the islands of tooth tissue or core material between the depth cuts, the fissure bur should be used at a slightly different angle to the initial depth cuts. In this way the bur is prevented from re-entering the depths of the initial cut and forming a rippled occlusal reduction.

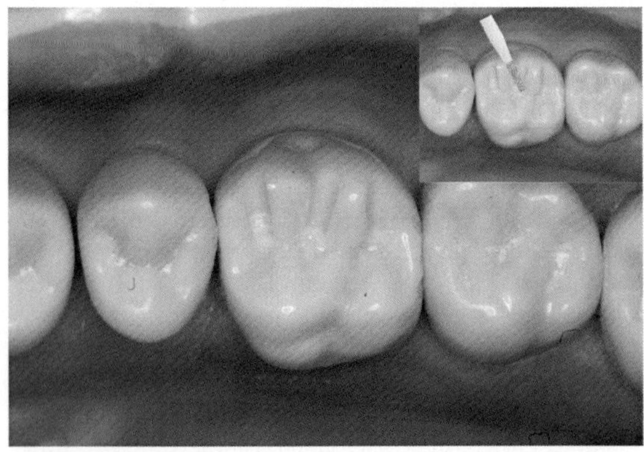

Figure 8.8 Depth cuts on the occluso-buccal surface ensure an even and adequate occlusal reduction. The islands of tooth tissue between should be removed with the bur at a different angle (inset).

What is the functional cusp bevel and why should it be prepared?

Once the basic occlusal reduction has been carried out, further reduction over the functional cusp should be undertaken. This is termed the functional cusp bevel and provides sufficient thickness of gold over the functional cusp during mastication and in some patient's parafunction. This gives strength to the restoration where occlusal forces are highest and allows for some degree of wear of the crown with time. So is this necessary if the patient has incisal/canine/anterior guidance and posterior disclusion in lateral excursion? It is controversial as to whether or not those with anterior guidance can exhibit bodily lateral movement of the mandible and the potential for increased wear. The argument is perhaps academic and clinically all that is needed is to ensure sufficient occlusal clearance between the preparation and opposing teeth, both in intercuspal position and excursive movements.

Confirming that sufficient occlusal reduction has been carried out

The most satisfactory way is to look clinically, as this can check out dynamic excursions (Figure 8.9). Another reliable method is to evaluate the thickness of correctly made provisional restorations which have been adjusted to fit the patient's occlusion. This can be achieved by looking for the transmission of light when holding the restoration up at the light or measuring the thickness of the provisional restoration using an Iwanson gauge (see Chapter 9). The other common method is to ask the patient to close against soft wax (Occlusal Indicator Wax, Kerr Hawe) and make excursive movements. This

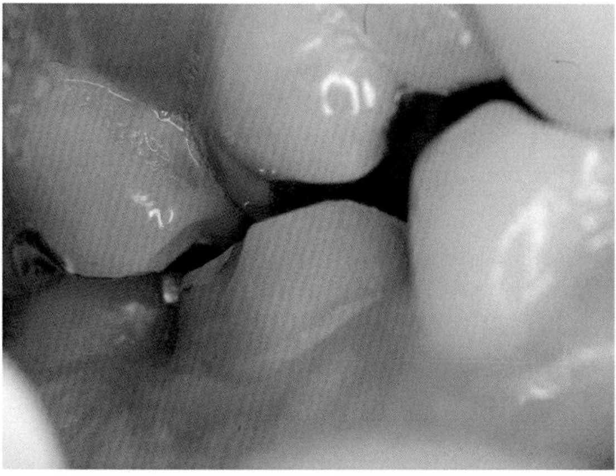

Figure 8.9 Visual evaluation of occlusal clearance for a full gold crown preparation on the endodontically treated lower right first molar tooth. Sufficient occlusal clearance between the buccal cusp and opposing tooth has been created. Altering the angulation with which the tooth is viewed will allow assessment of clearance lingually.

can be removed from the tooth and examined for excessively thinned areas against light (Figure 8.10). The use of a putty stent taken before tooth preparation is also useful (see Chapter 10). Whatever method is used, if it has been shown that there is inadequate occlusal reduction, the preparation must be refined until sufficient reduction has been achieved.

Should an occlusal offset groove be prepared?

Before this issue is discussed, familiarize yourself with this preparation characteristic (see Figure 8.5). Generally these are not required in full coverage crowns, and where overlays and three-quarter gold crowns are concerned there is no evidence that those restorations incorporating such design characteristics have a superior outcome to those that do not. However, indisputably they permit location and seating of the casting, particularly when using some of the adhesive cements that act as lubricants in their unset state. They also allow increased thickness of gold and strength in otherwise weak areas of the restoration (see later for discussion of three-quarter gold crowns).

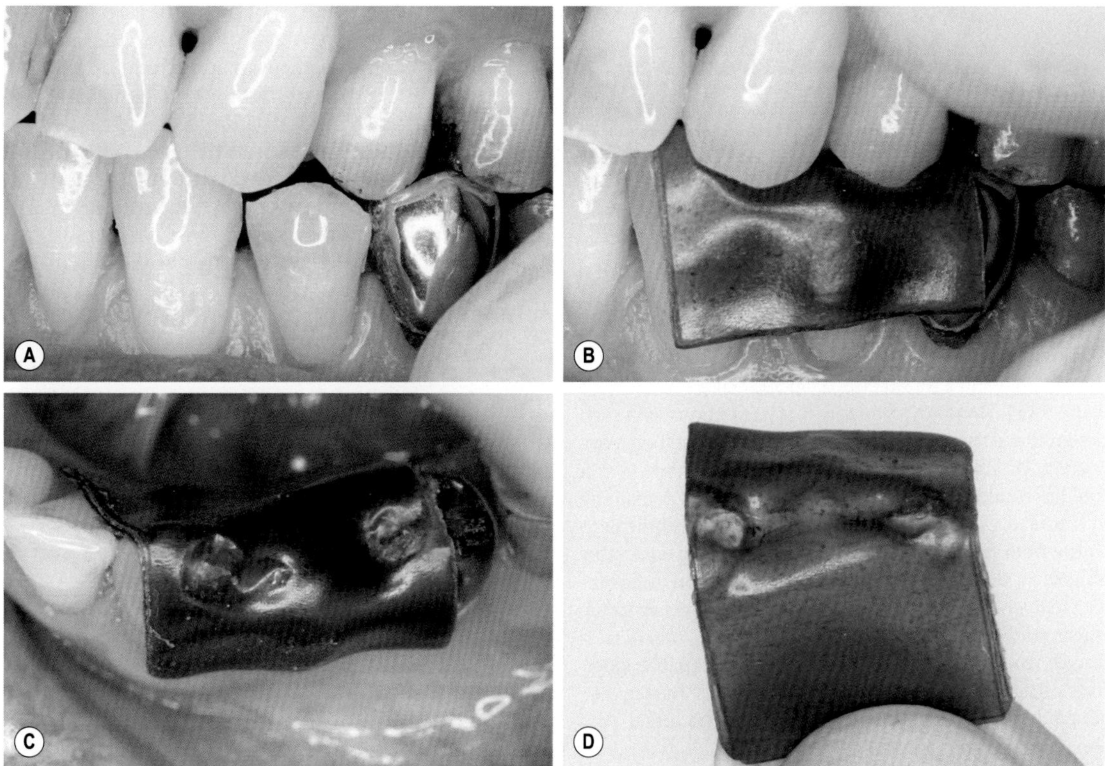

Figure 8.10 Wax used to determine the amount of occlusal clearance for a three-quarter crown preparation on the lower left first premolar tooth (**A**). The wax is 0.5 mm thick and has been doubled over. The patient bites into ICP and excursive movements (**B**). The wax is pierced where there are occlusal contacts on the teeth either side (**C**). The wax should not be thinned where the preparation is; this can be assessed by removing the wax and holding it up to the light (**D**).

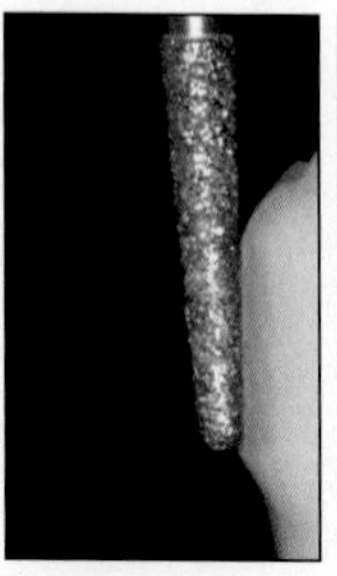
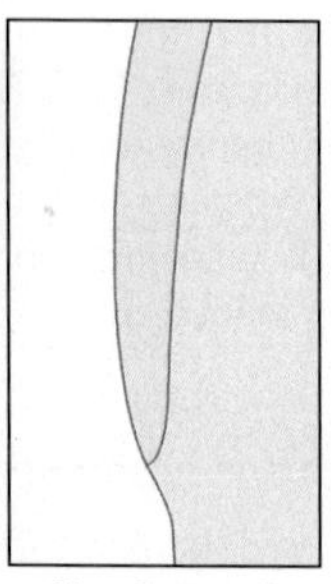
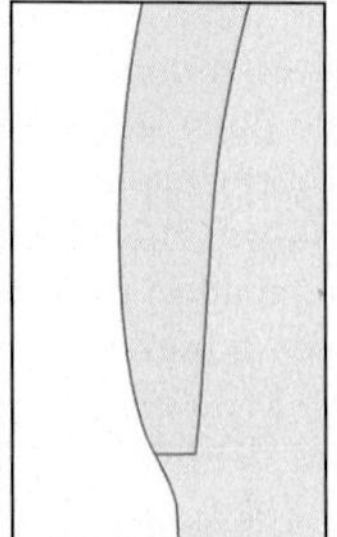
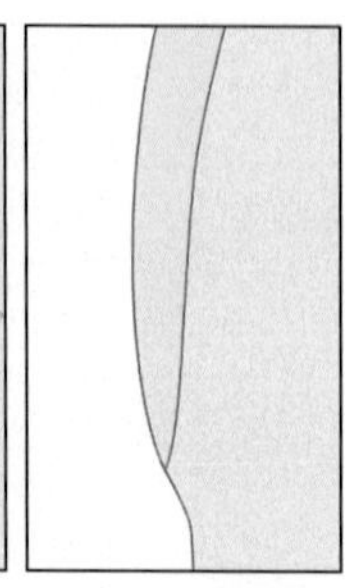

Chamfer margin and round ended blur | Chamfer margin | Shoulder margin | Knife edge margin

Figure 8.11 The chamfer margin is the most appropriate for gold. It allows for adequate thickness of gold and is easily seen clinically, in the impression and on the stone model in the laboratory. The shoulder margin is too destructive for gold castings and the knife edge margin is difficult to determine. The round ended tapered bur is best for creating a chamfer.

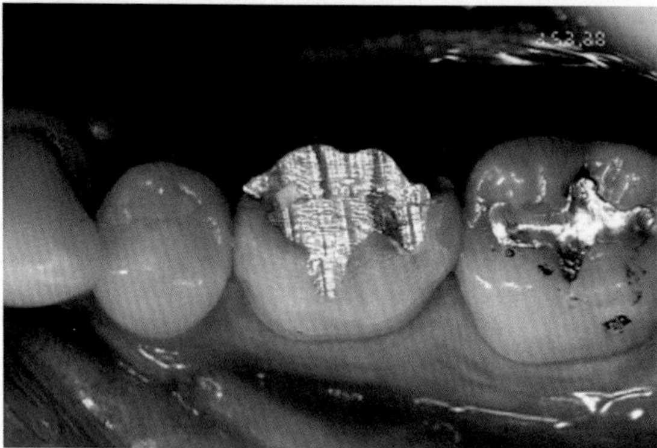

Figure 8.12 Occlusal reduction and buccal and lingual chamfer preparations in the lower left first molar tooth.

Axial reduction

Buccal and lingual preparations (Figures 8.11 and 8.12)

Cervical finishing lines

Traditionally a chamfer is prepared to accommodate the finishing margin and a round-ended tapered bur is ideal for this (Figure 8.11). There is no evidence that restorations with such a design characteristic have a better outcome in the long term. However, it would seem reasonable to use a chamfer as a shoulder would be unnecessarily destructive of remaining tooth structure and a knife-edge finish is not only difficult to identify both clinically and in the laboratory but invariably results in an overbuild of the crown margin and an unfavourable emergence profile. The emergence profile relates to the contour and angle that the tooth (and crown) makes as it emerges from the gingival tissues. An unfavourable emergence profile could lead to gingival trauma if inadequate, and plaque accumulation and potential periodontal problems if too great.

'Parallel belt'

This is in order to create both retention and resistance form. In addition, this characteristic should be of sufficient height to minimize the restoration 'rocking-off' the preparation (resistance).

Retention and resistance form

It is important to consider both the retention and the resistance form of tooth preparation, as it is these that ensure the restoration is not dislodged.

- *Retention form of the preparation*. To understand retention form, two definitions are required: total occlusal convergence and taper. Total occlusal convergence (TOC) is the angle of convergence of two opposing walls (e.g. mesial and distal walls) whilst the taper of a wall is the inclination of one wall in relation to the long axis of the tooth (Figure 8.13). The TOC of the preparation will largely dictate the resistance to dislodgment in an occlusal direction (retention). Surveys of tooth preparations have shown that generally posterior teeth end up with greater TOC than anterior teeth, mandibular teeth have greater TOC than maxillary teeth and bucco-lingual surfaces have a greater TOC than mesio-distal surfaces. These variations may be a direct result of access and vision in various areas of the mouth. The ideal taper has been stated to be in the range of 2–5°, giving a TOC of 4–10°. This is very difficult

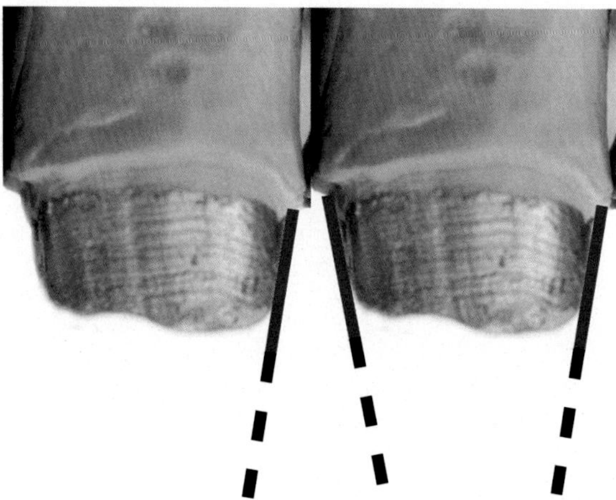

Figure 8.13 Taper, the inclination of one wall to the long axis of the tooth (left) and total occlusal convergence, the angle of convergence of two walls (right).

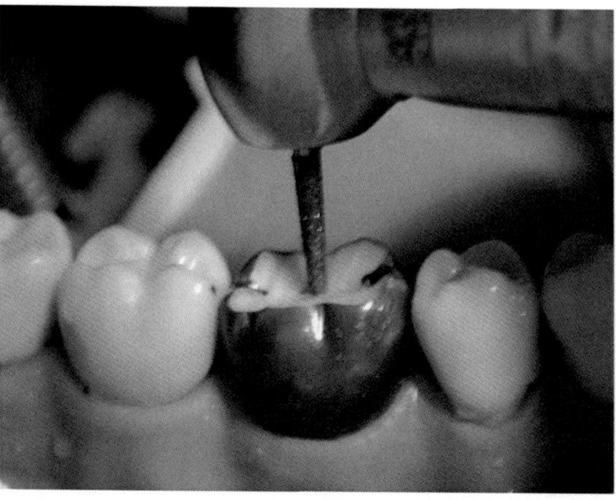

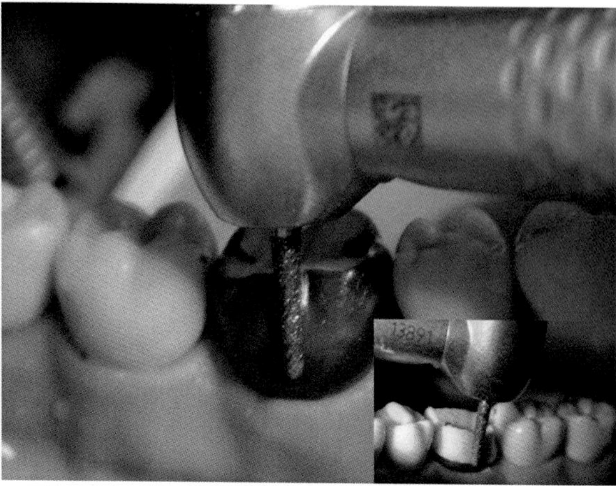

Figure 8.14 For the axial reduction, visualize the long axis of the tooth (left) and without tilting the bur, move it to cut the buccal (right) and lingual reduction (inset).

to achieve clinically and the more realistic range of 10–20° has been suggested; however, assessment of the TOC has been shown to be greater than this in many instances. Clinically, the TOC is usually assessed by visual means with monocular vision; this often produces preparations with a greater than ideal TOC. At a distance of 30 cm the use of binocular vision can result in areas of the preparation that are undercut not being identified.

- *Resistance form of the preparation*. Resistance to dislodgement in a non-axial direction (resistance) is provided by the TOC, height of preparation (parallel belt) and the ratio of occluso-gingival height to bucco-lingual width. It has been estimated that only 46% of molar preparations have adequate resistance form compared to 96% of incisor preparations. This has been attributed to a general increase in TOC of posterior preparations, the smaller occluso-gingival height of molars and the smaller occluso-gingival to bucco-lingual height ratio.

Where the TOC is inadequate, auxiliary retentive features such as grooves can be prepared. Placement of grooves essentially bisects the TOC, giving greater retention and resistance form. Consider Figure 8.13 for example, placement of a longitudinal groove down the buccal and/or lingual surface would effectively bisect the mesio-distal TOC. If the tooth preparation is more tapered bucco-lingually, the grooves would need to be placed on the mesial and distal surfaces. Much of a crown preparation will involve removal of core material, but if the preparation of grooves would remove sound tooth unnecessarily and weaken the tooth further, consideration should be given to cementing the crown in place with an adhesive luting cement.

To achieve the optimum TOC, a tapered bur should be used and the long axis of the tooth visualized. Keeping the bur in exactly the same plane and resisting the temptation to tilt the bur as the buccal and lingual reduction is carried out will ensure the optimum TOC (Figure 8.14). A useful analogy is as if the handpiece was held by a jig. Ideally the 'parallel belt' or axial preparation should be 3–4 mm in height (Figure 8.15). If its dimension is excessive the restoration would be difficult, if not impossible, to seat.

Parallelism is best gauged by adopting the mantra of: (1) one eye; (2) head still; and (3) the use of a photographic mirror (a hand mirror is easily tilted when viewing single preparations and is always too small to confirm parallelism between preparations when teeth are prepared

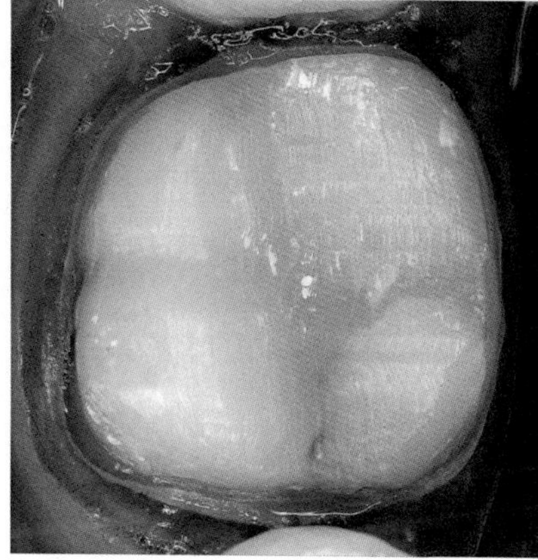

Figure 8.15 Full gold crown preparation, lower right first molar tooth. Note the 'ring' formed by the occlusal reduction and chamfer. This would imply a satisfactory 'parallel belt' has been prepared.

for bridges). Parallelism is then confirmed by small movements of the head.

Some, instead of referring to this design characteristic as a 'parallel belt', call this component of the preparation that which accommodates the ferrule. However, in dentistry, a ferrule usually refers to that part of the remaining tooth structure encompassed when providing post crowns (see Chapter 7).

Protecting the soft tissues

The final issue to be highlighted is protection of the soft tissues, particularly a lolling tongue when preparing the lingual cut in the lower posterior sextants. A Svedopter saliva ejector is impregnable whereas disposable flange saliva ejectors (Linguaflex) offer little protection (Figure 8.16). Lingual aspiration with a high volume aspirator tip is the only other way of protecting the tongue when preparing teeth in this sextant. For this you require excellent and reliable four-handed dentistry.

Approximal preparation

The traditional finishing margin for a full gold crown is a chamfer around the complete perimeter of the preparation. This is relatively straightforward to prepare for the buccal and lingual surfaces. However, in order to avoid damage to the adjacent tooth, preparation of an interdental chamfer may be difficult and result in an unacceptable amount of tooth preparation; a knife-edge preparation interdentally may have to be accepted.

As this is the most exacting cut when preparing a tooth for a crown, it will be described in more detail. The most controlled way in order to achieve this is as follows:

- Use direct vision. The patient's head should be moved to the side.
- Cut the knife-edge to the full depth below the contact point, moving the bur from the buccal to the lingual surface in one continuous motion, leaving a thin slither of tooth or core material between the bur and the adjacent teeth (Figure 8.17). This will fall away when the interdental preparation has been completed.
- When 'cutting-out', particularly palatally, the disto-palatal angle is further distally than one anticipates. If prepared more mesially, a destructive groove is made into the core/tooth.
- In order to avoid damage to the adjacent tooth, focus on the adjacent tooth and not the tooth being prepared.

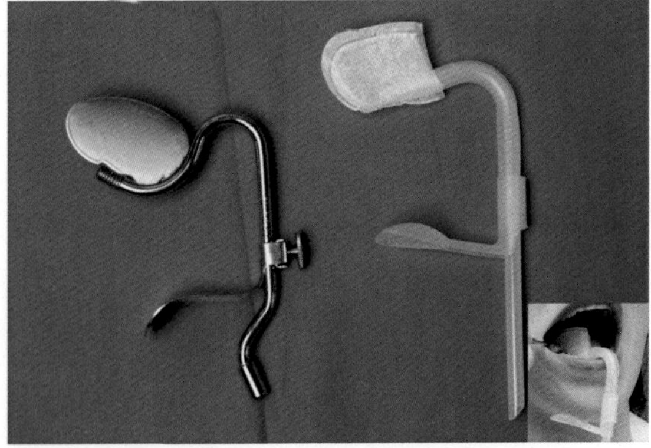

Figure 8.16 The Svedopter (left) and plastic Linguaflex saliva ejector (right and inset) both allow protection of the tongue when preparing lower posterior teeth.

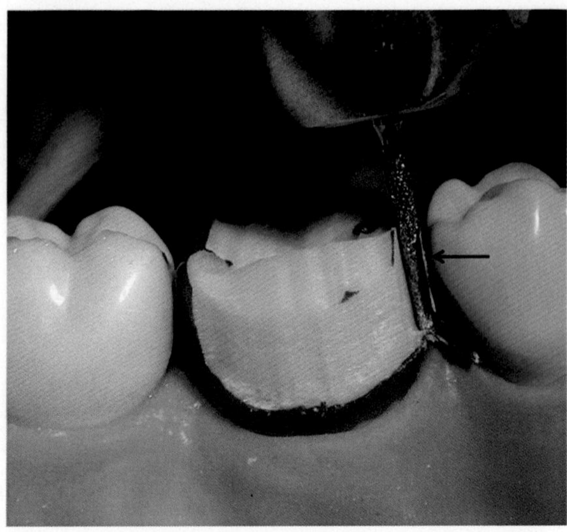

Figure 8.17 The interdental cut is best carried out by a narrow tapered diamond bur leaving a thin slither of tooth between the bur and the adjacent tooth for protection. This will fall away once the cut is complete.

Once the tooth preparation is complete it is important to check that there are no sharp internal line angles and that the margins are smooth and flowing with no steps as the individual aspects to the preparation are merged (Figure 8.18). Sharp internal line angles pose difficulty in the laboratory: it is difficult to pour die stone material into these aspects of the impression and if successful in this, the die stone is liable to wear or chip in these areas, leading to a casting that will not seat fully.

PREPARATION/DESIGN CHARACTERISTICS SPECIFIC TO A THREE-QUARTER GOLD CROWN

As implied earlier in this chapter, it is unclear as to the future role of gold crowns, let alone the three-quarter gold crown. Older members of the profession assert that the

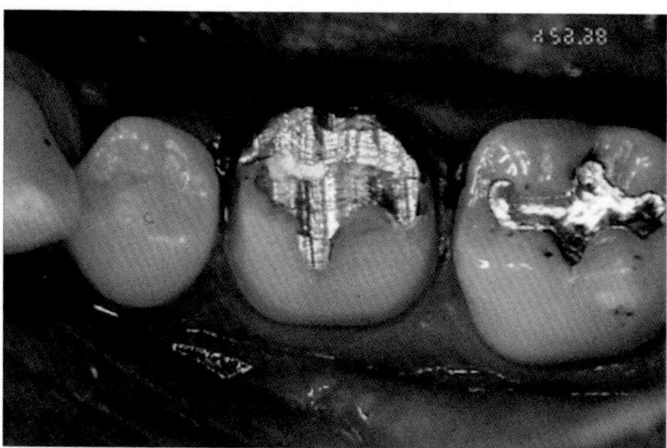

Figure 8.18 Completed full gold crown preparation, lower left first molar tooth. The patient, who is a dentist, did not want the amalgam core replaced with resin composite unless the restoration catastrophically failed during the preparation stage. It is understood the casting that was placed has been satisfactory for more than 10 years.

three-quarter gold crown is a superb restoration. However, many patients are unhappy to show any gold, even if it is only a thin line of gold bucco/occlusally. This textbook marks a transition period in indirect restorations with a move toward more aesthetic tooth-coloured restorations. All-ceramic or resin-based restorations are not, however, a panacea solution; in certain circumstances they do not have the physical properties for longevity and tooth preparation for such restorations is often less conservative of tooth tissue. For this reason the three-quarter crown preparation is described here.

It is a myth to suggest that this preparation is the most demanding to prepare – a perfectly executed posterior resin composite is more difficult. Before listing a summary of key design characteristics, the reader is invited to study carefully two illustrations showing this preparation (Figures 8.19 and 8.20).

The design characteristics have evolved from the necessity, in bygone days, to cut grooves in order to provide 'struts' to improve the structural integrity of such restorations where the fourth 'wall' of the crown is missing. The key features are as follows:

- Occlusal and palatal reduction is carried out as for a full coverage crown.
- Both interdental cuts should extend beyond the contact areas in order that the technician can section the resultant model in the laboratory and remove the die to work on.
- The mesial interdental cut should only extend sufficiently to clear the contact area so as not to compromise further the dental aesthetic.
- The distal interdental cut extends buccally in order to afford 'wrap around' to prevent the casting dislodging palatally.

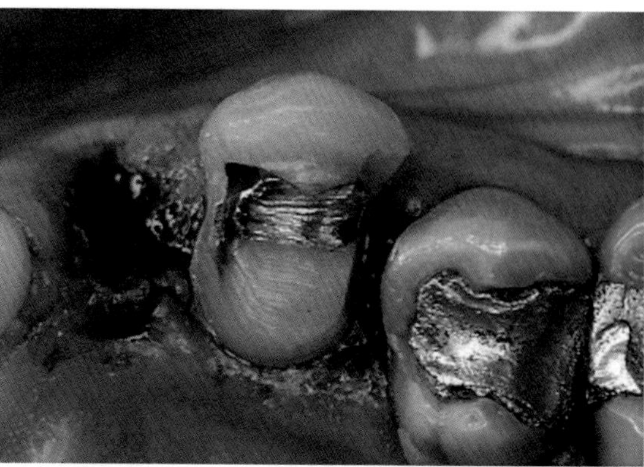

Figure 8.19 A very old image illustrating a three-quarter gold crown preparation for an upper left first premolar tooth. This preparation was in order to provide a retainer for a conventional cantilever bridge to replace an extracted deciduous upper canine tooth. The restoration met the patient's high dental aesthetic need within the constraints of this traditional treatment approach.

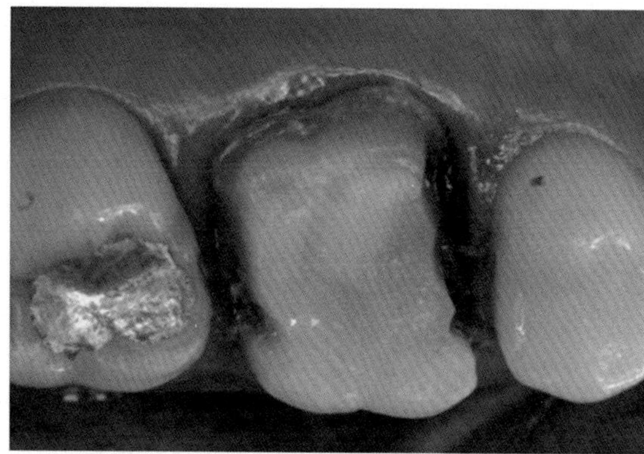

Figure 8.20 Three-quarter gold crown preparation, upper left first molar tooth. A mesial concavity was prepared in the core to accommodate the furcal groove between the mesio-buccal and palatal roots.

- Traditionally, mesial and distal grooves are prepared as far buccally as the interdental cuts will contain.
- Traditionally, an occlusal off-set groove extends between the mesial and distal grooves. This produces an arch of thickened gold buccally, giving the casting strength where the fourth buccal facing to the crown is missing. This preparation characteristic should be adopted judiciously as a compromised cusp could be further weakened.

Figure 8.21 shows the cemented three-quarter crown on the tooth seen in Figure 8.20.

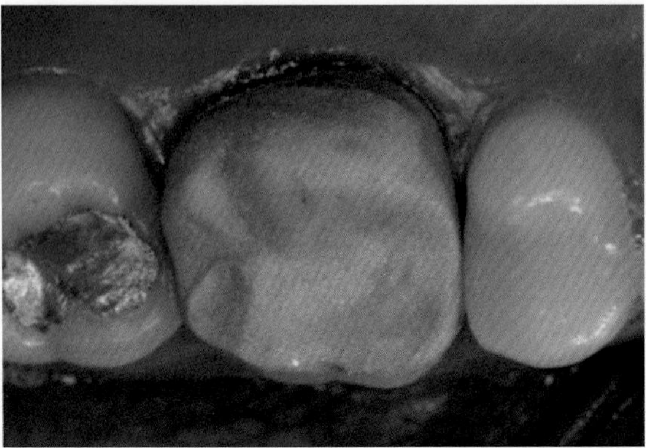

Figure 8.21 Three-quarter gold crown, upper left first molar tooth. Note: (1) satisfactory contact areas; (2) how the palatal margin has been 'thinned' to achieve a satisfactory emergence angle; and (3) polishing of the cervical 2 mm to facilitate optimum home care.

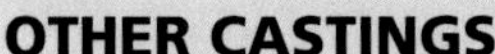

OTHER CASTINGS

Occasionally full coverage castings can have their external surfaces milled and prepared as abutments for a removable or fixed partial prosthesis (Figure 8.22). In the latter situation the bridge can be cemented with temporary cement for ease of removal and maintenance. The problem here is that to allow sufficient thickness of gold to the casting, which is cemented permanently onto the tooth, and then allow space for the overdenture/bridge materials, the tooth preparation is extensive. As a result these are rarely carried out today.

MAKING THE PROVISIONAL RESTORATION

Making a provisional restoration is extremely important. Why and how this is done is described in Chapter 14. In most instances the provisional restoration should be made before the impression is taken. There are two reasons for this:

- The provisional can be used to indirectly assess your tooth preparation. For example, if you are unable to remove the provisional restoration from the preparation or reseat it once fully set, the preparation might be undercut. If the tooth is inadequately prepared in areas, the provisional restoration will be too thin. The tooth preparation can then be modified and a new provisional restoration made if necessary before taking the impression.
- Time management. If you run out of time you have the temporary already made for cementation and the impression can be taken at a subsequent visit.

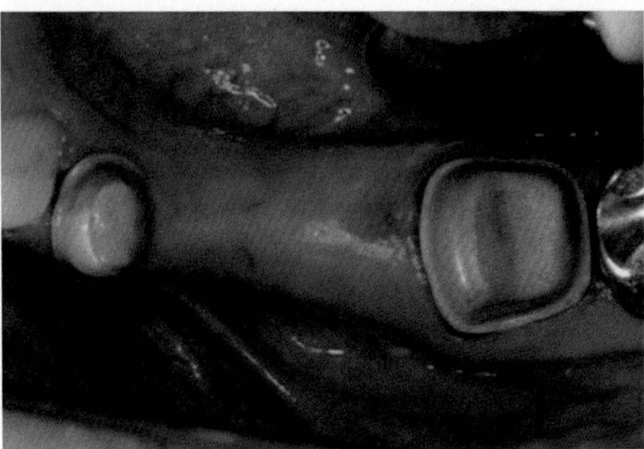

Figure 8.22 Full coverage telescopic crowns luted permanently, that form abutments for a fixed prosthesis that will be cemented temporarily.

IMPRESSION TAKING

It is pointless to try to take an impression of the preparation if all the margins cannot be identified. Chapter 13 discusses the management of soft tissues to ensure that preparation margins are accessible for taking an impression and it describes the impression materials and techniques used for indirect laboratory-made restorations.

RECORDING THE OCCLUSION

How the occlusion is recorded and whether casts should be mounted on an articulator will depend on how many units of crown or bridges are being placed, the occlusal scheme and the number of remaining teeth. If casts are mounted on an articulator, the type of articulator will be dictated by the complexity of the reconstruction. When there are sufficient index teeth and a single unit is being restored according to a conformative scheme, it is acceptable for the laboratory technician to 'hand-hold' the casts in maximum interdigitation. The reader should refer to Chapter 6 on when and how to articulate casts.

SUMMARY

This chapter has described how teeth are prepared for gold crowns. The subsequent chapter will discuss the materials used in making metal castings, how the crown is made in the laboratory, how the crown is checked for fit in the mouth, how the restoration is cemented and the supportive aftercare.

FURTHER READING

Blair, F.M., Wassell, R.W., Steele, J.G., 2002. Crowns and other extra-coronal restorations: preparations for full veneer crowns. Br. Dent. J. 192, 561–564, 567–571.

Donovan, T., Simonsen, R.J., Guertin, G., Tucker, R.V., 2004. Retrospective clinical evaluation of 1,314 cast gold restorations in service from 1 to 52 years. J. Esthet. Restor. Dent. 16, 194–204.

Lynch, C.D., Allen, P.F., 2005. Quality of communication between dental practitioners and dental technicians for fixed prosthodontics in Ireland. J. Oral Rehabil. 32, 901–905.

Stoll, R., Sieweke, M., Pieper, K., Stachniss, V., Schulte, A., 1999. Longevity of cast gold inlays and partial crowns – a retrospective study at a dental school clinic. Clin. Oral Investig. 3, 100–104.

Wassell, R.W., Walls, A.W., Steele, J.G., 2002. Crowns and extra-coronal restorations: materials selection. Br. Dent. J. 192, 199–202, 205–211.

Chapter | 9 |

Gold restorations: the metals, the manufacture and the fit

Graham Chadwick, John Radford, David Ricketts

CHAPTER CONTENTS

GOLD ALLOYS

Applications and constituents

The restoration of teeth with gold in the form of crowns, inlays, onlays and palatal veneers has considerable historical pedigree and should still be considered in treatment planning for reasons outlined in the preceding chapter. Although, in the past, pure gold has been used to restore cavities directly by the process of cold welding, this is no longer taught as the gold foil used is considered too soft for general application.

The International Organization for Standardization (ISO) defines four types of gold alloy: 1, 2, 3 and 4. They all contain gold, silver and copper in various amounts, with platinum and palladium also present in types 2, 3 and 4. The inclusion of all these metals enhances the physical properties of the gold, rendering the alloys suitable for a wider range of clinical applications. With increasing gold alloy type number, the content of gold (85% to 65%) and silver (11% to 9%) decreases and the proportions of copper (3% to 15%) and those of platinum or palladium (2% to 10%) increase. The effects on the physical properties of the alloy, with increasing alloy type number, are to increase strength and hardness, and to decrease ductility and corrosion resistance.

Type 1 gold alloys are recommended for use in clinical situations of low functional stress such as simple inlays. Situations where an inlay involves cuspal coverage require higher stress-bearing capability and so Type 2 gold alloy is recommended. Types 3 and 4 gold alloys are used where high strength is required such as in crown and bridgework. Both of these alloy types, by virtue of their relatively high copper content, may also be used to fabricate onlays or palatal veneers where adhesion to tooth substance, by use of a chemically adhesive luting resin, is required. Such adhesion can be enhanced by, following try-in, returning the restorations to the furnace for oxidation for a period of 10 minutes at 400°C.

Biocompatibility

The biocompatibility of gold alloys is considered to be good. Although gold allergy is rare, technicians with a known sensitivity to nickel are thought to be at heightened risk of palladium allergy.

FABRICATION OF GOLD RESTORATIONS

The majority of gold restorations are manufactured indirectly in the dental laboratory. This involves a series of stages which, in industrial terms, form a total process chain. Associated with each stage are losses in dimensional accuracy. It is important to realize that such losses may occur as both increases and decreases in dimensions; however, when the whole process chain is taken into account these balance out, culminating in a restoration that fits. A point often misunderstood by the public is that this manufacturing process is bespoke. Each restoration is made on an individual basis and is therefore unique. It is well established in general industrial production that this is the most expensive method of manufacture. The laboratory stages described for the production of a gold restoration in this chapter are common to many other materials and restorations.

Once tooth preparation has been completed by the dentist (Figure 9.1), an impression of the tooth is recorded, decontaminated and disinfected (see Chapter 13). Upon receipt of this, the dental laboratory technician casts an accurate die stone model of the preparation (Figure 9.2). Die stone is a gypsum-based material (calcium sulphate dihydrate) which has undergone a treatment process to make it harder and have a lower expansion on setting than conventional plaster. Die stones expand by 0.05–0.10% on setting compared to plaster's 0.2–0.3%. This small amount of expansion therefore produces a microscopically larger crown than the tooth preparation, ensuring a full seat at try-in.

Once the die stone has set, the technician has to section the model so that the master die of the prepared tooth can be removed to allow a wax pattern to be built up (Figures 9.2 and 9.3). It is therefore critical that the clinician clears the contact point during tooth preparation, not only to allow an impression to be taken of the margin but also to allow the model to be sectioned. Failure to do this will lead to the laboratory not being able to proceed with the work or, worse still, attempting to proceed and working on a die and contact damaged in the sectioning process. Once the model has been sectioned, the master die is covered with die spacer, a paint that is applied in coats to the master die (Figure 9.3). Two to three coats of conventional die spacer amount to a thickness of about

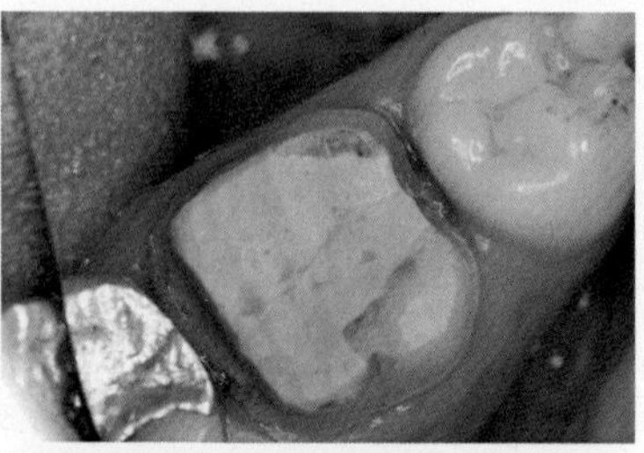

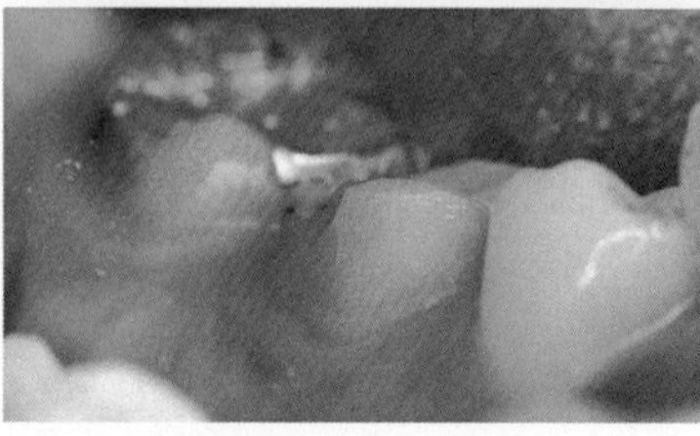

Figure 9.1 Occlusal (top) and buccal (bottom) view of a full gold crown preparation; the distal margin is deep. This has resulted from the operator's attempt to avoid damage to the adjacent gold restoration.

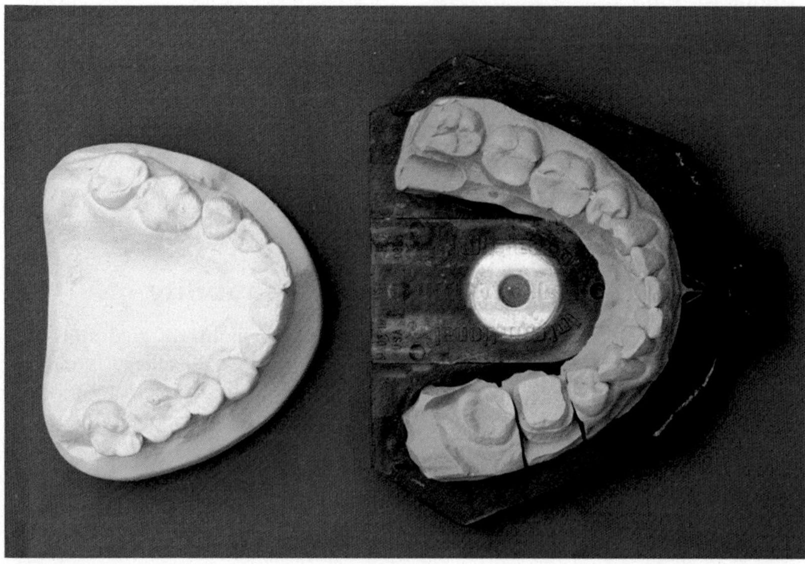

Figure 9.2 Lower die stone model cast from an impression taken of the tooth preparation seen in Figure 9.1 (right). Note the model has to be sectioned to allow the master die of the lower right first molar crown preparation to be removed from the model to build up the wax pattern. The upper model (left) is used to check the occlusion and create the occlusal form of the crown.

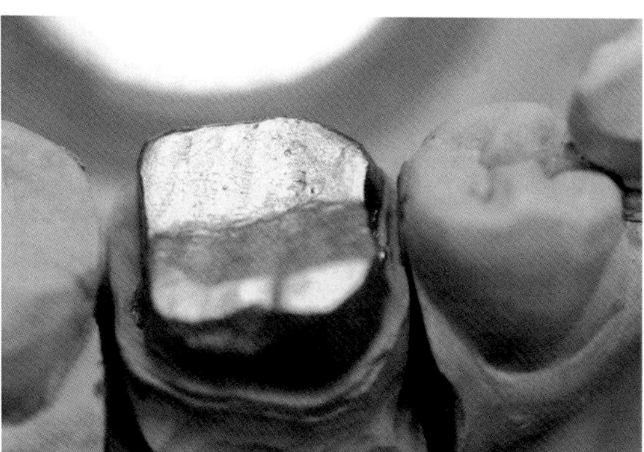

Figure 9.3 Sectioned model with the master die coated in die spacer.

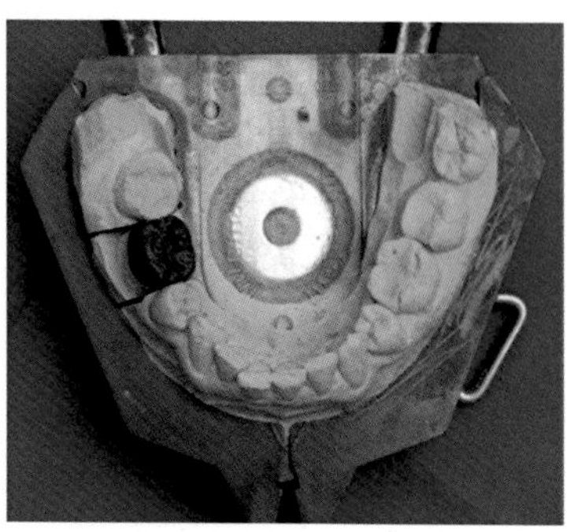

Figure 9.4 Wax pattern of a full gold crown built up on the model of the lower right first molar tooth.

25–30 μm. Ideally, the die spacer should be painted to just short of the preparation margin. The die spacer is placed to allow for an adequate layer of luting cement and full seat of the crown at fit.

Once the master die has been prepared, a wax pattern of the restoration is built up using the wax additive technique (Figure 9.4), checking that all contours are correct, all contact points are tight, and the occlusal surface and contacts conform to the existing occlusion; articulated study models facilitate this (Figure 9.5). It is also possible with the advent of computer-aided design and computer-aided manufacture (CAD-CAM; see Chapter 11) technology to computer design and mill wax blocks to form wax patterns of crowns. Once the wax pattern has been made, it is then removed from the die and a wax sprue attached (Figure 9.6). The sprued pattern is then placed

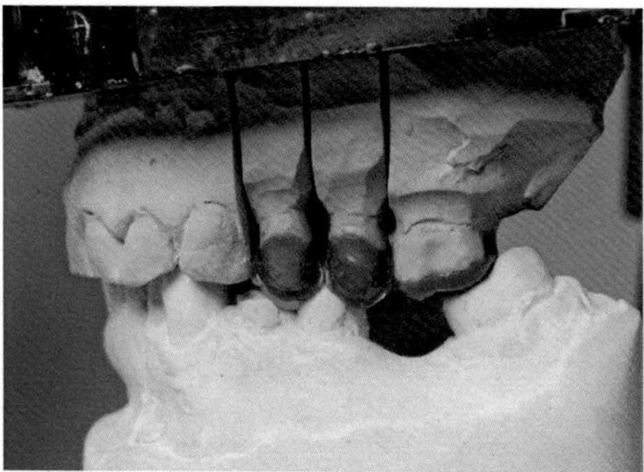

Figure 9.5 Articulated die stone model being used in the wax-up of the metal substructure for metal–ceramic crowns on the upper premolar teeth and a gold cuspal overlay on the molar tooth.

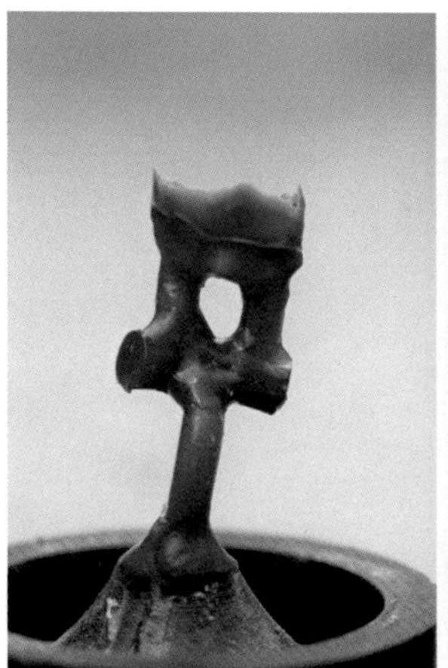

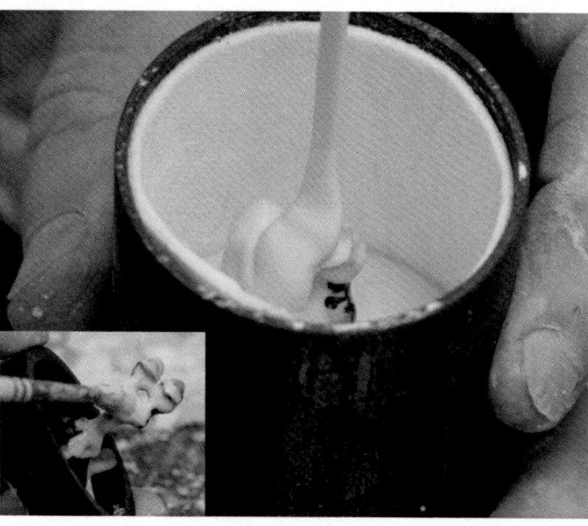

Figure 9.6 Cuspal overlay wax pattern seen in Figure 9.5 being sprued (left) and being invested in investment material (right). The sprued wax pattern is placed in an investment cylinder and the investment material is poured over – initially a small paintbrush is used (inset) to coat the wax pattern and to ensure no air bubbles attach to the wax surface.

in a lined investment cylinder and invested in an investment material which is mixed under vacuum so as to avoid the incorporation of air and hence porosities in the investment mould (Figure 9.6).

Thereafter, once the investment has set, the wax is removed from the mould by burning it off. For gold alloys this is achieved by placing the investment mould in a furnace at either 450°C (slow burn out) or 700°C (fast burn out). The mould is then placed into a casting machine and gold alloy, in molten state, is forced into it using centrifugal force. Once cooled, the surrounding investment is removed, the sprue is cut off the restoration and the resultant alloy casting trimmed and polished (Figure 9.7).

Clearly in such an elaborate process faults in the casting may occur. Common faults include:

- *Incomplete casting* – where there has been incorrect spruing or lack of either molten alloy or applied centrifugal force. This prevents the flow of sufficient gold into the investment mould.
- *Porosity and pitting* – these are seen as bubbles or pitting upon the casting surface. They may arise from porosity in the investment mould itself, the incorporation of investment material in the casting or the liberation of gases from the investment material.
- *Incorrect dimensions of restoration* – these may arise from insufficient expansion of the investment mould or other errors in the process chain.

Fitting the completed restoration to the die minimizes the chances of such a flawed casting reaching the patient for try-in.

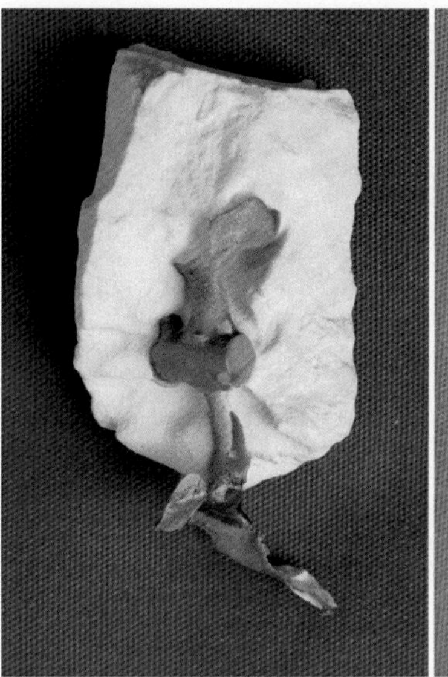

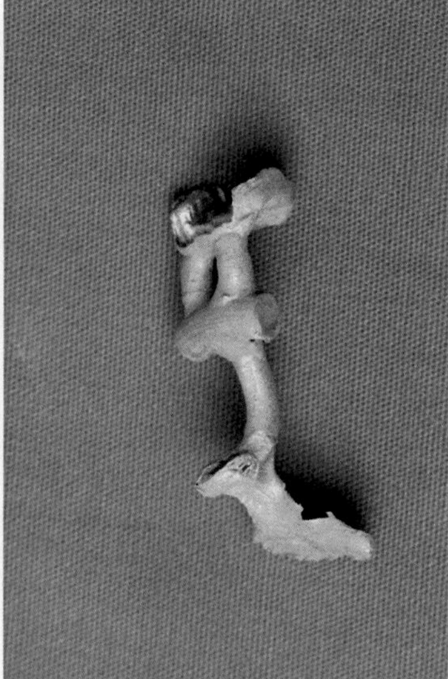

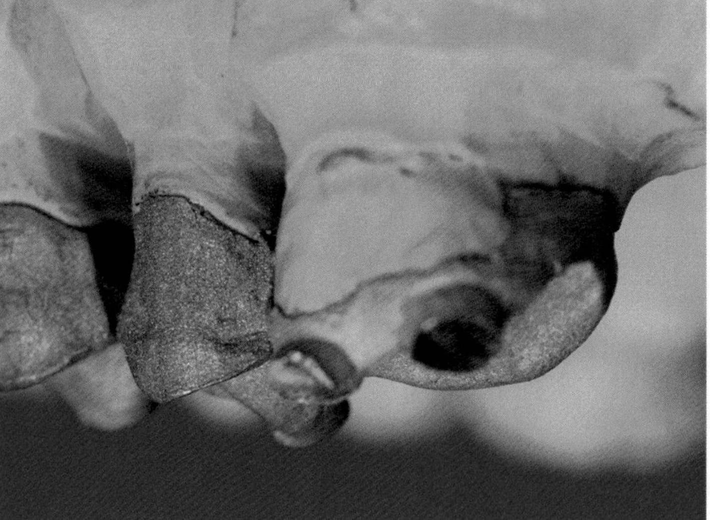

Figure 9.7 Gold casting being removed from the investment material (top left), completely removed from the investment (top right) and being tried onto the model once the sprue has been cut off (bottom).

CHECKING THE RESTORATION

On receipt of the casting, the dentist should examine it meticulously, both on and off the master die, checking for the aforementioned flaws. As the laboratory technician would have had to trim the master die in order to capture the margins, errors can occur in over- or under-trimming, leading to negative and positive ledges respectively when tried in the mouth. In addition, damage can occur to the master die during the fabrication of the restoration. Sometimes the casting may fit on the master die and not on the tooth, but this is the exception, not the rule. Similarly, damage can occur to the opposing cast resulting in occlusal discrepancies. Such errors may not be evident on the cast. Trying-in the restoration at the chairside is therefore essential before the restoration is cemented.

Refining the casting before the patient's appointment (Figure 9.8)

Prior to the patient's appointment the laboratory work should be checked for obvious errors:

- *Fit surface.* Castings with significant deficiencies or defects on the fit surface should be remade.
- *Contact areas.* The master die with the casting should be held up to the window. If daylight is visible between it and the adjacent tooth, the casting should be returned to the laboratory for a remake or possibly soldering.
- *Emergence angle.* Bulbous crowns may compromise effective home care. In order to shape these to make them more favourable, remove the casting from the working die and hold it such that the fit surface is being examined and thin the bulbosity with a green stone in a slow handpiece. An over-contoured crown is not necessarily a laboratory fault as it might occur following insufficient tooth preparation by the clinician.
- *Occlusal table.* After removing the casting from the master die, confirm centric stops on other teeth by pulling through thin articulating paper or Shimstock foil (Roeko, Germany; see later). Where there are centric stops the paper or foil will not pull through. Then place the casting on the master die and repeat the process. If there are any prematurities in intercuspal position on the restoration, the articulating paper or Shimstock foil will pull through where the previous centric stops were identified. The occlusal prematurities on the casting can then be identified using articulating paper and removed by using a stone. This is easier to do if the models have been articulated.

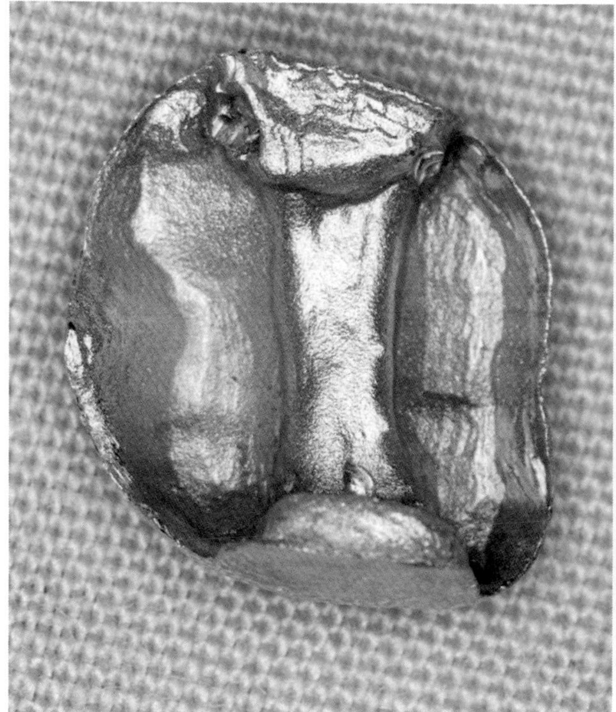

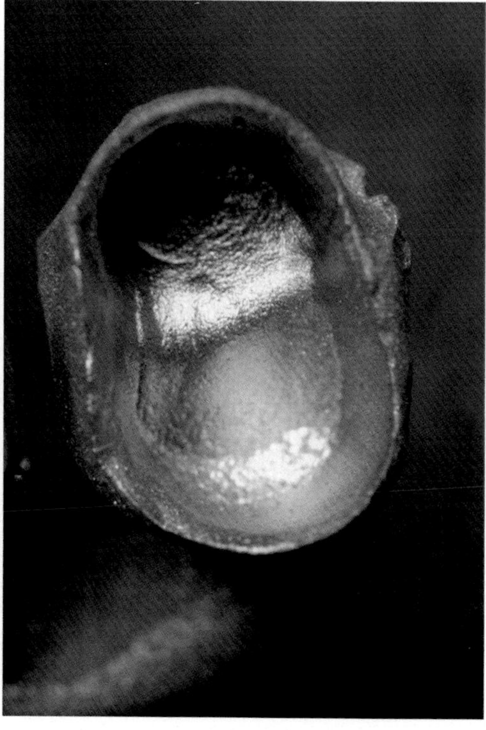

Figure 9.8 Fit surface of castings being checked for any defects and retained investment material. Both are satisfactory.

Refining the casting at the chairside

The most satisfactory and safest method is to try the restoration in the mouth, identify any problems or adjustments required and then remove the restoration from the mouth to carry out the adjustment.

- *Checking the marginal fit*. This should initially be assessed visually and with the use of a dental probe. The margin of the crown should seat fully with no space between the crown margin and tooth preparation margin. If a gap exists it should be established if it is localized or generalized around the whole perimeter of the restoration. In the former this is likely to be due to a local error, which could have occurred at any stage in the process from taking the impression; if this is the case, a remake is usually indicated and a new impression should be taken. The latter would indicate that the casting is not seating fully and in these circumstances the tooth preparation should be checked for any remaining temporary cement. The casting should be rechecked for bubbles of gold (where air bubbles in the investment sat at the wax pattern surface) or retained investment material. The master die should be checked for any damage, typically at any internal line angles, comparing the model with the tooth preparation; rounding internal line angles at the end of tooth preparation reduces the risk of this. Overbuilt contacts might also be the cause of the gold casting not seating fully. Tight contact points can be checked with indicator die spray such as Occlude (Pascal Co., Inc.) (Figures 9.9–9.11). This spray can be used in a similar manner to check the fit surface of the crown for any tight areas which might be preventing the crown seating and can also be used to check the occlusion for premature contacts.

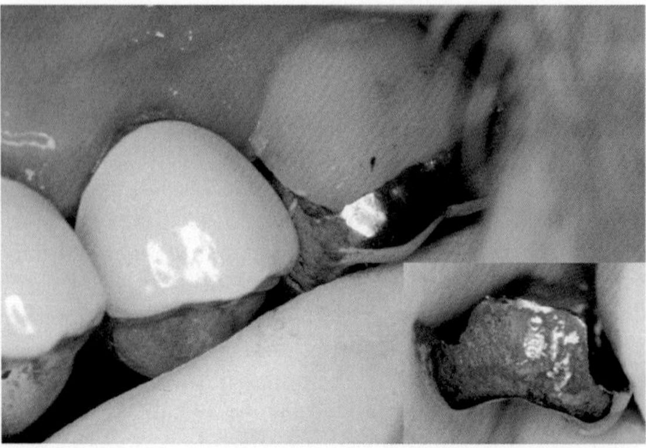

Figure 9.10 The Occlude-coated overlay is seated. The poor seating is evident as a large marginal gap. Where the contact point is tight, the Occlude spray has been worn away, indicating where the crown needs adjustment.

- *Contact areas*. These should be confirmed by using waxed floss. It is essential when checking the contact areas to secure the casting against the preparation with, for example, a firmly positioned ball-ended burnisher; holding the ball-ended burnisher against the casting is best carried out by a dental nurse. Check the contact areas by moving floss gingivally, not coronally as this will dislodge the restoration with potentially catastrophic consequences. The floss should meet with resistance when passing it through the contact area. Once checked, the floss can be

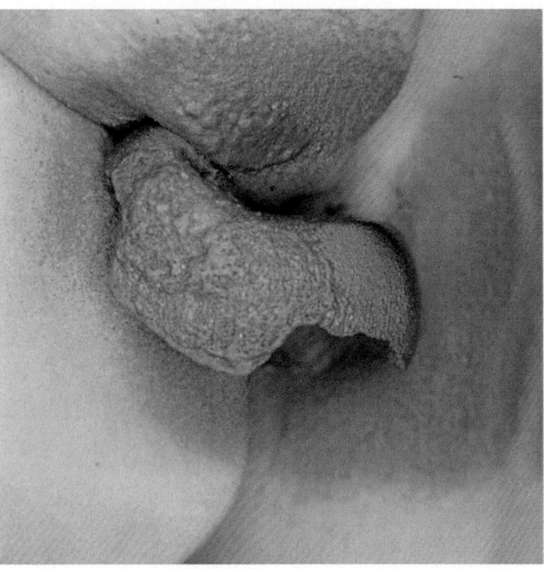

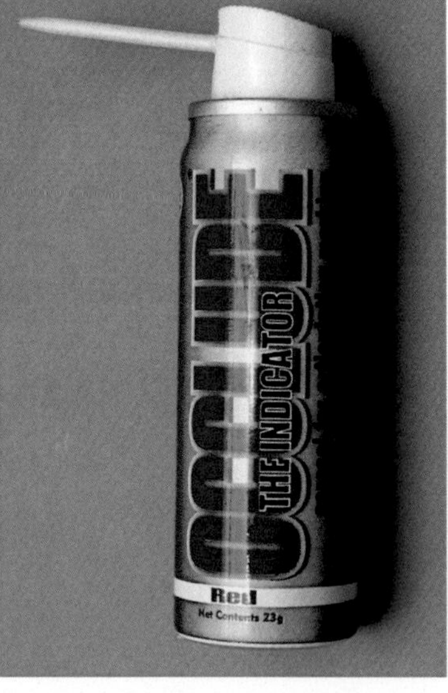

Figure 9.9 Occlude indicator spray has been sprayed onto the proximal surface of the gold cuspal overlay seen in Figures 9.5–9.8.

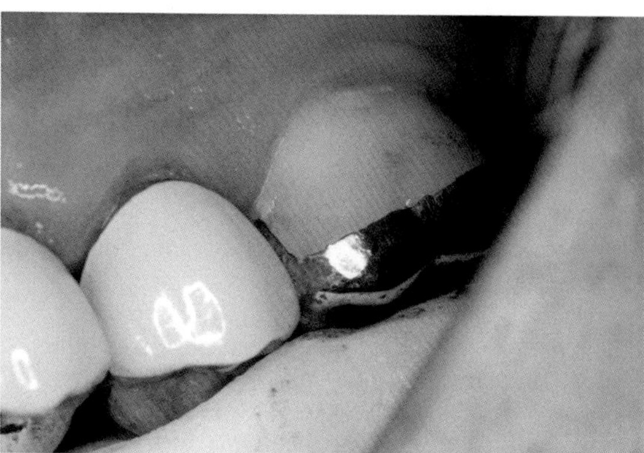

Figure 9.11 After adjusting the contact point on the overlay seen in Figures 9.5–9.10, the overlay seats down further.

removed from beneath the contact by pulling it through the interdental space in a buccal direction.

- *Interdental fit*. Again this is checked with waxed floss. If the margin has a positive ledge the floss will catch. Any overbuilt margins can be thinned first by using green stones and then abrasive discs and finally rubber points (Figure 9.12), all with decreasing abrasiveness. Final adjustment and polishing of accessible margins can be carried out after the restoration has been cemented onto the tooth but care should be exercised so as not to remove any gold bevel which would result in an unacceptably thick exposed cement lute.
- *Checking the occlusion*. This is carried out in a similar way to that detailed above when the restoration is checked on the cast (master die) prior to the patient's visit. Articulating paper can be used to mark up any premature contacts or high spots (Figure 9.13). Shimstock foil can be used to ensure that the restoration remains functional, in at least maximum intercuspation, if not other excursions depending on the occlusal scheme; the restoration should not be adjusted until it is not in occlusion (Figure 9.14).

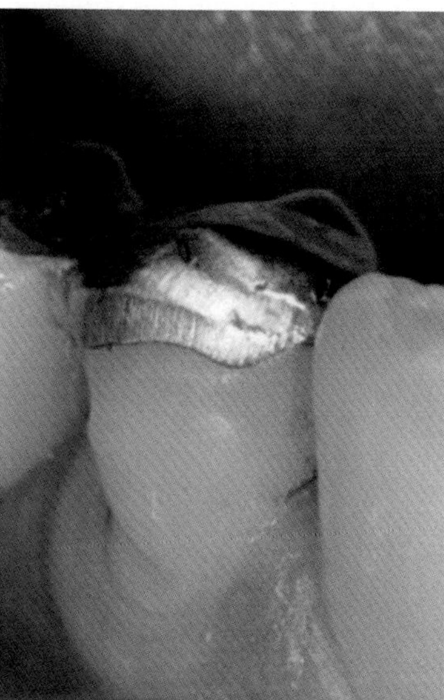

Figure 9.12 Use of abrasive discs in order to achieve a satisfactory buccal margin. The grit marks are now removed with rubber cups/wheels before cementation.

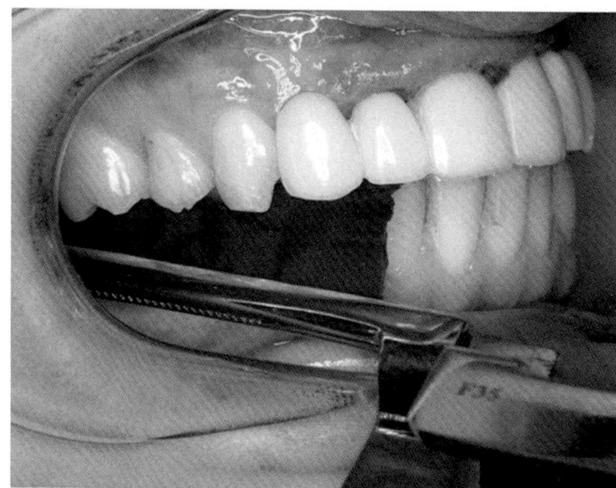

Figure 9.13 Articulating paper being used in a Miller forceps to check the occlusion. Provisional restorations have been placed in the upper anterior region; the articulating paper is being used to check that there are posterior occlusal contacts as well as even occlusal contacts on the anterior provisional restorations.

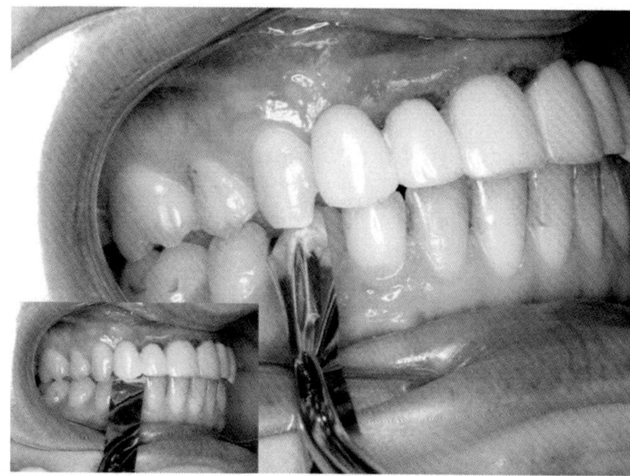

Figure 9.14 Shimstock foil being used to check the occlusion on the provisional restorations seen in Figure 9.13. A tight occlusal contact exists between the premolar teeth which resist the withdrawal of the foil, hence the provisional restorations are not 'high'. When placed between the provisional restorations and the opposing teeth, resistance to withdrawal is also found, indicating that they are also in functional occlusion (inset).

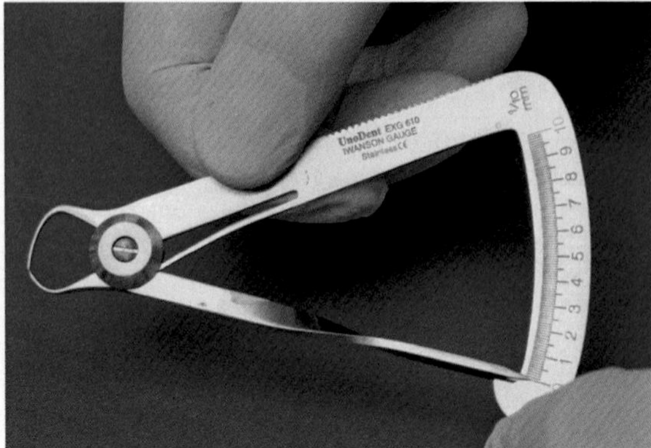

Figure 9.15 An Iwanson gauge. Ensure that when the tips of the gauge are in contact (left) the pointer reads zero (right).

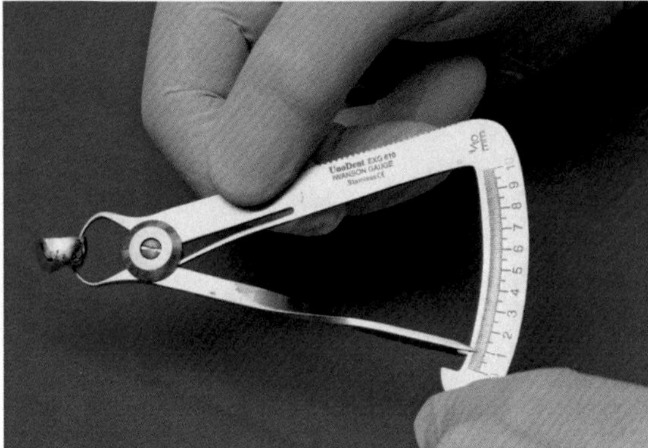

Figure 9.16 An Iwanson gauge being used to measure the thickness of a gold crown. At the point in question the gold is 0.9 mm thick.

When adjusting the casting it is important that the gold does not become too thin (<0.3 mm) as there is a risk of perforation after years of function. An Iwanson gauge (UnoDent) is essential in determining the thickness of the crown material (Figures 9.15 and 9.16).

CEMENTATION OF THE RESTORATION

Before the gold restoration is prescribed the dentist must decide how it is to be cemented. This is because if adhesive cementation is required the correct alloy type needs to be specified. In any regard the cement used should be non-irritant and have sufficient working time to allow manipulation of the restoration into place. Cementation is helped if the material used is pseudoplastic, as such materials coat the fit surface well with no slumping, yet flow readily on seating the restoration home. Once set, the cement should seal the interface between the restoration and the tooth/core and demonstrate high compressive strength. In order to prevent microleakage at the restoration margins, it is also desirable that the cementing agent should have low solubility in the oral environment. Over the years a wide range of materials have been developed for this purpose. These include the following:

- *Zinc phosphate cements*. These cements are formed from the reaction of zinc oxide with phosphoric acid. They are generally presented as powder (ZnO) and liquid (H_3PO_4; 45–64%) and the key to their successful application is to observe the correct powder to liquid ratio upon mixing. Although successfully used over many years, they are non-adhesive and considered to be irritant to the pulp due to their initial high acidity and with time they are soluble in oral fluids. Whilst cheap and still widely available, zinc phosphate cements have been superseded by more modern adhesive materials and hence not discussed further in this text.
- *Polycarboxylate cements*. These arise from the reaction of zinc oxide powder with an aqueous solution of polyacrylic acid (30–40%). Some formulations have the acid freeze dried and added to the powder, which is then mixed with water. They are adhesive to tooth substance and form a weak bond to gold but not to porcelain. They are not considered to be irritant to the pulp. Clinical experience suggests that their higher solubility, compared to zinc phosphate, does not pose a significant clinical problem. The main disadvantages of these cements are that they have a short working time and crown placement needs to be quick. When mixed in the correct proportions, the cement initially appears too thick to flow and it is tempting to add more liquid to thin it down. This should be resisted as the cement is pseudoplastic and will flow well under pressure; in addition, adding more liquid will adversely affect the physical properties of the cement.
- *Glass polyalkenoate cements, e.g. AquaCem (Dentsply)*. These cements are more commonly known as glass ionomers and the luting cement is derivative from the filling material of the same name. In common with these they are a reaction product of fluoroaluminosilicate glass and an aqueous solution of either acrylic acid or of a maleic/acrylic acid copolymer to which, in order to control the setting reaction, the manufacturer has incorporated tartaric acid. Some manufacturers, as with the polycarboxylate, have freeze dried the acids and added them to the powder, which is then mixed with water. It should be noted that in order to produce a film thickness amenable for luting, the particle size of the glass is less than in the filling material version. Such cements are adhesive to tooth substance and less soluble than the polycarboxylate cements. They are, however, susceptible to moisture contamination during the first few hours of placement. Any benefits of fluoride release and reduction in secondary caries are unlikely to play a significant clinical role (see Chapter 7).

- *Resin modified glass polyalkenoate cements and compomers, e.g. RelyX Luting Cement (3M ESPE).* These may simply be considered as a blend of glass ionomer and resin composite technology. They are less soluble than conventional glass polyalkenoate cements due to the incorporation of resin into these materials. Some concern has been expressed about the possibility of hygroscopic expansion in a moist environment. Whilst this is not a problem with metal-based restorations, its use with all-ceramic crowns should be avoided, perhaps with the exception of zirconia-based crowns.
- *Chemically adhesive luting resins, e.g. Panavia F (Kuraray Dental) and RelyX ARC (3M ESPE).* These are suitable for adhesive luting of Type 3 and 4 gold alloys. They derive from resin composites with the active constituent being either 4-META (4-methacryloxyethyl trimellitate anhydride) or MDP (10-methacryloyloxydecyldihydrogenphosphate). If oxidation of the gold restoration is enlisted to enhance its retention, the cemented, oxidized and blackened restoration must be polished by the dentist in situ. If metal-based crowns have been cemented with these cements, retrieval can be extremely difficult and principles of tooth preparation and conventions of retention and resistance form should be preferred.
- *Resin luting cements, e.g. RelyX Unicem (3M ESPE).* There is a distinction between these cements and the preceding group of cements in that this group does not bond chemically to metal. Some, like RelyX Unicem, are self-adhesive (etching and bonding) to tooth tissue and do not require a separate etching and bond application. These materials, like their restorative counterpart, also have good aesthetic properties if used in conjunction with indirect composite or ceramic restorations.

Luting the restoration

There is an abundance of in vitro product testing studies comparing the mechanical and biological properties of different luting cements. However, there are no known randomized controlled studies of sufficient duration to demonstrate that one cement results in a superior clinical outcome to another. Anecdote would suggest that a glass ionomer luting cement or resin-modified glass ionomer luting cement is appropriate for all metal-based restorations apart from those where the dentist considers the preparation lacks adequate retention and resistance properties. For these preparations an adhesive resin composite should be used.

Regardless of which luting material is chosen, the most important factor in carrying out this stage predictably is to follow the manufacturer's instructions. Other tips are:

- The dentist should repeatedly rehearse the path of insertion of the restoration.
- Complete moisture control with cotton wool rolls and aspiration – a saliva ejector or a Svendopter or Linguaflex suction and tongue retractor should be used (see Chapter 8). Rubber dam placement which allows a crown to be cemented unhindered is often difficult and unrealistic; a split dam may be the only option.
- The dental nurse mixes the correct ratio of materials according to manufacturer's instructions; no attempt should be made to alter this as it will adversely affect the properties of the material (Figure 9.17).
- With the restoration held by the dentist in the same manner as when establishing the correct path of insertion, the fit surface of the restoration is presented to the dental nurse.
- The nurse then carefully works/agitates the mixed cement over the entire fit surface (Figure 9.18) and the dentist seats the restoration.
- Before the cement is set, the occlusion is checked in intercuspal position to ensure complete seating.
- While the cement sets, the patient can gently close on a cotton wool roll placed between the restoration and the opposing tooth.
- When the cement is set partially, excess is removed (Figure 9.18).
- When fully set, the margins are examined meticulously. Every speck of excess cement is removed. Interdental excess cement is removed with dental floss.
- Accessible margins can be further finished with appropriate rubber points if necessary.
- If a glass ionomer luting cement is used, an unfilled resin can be applied to the margins to prevent any premature dissolution or drying out of the cement (Figure 9.18). This may be unnecessary with newer glass ionomer formulations.

Figures 9.19 and 9.20 show cemented gold crowns for patients illustrated in this and the preceding chapter.

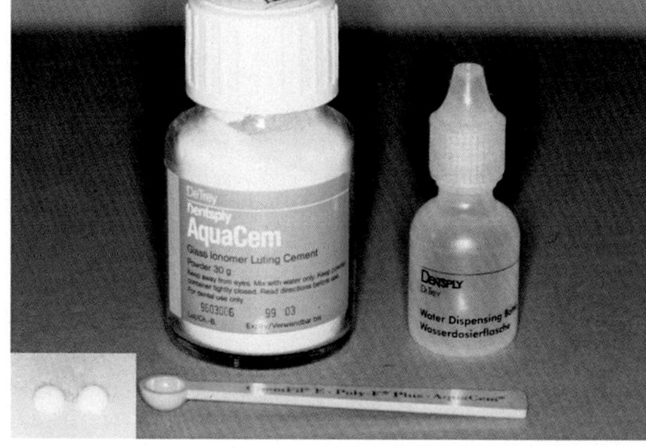

Figure 9.17 A glass ionomer luting cement with water dispenser and scoop to ensure an accurate and reproducible ratio of powder (inset) to water.

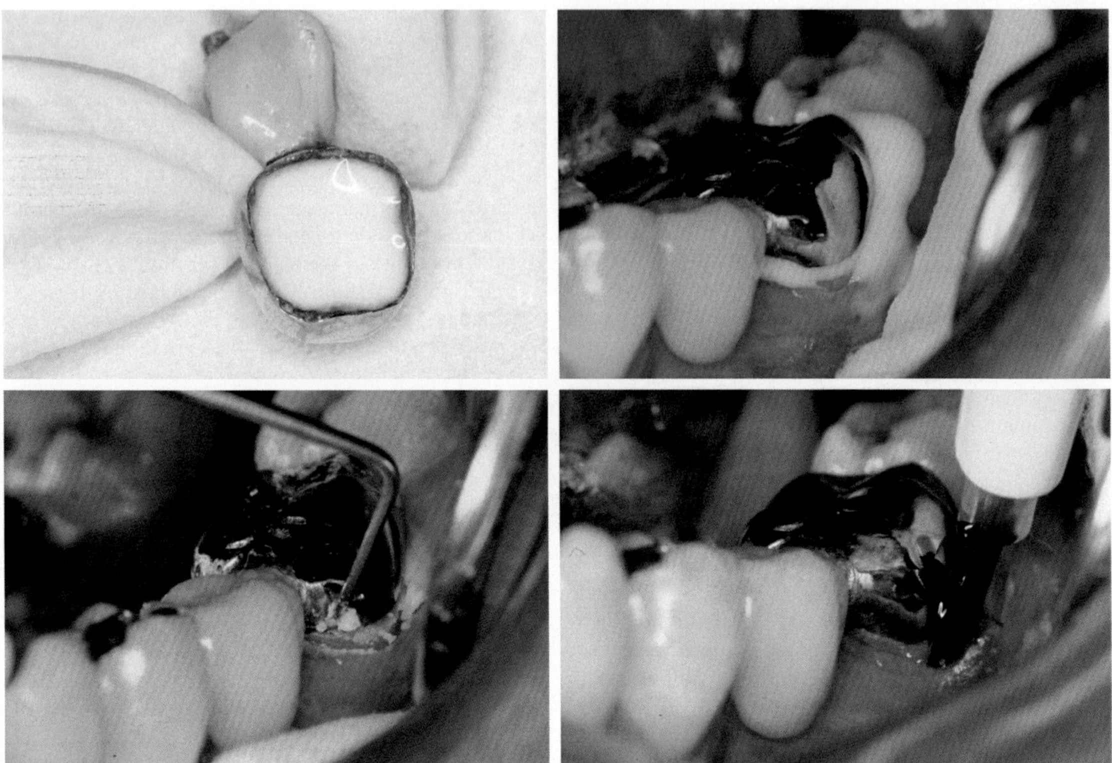

Figure 9.18 From top, left to right. A gold full coverage bridge retainer is filled with a glass ionomer luting cement (the retainer only needs a complete lining), the bridge is completely seated, the excess cement allowed to reach the setting (gelation) stage and the excess gently removed with a probe. Excess interdental cement should always be removed by passing dental floss between the restoration and adjacent teeth. Finally, resin is applied to the margin to prevent premature dissolution of the cement.

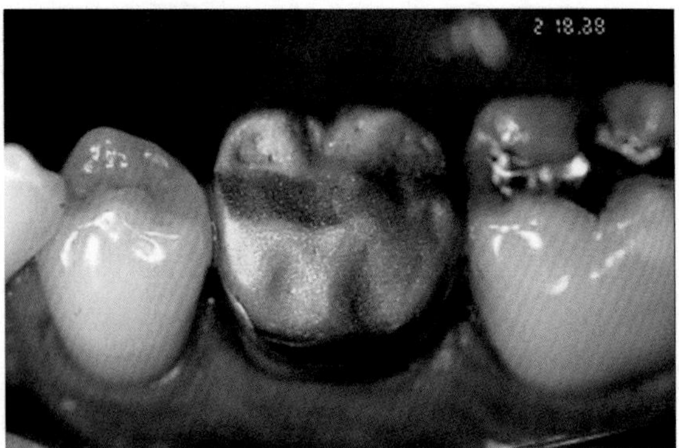

Figure 9.19 Completed gold crown lower left first molar for patient seen in Figure 8.1B, Chapter 8. Note how the occlusal morphology has been refined to accommodate the group function and the gingival one-third has been polished to facilitate optimum oral hygiene.

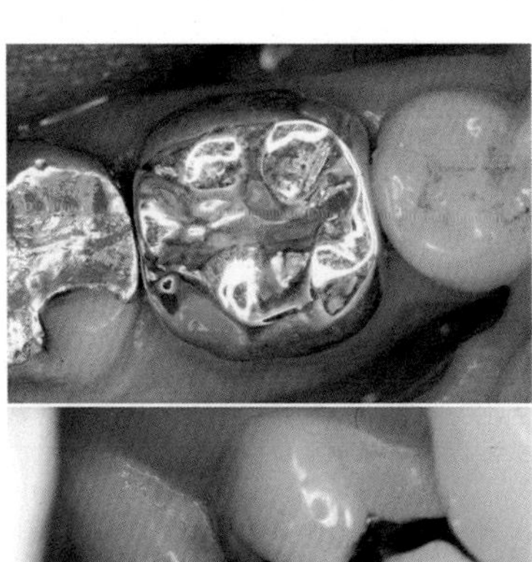

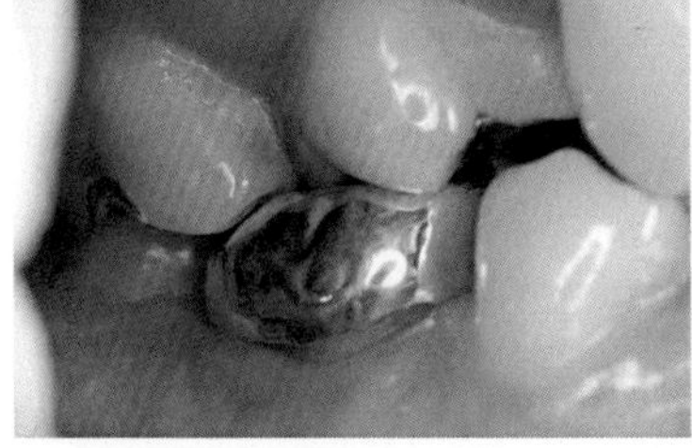

Figure 9.20 Cemented full coverage gold crown for the patient seen in Figures 9.1–9.4.

SUPPORTIVE PHASE

Following the 'fit appointment', it is good practice to arrange a further visit to review the completed restoration. Not only can the restoration be reassessed after a period of function, but a dental carer can also encourage and reinforce oral health, lifestyle changes and aspects of home care that were discussed during the preparatory phase. Specifically, the patient should be asked whether or not they have been able to resume their normal home care, particularly interdental cleaning. Evidence of effective plaque removal and periodontal health should be confirmed by a clinical examination. At this appointment, it is occasionally necessary to refine the occlusion as the patient may have had local anaesthetic at the fit appointment and found it difficult to assess the occlusion accurately.

SUMMARY

Undergraduate students in many dental schools worldwide do not have the opportunity to make metal-based crowns for patients; however, knowledge of the materials and the laboratory techniques used is important. This knowledge will allow dentists to critically analyse these bespoke restorations, especially when castings do not appear to fit immediately. Whilst great care is taken over tooth preparation, impression taking and manufacture of metal crowns, little credence is given to cementation. This final stage in providing the patient with an indirect restoration is equally important. These important issues have been addressed throughout this chapter.

FURTHER READING

Burke, F.J., 2005. Trends in indirect dentistry: 3. Luting materials. Dent Update 32, 251–254, 257–258, 260.

Van Noort, R., 2007. Introduction to dental materials, third ed. Mosby, Edinburgh. Section 3.

Chapter 10

Metal–ceramic crowns

Brian Stevenson

CHAPTER CONTENTS

INDICATIONS FOR METAL–CERAMIC FULL COVERAGE CROWNS

If a tooth requires a full coverage indirect restoration and there is a need for an aesthetic restoration, a metal–ceramic crown can be considered. However, all-ceramic restorations may be more appropriate in patients with extremely high aesthetic demands and these are increasingly being used by some clinicians. There are also special circumstances that require specific modifications to the standard metal–ceramic crown detailed throughout this chapter. Metal–ceramic restorations can be waxed-up or milled to provide space for a movable component of a fixed prosthesis (Figure 10.1; see also Chapter 19) or a rest for a removable partial denture (see Chapter 8). These must not be confined to ceramic as this can lead to catastrophic fracture and failure. In addition, guide planes and undercuts to aid the retention of a removable prosthesis can be incorporated into the restoration.

METAL–CERAMIC FULL COVERAGE CROWNS

Metal–ceramic crowns consist of:

- A metal substructure
- An opaceous ceramic layer
- A veneering ceramic layer (Figure 10.2).

The rationale for this restoration is to combine the strength of a metal substructure with the aesthetic qualities of dental porcelain. However, tooth preparation for

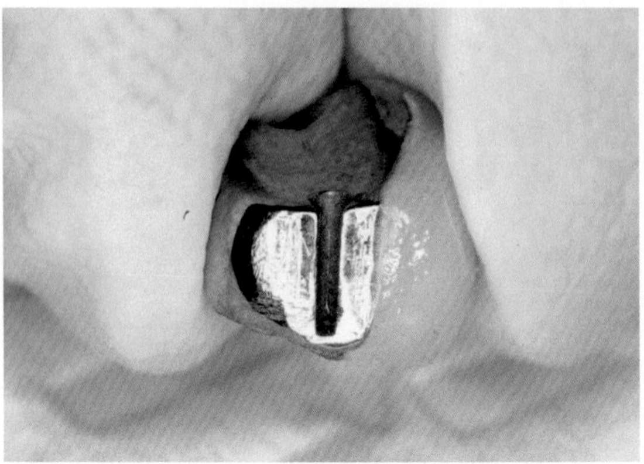

Figure 10.1 Female component of movable connector that is incorporated into a fixed prosthesis. The component is confined to metal within the restoration.

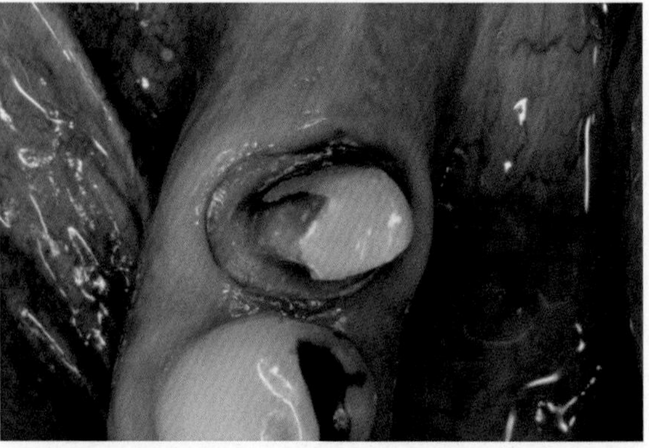

Figure 10.3 Metal–ceramic crown preparation with shoulder buccally merging into a chamfer lingually. Reduction of the buccal cusp has significantly reduced the amount of remaining tooth tissue.

a full coverage metal–ceramic restoration is destructive of tooth substance (Figure 10.3) as clearance needs to be created not only for the metal but also for the opaceous ceramic and the dentine and enamel effect veneering ceramics. To provide sufficient strength the metal substructure should normally be between 0.3 and 0.7 mm thick; ideally this should be at least 0.5 mm thick with a greater thickness on the occlusal surface.

The metals

Metal alloys used in dentistry fall into three groups:

- *Gold alloys*. These have been described in the previous chapter.
- *Base metal alloys*. These are usually alloys of nickel and chromium, some with small amounts of other metals (e.g. molybdenum). Some patients may be allergic to nickel and these alloys should be avoided in such patients.
- *Titanium alloys*.

Any of these metals can be used for metal–ceramic restorations, providing their melting point is above the sintering temperature of the ceramic. If the two are too close, thin sections of the metal might melt and the metal framework may warp or sag when it is placed in the ceramic furnace.

The price of metals fluctuates and therefore prescribing patterns often vary depending on the cost of the constituents of these metals. Precious metal alloys have a long clinical track record with good longevity in longitudinal studies. Titanium alloys have recently been used with some short-term clinical success; however, their long-term effectiveness remains unproven.

The metal–ceramic bond

The opaceous ceramic layer masks the colour of the underlying metal and should be 0.2–0.3 mm in thickness. Once the metal substructure has been cast, several processes prepare the metal surface to enable reliable bonding of the ceramic layers:

- Smoothing is completed in one direction, usually using a brown stone.
- The coping is sandblasted (usually with 50 μm aluminium oxide particles) and cleaned using a steam cleaner.
- Formation of an oxide layer. The exact process is often specific to the alloy used due to the varying amounts of base metal alloy present. The oxide layer can usually be formed by placing the substructure back into the furnace to complete a de-gassing (oxidization) cycle.

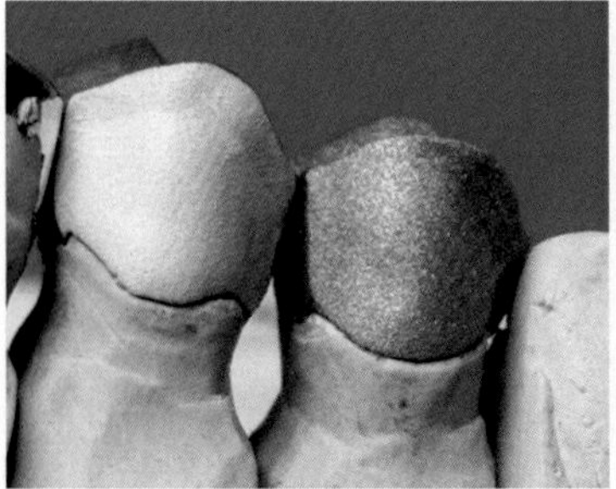

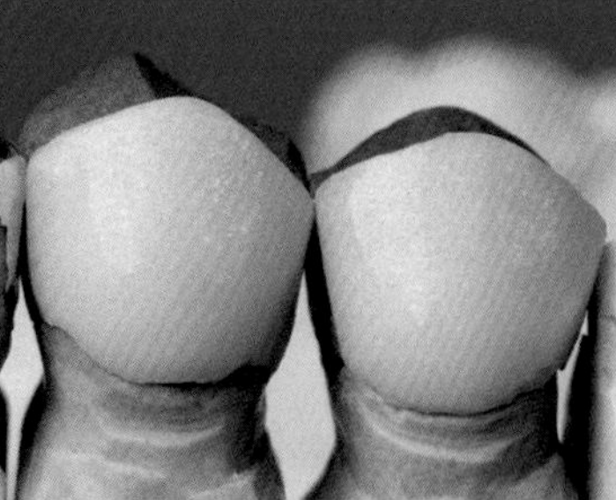

Figure 10.2 The making of a metal–ceramic crown, showing the metal substructure (cast using the lost wax technique) and the opaceous ceramic layer (left) and the veneering ceramic layer in its unglazed state (right).

The mechanism(s) by which the ceramic bonds to the metal coping has been a matter for debate. However, it is now generally accepted that the total bond is created by different mechanisms, with the chemical bonding thought to be most important. The total bond between the ceramic and metal substructure is thought to consist of:

- *Van der Waals forces*. The forces that attract (or repulse) molecules, but where no electrons are exchanged between the molecules (covalent bonding).
- *Mechanical interlocking*. The coping surface will have small irregularities on its surface. These provide a surface in which micromechanical interlocking, or retention can occur. The surface of the metal is often treated (e.g. sandblasted with Al_2O_3) to increase the surface area available for bonding.
- *Compression bonding*. The metal coping should expand slightly more than the overlying ceramic when heated to place the ceramic interface under compression when cooled down. In addition, the ceramic will shrink more than the metal once sintered and cooled, thereby allowing the ceramic to 'wrap-round' the metal coping.
- *Chemical bonding*. Thought to be created by the partial dissolution of the porcelain at the metal–ceramic interface causing saturation of the porcelain with metal oxides and the subsequent intimate atomic contact between the metal and porcelain.

The ceramic

The types of dental porcelain available are discussed in Chapter 11 and are used to provide the aesthetic component of these restorations. Usually glass ceramics are used for metal–ceramic restorations; these ceramics must be thermally compatible with the specific alloy being used. The difference in coefficient of thermal expansion between the ceramic and metal is important; if the difference is too great, stresses will be introduced into the ceramic, leading to crazing, cracking and ceramic fracture. Ideally, the coefficient of thermal expansion of the metal should be slightly higher than that of the ceramic (see compression bonding above). The thickness of the veneering ceramic should allow the dental technician to match the colour of the restoration to the desired shade (Figure 10.4). However, it should not be more than about 1 mm thick as the ceramic has a relatively low flexural strength and may fracture if not adequately supported by the metal framework, although newer ceramics have improved physical properties.

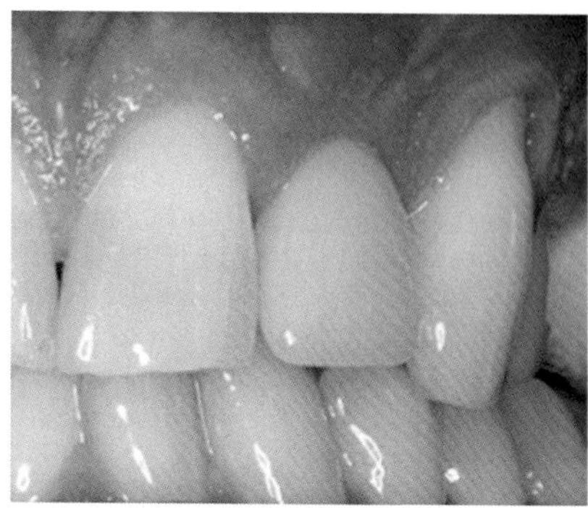

Figure 10.4 Shade match of a metal–ceramic restoration placed on the upper left lateral incisor.

Advantages of metal–ceramic full coverage crowns

- *Strength*. Laboratory studies have shown metal–ceramic restorations to be stronger than conventional all-ceramic restorations. However, it must be borne in mind that bespoke all-ceramic crown materials (e.g. zirconia-based restorations) have improved physical properties compared to the conventional porcelains.
- *Fit*. Different materials produce crowns with different marginal gaps. In laboratory studies, high gold alloys often produce restorations with the smallest gaps.
- *Metal lingual and occlusal surfaces*. This reduces the amount of tooth preparation required. It is important, where possible, that occlusal surfaces are covered in metal only, not only to reduce the amount of tooth reduction required but also to reduce the potential adverse effects of having a ceramic occlusal surface: ceramic that has not been adequately polished or glazed, or subsequently been ground/worn, has been shown to accelerate the wear of the dentition opposing the ceramic. Additionally, increased plaque accumulation and a reduction in the strength of the restoration have been found following wear/grinding of the ceramic. For some patients the appearance of a metal occlusal surface may be unacceptable; for example, a lower premolar crown may be very visible and a pragmatic approach is required provided the patient is fully informed of the potential pitfalls. Metal occlusal surfaces are generally better accepted in the maxilla than the mandible where they tend to be visible.

Disadvantages of metal–ceramic full coverage crowns

- *Extensive tooth preparation*. All full coverage preparations and their restorations have the potential to be the final insult to a stressed pulp, resulting in loss of vitality. The rate at which this occurs is a matter for debate (see Chapter 3). Systematic reviews of the literature have demonstrated the single crowns have a lower incidence of pulp necrosis than fixed bridgework. It must be stressed that many of these teeth may have become non-vital without crown preparation due to the various carious and restorative insults over a prolonged number of years. It has been estimated that an anterior metal–ceramic crown preparation removes 72% of the remaining tooth volume by weight (Edelhoff & Sorensen, 2002).

- *Fit.* Metal–ceramic restorations tend to have larger marginal gaps when compared to all-metal crowns. These gaps are related to the finish line configuration and internal line angles. However, the clinical significance of these gaps in relation to caries, periodontal disease and sensitivity has never been established. However, good clinical practice is to make the marginal gap as small as possible to eliminate any potential adverse effects.
- *Aesthetics.* If a metal collar has been used, the metal substructure may be obvious at the cervical margin, either immediately or over time (Figure 10.5A). The metal and opaque ceramic layer may make it difficult to attain the translucency of natural teeth (Figure 10.5B). In addition, the value (brightness) of these restorations is often higher than that of natural teeth, reducing their aesthetic integration (Figure 10.5C).
- *Cost.* In addition to clinical time, the cost both in terms of the monetary value of the metal alloys and ceramics and the technical time (waxing-up, casting and surface treatment of a metal substructure, in addition to ceramic build-up and finishing of the ceramic layers) is considerable for these restorations.
- *Substructure design.* The metal substructure has to be designed to support the veneering ceramic, otherwise the ceramic may fracture (Figure 10.5D).
- *Strength.* Due to their high strength the remaining coronal tooth structure may fracture before the restoration following direct trauma.

PATIENT CONSENT

The longevity and possible complications associated with full coverage restorations need to be discussed together with possible alternatives (partial coverage crowns, bonded direct restorations). Ideally metal–ceramic crowns should be prescribed with metal occlusal and lingual/palatal

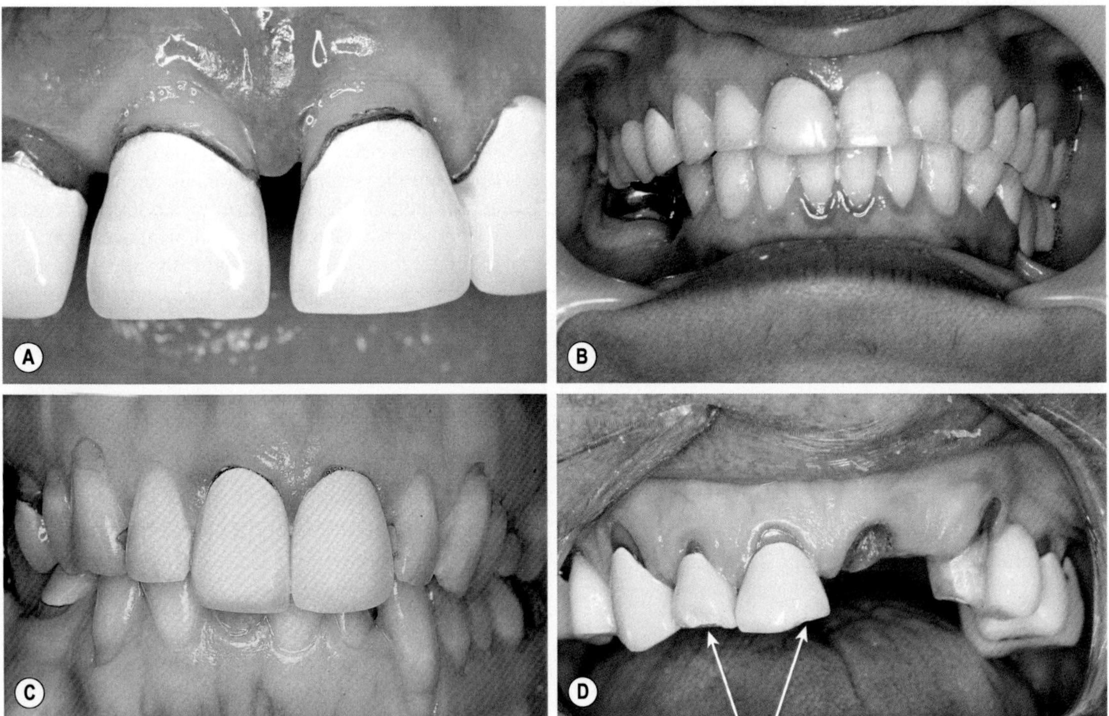

Figure 10.5 Problems of metal–ceramic restorations. **A** Metal margin exposure and discolouration. **B** Poor translucency, shape and shade of metal–ceramic crown on the upper right central incisor. **C** High value (brightness) of metal–ceramic restorations on the central incisors. **D** Ceramic fracture due to increased occlusal forces (bruxism) and incorrect metal coping design.

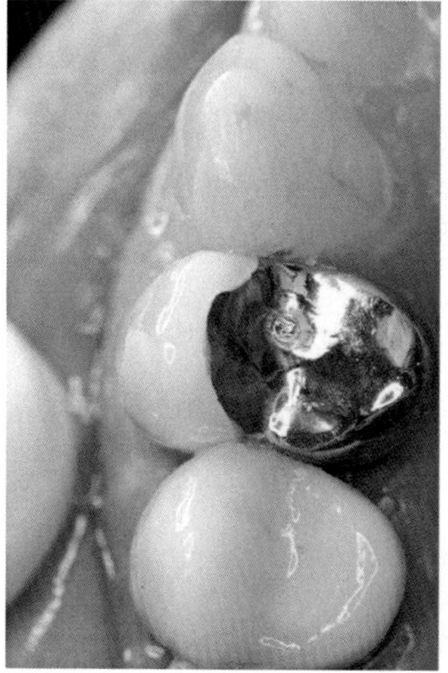
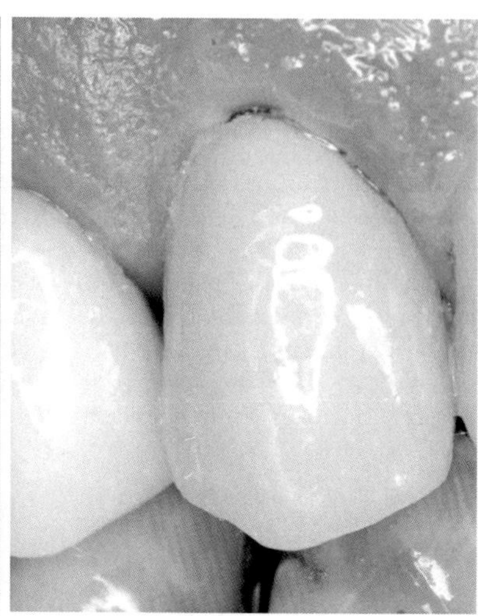

Figure 10.6 Metal–ceramic full coverage crown. The occlusal view demonstrating metal occlusal surface with small ceramic overlay for aesthetic reasons (left) and buccal view showing buccal ceramic facing prior to excess cement removal (right).

surfaces (Figure 10.6) for reasons outlined earlier in this chapter. Patients should be informed of this and the fact that they contain a metal alloy as part of the consent process. If a patient wishes a full coverage crown to be wholly tooth coloured or metal-free, then the advantages and disadvantages of all-ceramic crowns should also be addressed (see Chapter 11).

GENERAL PRINCIPLES OF TOOTH PREPARATION

Many of the general principles underlying the preparation of posterior teeth for metal–ceramic crown preparations are similar to those for full coverage gold (metal) crowns. The salient details that are common will be reiterated in this chapter to avoid excessive cross-referencing and to enable this chapter to be read independently; emphasis will be placed where they differ. Preparation of anterior teeth for metal–ceramic crowns is slightly different and this will be described separately in this chapter.

The burs used for a metal–ceramic crown preparation are the same as those used for any other crown and bridge preparation (see standard bur kit, Figure 8.3, Chapter 8). Ideally a preoperative matrix of the tooth to be prepared should be made. This matrix can be made either from a diagnostic wax-up or from the tooth once the core has been built up to the correct anatomical contours (Figure 10.7). It should be noted that the amount of tooth reduction is not necessarily the same as the clearance that may be required. For example, if the incisal length of a maxillary central incisor is shorter than the contralateral tooth, less tooth reduction will be required than if it was the same length as the contralateral tooth to achieve the desired 1.5–2 mm of clearance incisally.

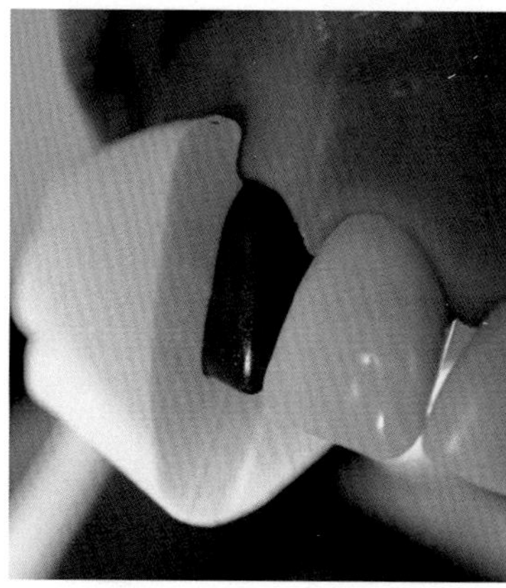

Figure 10.7 Putty matrix adapted to the teeth by hand and sectioned with a scalpel blade (out of the mouth) midway over the tooth to be prepared. This can be reinserted intermittently throughout the tooth preparation to assess the amount of tooth reduction (see Figure 10.17B).

Occlusal reduction

Depth grooves are used by many clinicians to guide the amount of reduction where the original contours of the tooth and core are correct. As with all depth cuts, care must be taken when removing the 'islands' of tooth tissue between the depth cuts to ensure that the bur does not 'bounce' from one groove to another, resulting in excessive tooth substance removal at the base of each groove and possibly inadequate reduction at their peaks, leaving a rippled finish. It can be advantageous to remove the islands of tooth tissue between the grooves with the bur held at an oblique angle to the grooves (see Figure 8.8, Chapter 8).

Axial reduction, retention and resistance form

Reduction of the axial walls should ensure appropriate clearance for the restoration. There is often a temptation to tip the bur away from the long axis of the tooth to gain the ideal finish line and depth cervically; however, this often leads to an undercut being formed and insufficient tooth reduction in more coronal areas. The overall preparation configuration must be considered and will vary between clinicians and in different areas in the mouth. It is important to consider retention form and resistance form as for the full gold crown preparation (see Chapter 8).

Cervical finishing lines

The gingival contour of a natural tooth is not flat but scalloped in its horizontal orientation and therefore a crown preparation should follow this contour. The amount of scallop depends upon the gingival biotype (thin, type I biotypes have a more pronounced scallop) and other factors such as previous subgingival restorations. The finish line almost without exception should finish on natural tooth throughout its circumference, ideally with a 2 mm collar of dentine being present to provide the ferrule effect. A chamfer finishing line should be present on the palatal/lingual aspects of a preparation whilst the labial/buccal aspects should be a rounded shoulder.

Finishing of preparations

When completed, the preparation should not have sharp angles or ridges present at internal line angles or at the preparation margin. A fine-grit, tapered diamond bur or a tungsten–carbide finishing bur may be used to smooth these irregularities.

POSTERIOR METAL–CERAMIC FULL COVERAGE CROWN

The general principles of tooth preparation for a metal–ceramic crown have been outlined in the preceding section; however, this section gives a step-by-step guide to the preparation of a posterior tooth. The subsequent section will deal with anterior teeth.

The preparation should combine the relevant aspects of a full gold crown preparation for the lingual and occlusal surfaces with those of a metal–ceramic crown preparation for the buccal surfaces and buccal cusps. The sequence of tooth preparation is decided by each individual; however, the authors recommend the following.

Occlusal preparation

The occlusal reduction is carried out in a similar manner to that of a full coverage gold crown. It is commenced by making depth-orientation grooves using a parallel-sided bur to guide the depth of the grooves, ensuring that the cuspal inclines are followed. The amount of reduction depends on several factors:

- Where ceramic coverage is required for aesthetic reasons there should be 1.5–2 mm of reduction to provide clearance for an adequate bulk of both metal and ceramic. In most situations the buccal cusps of both maxillary and mandibular teeth require this reduction. Where metal-only occlusal coverage is planned, a reduction of 0.5–1 mm is required.
- The concept of the functional cusp and increased occlusal forces is viewed by some to need greater tooth preparation to provide a larger bulk of material. If metal is covering the functional cusp, then 1.5 mm of reduction is required whereas 2 mm is needed if the functional cusp is covered by both metal and ceramic. In a Class I occlusion, the functional cusps are the palatal cusps of maxillary teeth and buccal cusps of mandibular teeth. This is reversed if there is a cross-bite. The rationale for the functional cusp bevel has never been proven but is supported by some clinicians. It is unlikely ever to be proven through clinical research and so remains a contentious issue. When the tooth reduction needed for a functional cusp bevel may weaken or reduce retention, careful thought should be given to its incorporation into a preparation.

The preparation of the occlusal surface is continued by removing tooth tissue between the depth grooves, again ensuring that the outline shape of the occlusal surface is followed. The occlusal surface should then be smoothed to remove any sharp angles and depressions. It is helpful to prepare one half of the occlusal surface first and compare the prepared half to the other to aid the clinician in the assessment of the correct amount of clearance. Alternatively, a sectioned matrix can be used to verify the amount of clearance. The stages of occlusal reduction are shown in Figure 10.8.

Buccal preparation

Buccal reduction should be completed after placement of depth grooves in at least two planes to mirror the buccal curvature of the tooth (Figure 10.9). Grooves should be placed to a depth of at least 1.5 mm to create clearance for both the metal and ceramic. The finish line should ideally be supragingival and be a rounded shoulder or a deep chamfer. For aesthetic reasons, however, the finish line is often placed just into the gingival sulcus.

A round-ended bur is often used to reduce the buccal surfaces and create the approximate finish line configuration

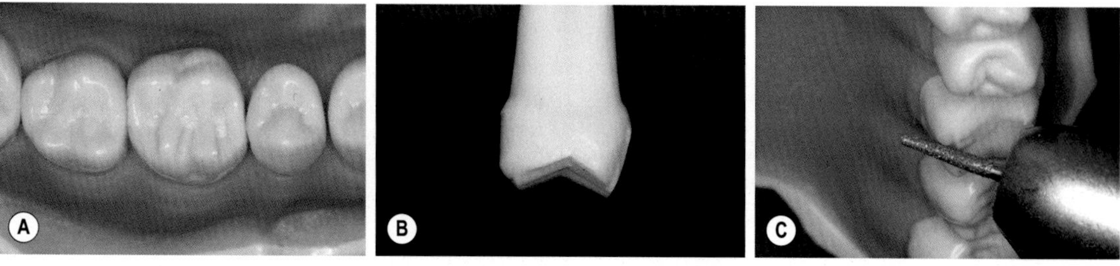

Figure 10.8 Occlusal reduction for a metal–ceramic crown. **A** Occlusal depth grooves. **B** Occlusal reduction. **C** Functional cusp reduction and bevel.

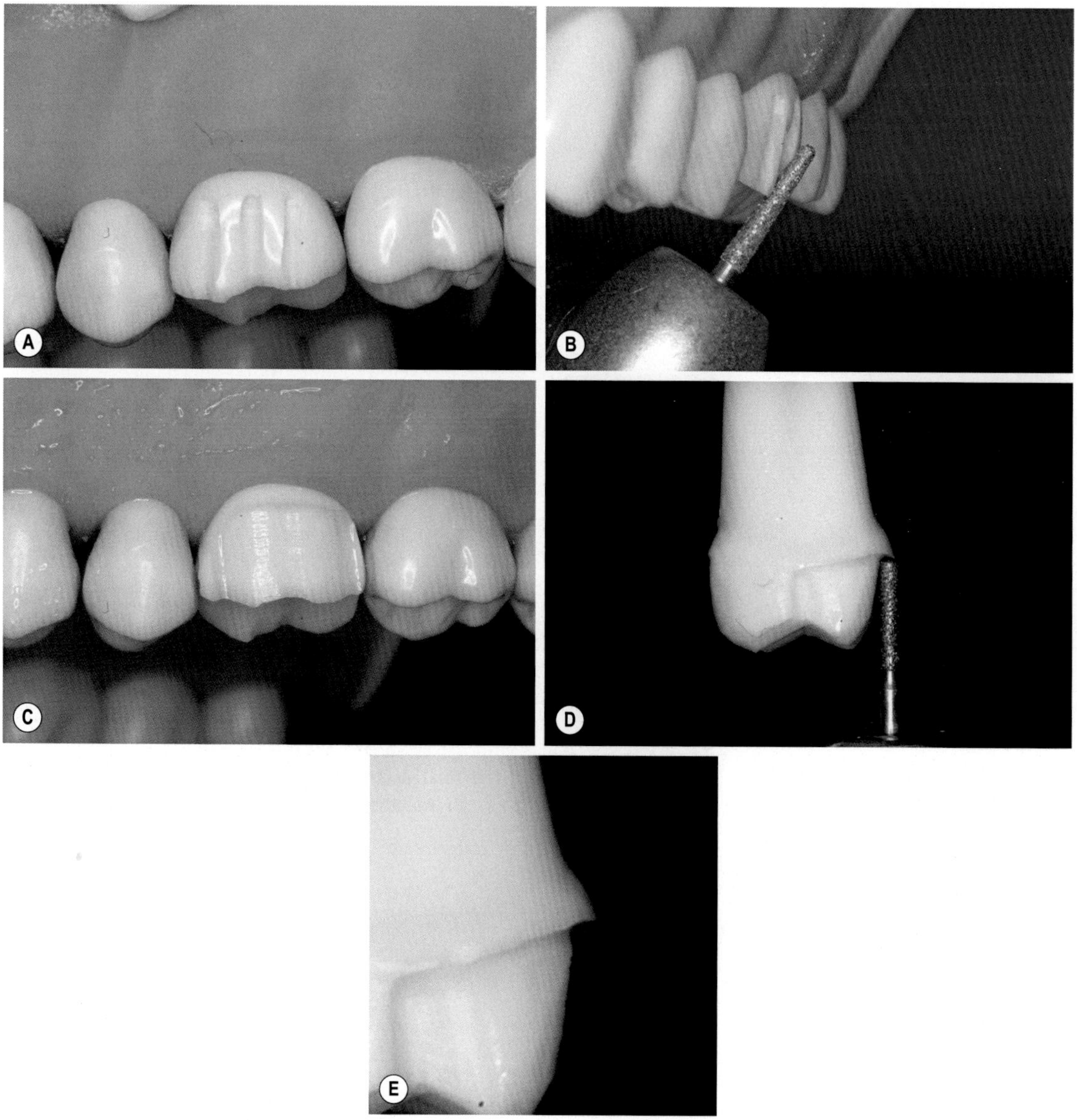

Figure 10.9 Buccal preparation for a metal–ceramic crown. **A** Buccal depth grooves parallel to the long axis of the tooth. Remember that at least two planes of buccal reduction are required. **B** Second plane of buccal reduction. **C** Buccal reduction with a supragingival finish line. **D** A round-ended bur may create a lip of enamel; observe the gap under the flat-ended bur. **E** A flat-ended bur allows for easier preparation of the desired finish line.

(Figure 10.9C). It should be noted that it is difficult to create a rounded shoulder finish line using a chamfer/torpedo bur alone as their shape will often leave a lip of enamel/dentine (Figure 10.9D). This lip is prone to fracture either intraorally or on the laboratory model, both of which will provide a restoration with an unacceptable marginal fit. A flat-ended bur should be used to finalize the desired margin (Figure 10.9E).

Lingual preparation

The lingual reduction is completed in the same manner as described for the full gold crown (Chapter 8). This provides a chamfer margin of approximately 0.5 mm depth. A chamfer or round-ended tapered bur is used to half its width, thus creating a margin with the correct shape and amount of reduction (Figure 10.10).

Approximal preparation

The buccal and lingual margins need to be joined in the approximal areas. Contact points are completely removed, creating separation of the teeth. It is important that adjacent teeth are not damaged at this stage and therefore a narrow, tapered bur is used in a bucco-lingual direction. The bulbosity of some teeth can be used to reduce the chance of damaging the adjacent teeth whilst maintaining the taper and finish line of the preparation (Figure 10.11). When separation is complete a chamfer/round-ended tapered bur is used to complete the approximal preparation in a similar fashion to that described for the lingual chamfer.

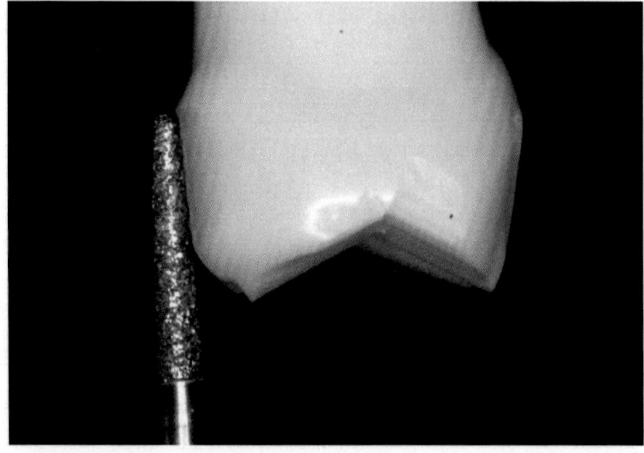

Figure 10.10 Lingual reduction using half the width of a round-ended tapered bur.

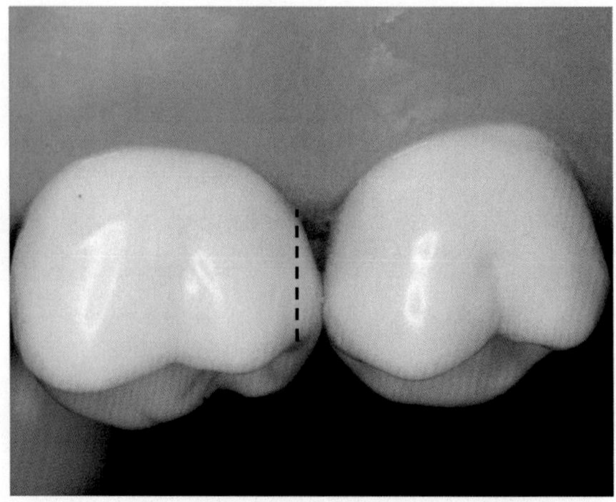

Figure 10.11 Approximal reduction. The risk of damage to adjacent teeth is aided by tooth bulbosity, the dotted line illustrates the intended wall after preparation.

There is debate as to the configuration of the approximal area. Some authors advocate a 'blending' of the buccal rounded shoulder/heavy chamfer to the smaller lingual chamfer, whilst others state a 'wing' should be present to demarcate the two marginal configurations (Figure 10.12). A 'wing' provides several advantages: firstly, it affords additional retention and resistance form that are often lacking in molar crown preparations, and secondly, the 'wing' indicates to the laboratory technician where the porcelain margin should finish. Authors that advocate the proximal 'wing' also state that this preserves tooth structure, but Figure 10.12 shows that this is minimal.

The final decision lies with the treating clinician; however, one must ensure that blending does not start too far

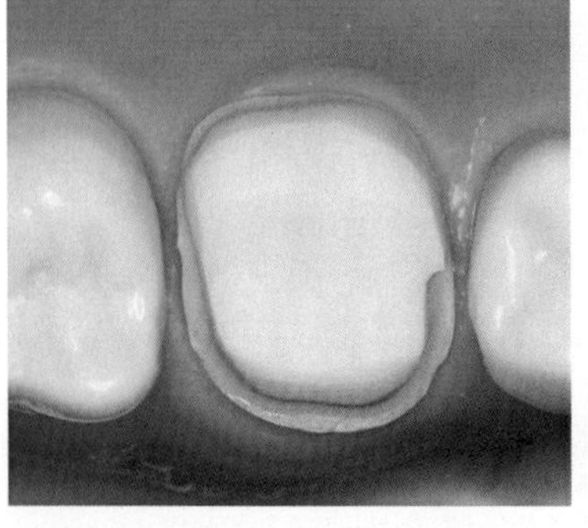

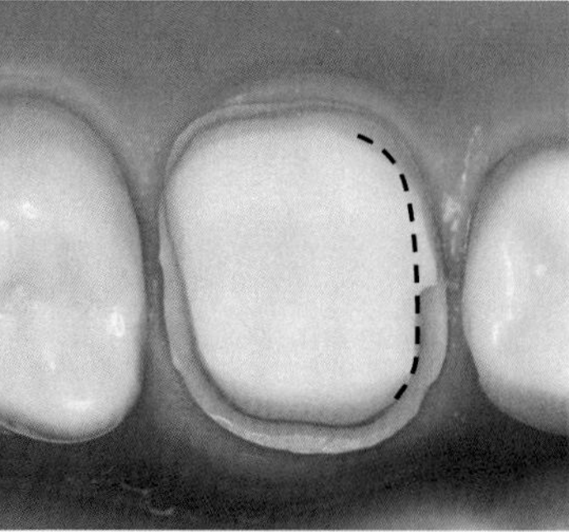

Figure 10.12 Approximal configuration. Distal wall: the buccal shoulder is 'blended' into the palatal chamfer, whereas the mesial wall has a 'wing' (left). An outline of the 'blended' margin is superimposed on the 'wing' (right), giving an indication of the relative amounts of tooth removal. It must be emphasized that this blended margin should provide the technician with sufficient space to provide an aesthetic restoration.

buccally as this will reduce the amount of clearance for metal and ceramic and may result in compromised aesthetics. Figure 10.13 demonstrates a crown with poor aesthetics on the mesio-buccal aspect of the second premolar tooth due to inadequate reduction; it is unknown what marginal configuration was present in this area.

Prior to making the provisional restoration and impression, the geometry of the preparation should be reassessed (Figure 10.14). Figure 10.15 shows typical metal–ceramic preparations on posterior teeth, with blended approximal margins.

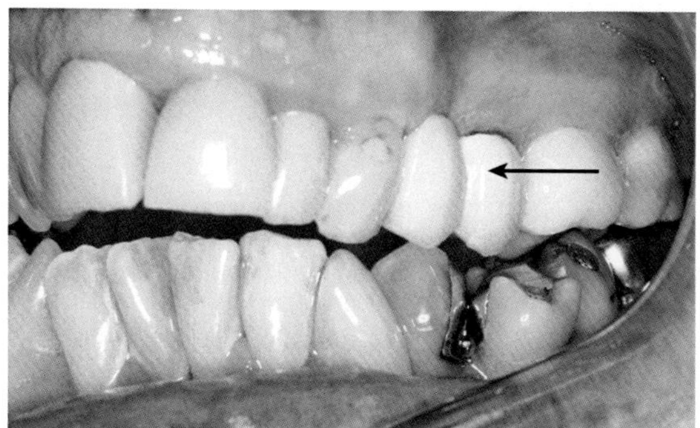

Figure 10.13 Inadequate reduction of the mesio-buccal aspect (arrowed) of the upper left second premolar tooth resulting in poor aesthetics due to the opaceous porcelain not being adequately masked by the veneering ceramic.

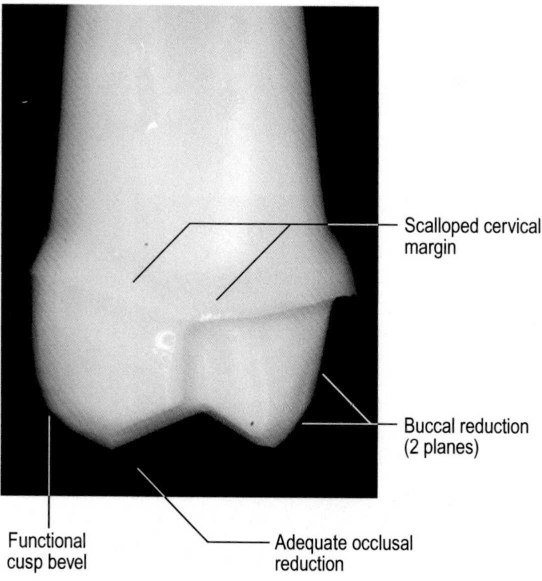

Figure 10.14 Overview of completed metal–ceramic preparation for posterior teeth.

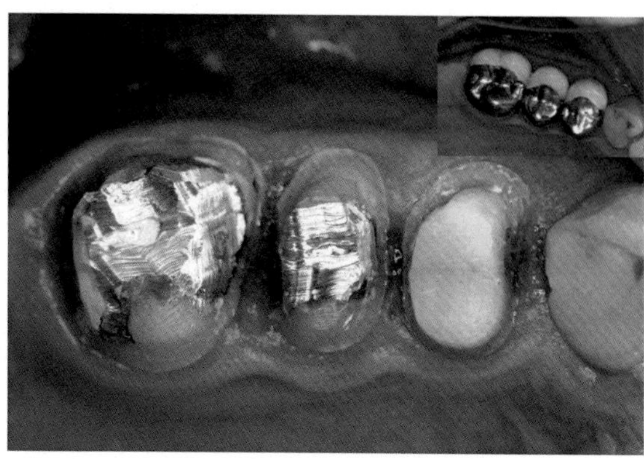

Figure 10.15 Typical metal–ceramic preparations of the posterior teeth in the upper right quadrant. Inset: the metal–ceramic crowns in situ.

ANTERIOR METAL–CERAMIC FULL COVERAGE CROWN

Incisal preparation

The incisal reduction is commenced by making depth-orientation grooves (Figure 10.16A) using a parallel-sided bur to guide the depth of the grooves. Reduction of the incisal edge should result in the tooth height being reduced by approximately 2 mm. The grooves should then be connected to each other (Figure 10.16B) to produce a uniform reduction of the incisal edge. The preoperative matrix can also verify the incisal clearance.

Labial preparation

The labial reduction should be in two or three different planes to allow the technician to create a restoration with the ideal emergence profile, contour and shape, and to match the selected shade. Depth orientation grooves and a matrix can be used to guide the clinician in the amount and location of reduction. These should result in a uniform reduction of the labial surface in the magnitude of around 1.5 mm (Figure 10.17).

Palatal/lingual preparation

The palatal reduction of anterior teeth is in two distinct stages:

- Palatal axial or palatal collar reduction (Figure 10.18A)
- Palatal cingulum reduction (Figure 10.18B).

These provide a uniform palatal reduction with 0.5 - 1 mm of occlusal clearance and a chamfer margin. The palatal

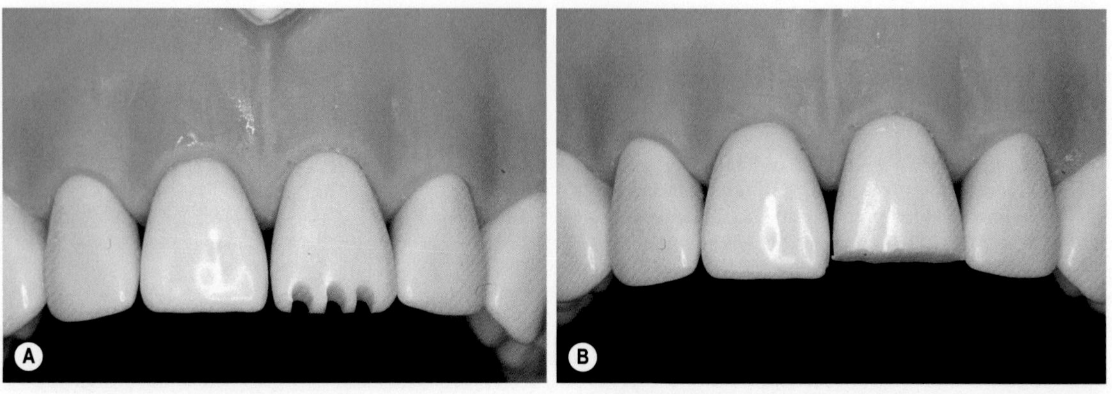

Figure 10.16 Incisal preparation for a metal–ceramic crown. **A** Depth grooves on incisal edge. **B** Uniform reduction of incisal edge.

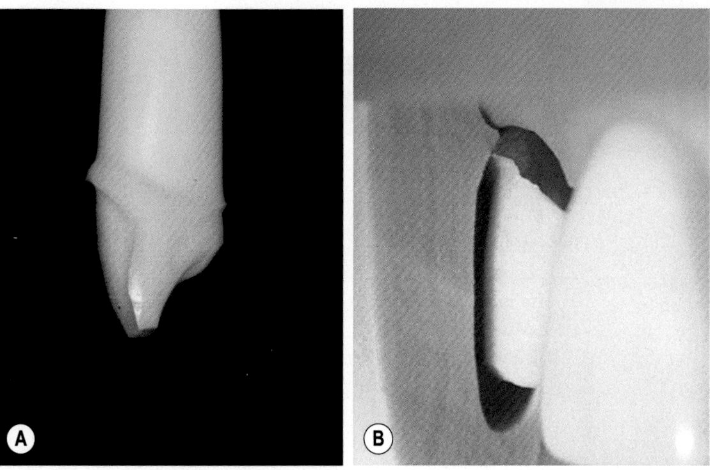

Figure 10.17 Labial preparation for a metal–ceramic crown. **A** Note uniform reduction of labial face in at least two planes. **B** Reinsertion of the putty matrix seen in Figure 10.7 shows adequate and uniform reduction.

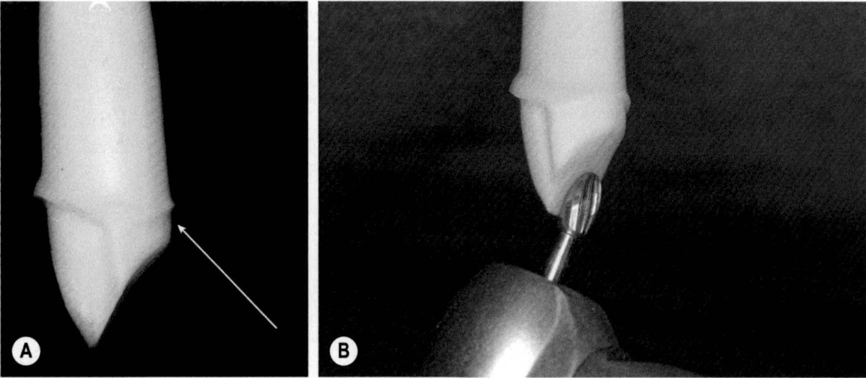

Figure 10.18 Palatal preparation for a metal–ceramic crown. **A** Stage 1: the cervical, palatal collar reduction using a round-ended tapered bur. **B** Stage 2: cingulum reduction using a round or rugby ball-shaped bur.

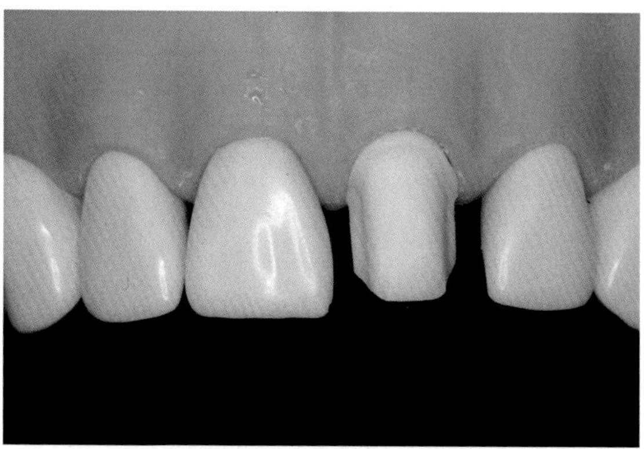

Figure 10.19 Approximal preparation with a 'wing' demarcating the transition from labial shoulder to palatal chamfer.

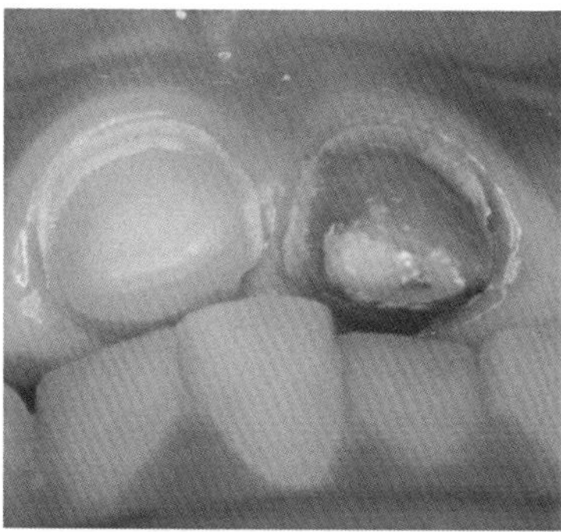

Figure 10.20 Two typical metal–ceramic crown preparations on anterior teeth. Note the labial shoulder, palatal chamfer and adequate occlusal clearance.

axial reduction should be as parallel to the cervico-labial reduction as possible to give the preparation good retention and resistance form.

Approximal preparation

The buccal and lingual margins again need to be joined in the approximal areas. The configuration of this junction has been discussed previously for the posterior preparation and these principles apply to anterior preparations (Figure 10.19). Figure 10.20 shows typical anterior metal–ceramic crown preparations.

LABORATORY PRESCRIPTION

Attention has been drawn to the fact that the quality of laboratory prescriptions is generally poor (Lynch & Allan, 2005). The basic prescription should include patient details, that a metal–ceramic crown is required, and the shade and characterization. When starting in a new practice and not knowing the technician, the importance of an accurate prescription is essential; however, as experience between the clinician and the technician improves, and each understands the other's needs, the detail of the prescription may change. Also, many technicians offer a shade-taking service which also allows them to see the tooth and so understand the situation better. In addition to the basic prescription details outlined, other pieces of information are needed to allow the technician to fabricate the desired metal–ceramic restoration.

Materials

- *Metal composition*. The classification of metal to be used has to be prescribed (precious, semi-precious, non-precious or titanium).
- *Ceramic type*. The ceramic types available are described elsewhere (feldspathic, pressable, etc.). The majority of metal–ceramic restorations utilize feldspathic porcelains, with some brands being considered as more aesthetic.

Design

- *Contact points*. The size and location of the contact point has to be considered. Contact points, from an aesthetic point of view, are found in pairs and ideally should show symmetry (e.g. the mesial surface of both upper lateral incisors). The exceptions are the contact between the upper and lower central incisor pairs. If one contact point of the pair is long and wide, the contralateral prosthetic contact should match. In the absence of a dental papilla, a long contact point may be used to improve the aesthetics by eliminating a black triangle; however, this can often be at the detriment of the emergence profile.
- *Gingival margin*. The type of gingival margin of metal–ceramic restorations has to be prescribed. It is usually either a porcelain butt finish or a metal collar.
- *Metal coverage*. The surfaces to be covered by ceramic should be described. Usual practice is to fabricate the occlusal and palatal/lingual surfaces in metal.
- *Occlusal factors*. Single crowns should provide even and holding occlusal contacts in the intercuspal position. Unless the crown is involved in guidance in lateral excursion (e.g. a premolar in group function), the posterior single crown should usually be free of contacts on both the working and non-working side in lateral excursions. If a custom incisal guidance table is not being used, then an anterior single crown should follow the anatomical contours of adjacent teeth to prevent it from providing an occlusal interference.

SUMMARY

Metal–ceramic crowns are an essential part of the dentist's armamentarium, allowing provision of high-strength aesthetic restorations with a history of longevity. The preparation of a tooth for such a restoration is, however, exacting, to allow the technician scope to provide a restoration with a good appearance and fit. This requires a very skilled technician and good three-way communication between the patient, clinician and technician.

FURTHER READING

Further details relating to the fabrication and technical aspects of metal–ceramic restorations can be found in W.P. Naylor's text, *Introduction to Metal–ceramic Technology* (Quintessence Publishing Company (Chicago), 1992) and J.W. McLean's book, *The Science and Art of Dental Ceramics* (Quintessence Publishing Company (Chicago), 1979).

Edelhoff, D., Sorensen, J.A., 2002. Tooth structure removal associated with various preparation designs for anterior teeth. J. Prosthet. Dent. 87, 503–509.

Lynch, C.D., Allen, P.F., 2005. Quality of communication between dental practitioners and dental technicians for fixed prosthodontics in Ireland. J. Oral Rehabil. 32, 901–905.

Chapter 11

All-ceramic crowns

Andrew Hall, Graham Chadwick

CHAPTER CONTENTS

INTRODUCTION

All-ceramic crowns developed from a desire to restore heavily broken down anterior teeth to a form and function that was aesthetically pleasing. Prior to the development of contemporary tooth-coloured direct restorative materials, and in place of gold or amalgam restorations, anterior teeth could be restored using all-ceramic restorations.

THE PORCELAIN JACKET CROWN

In initial attempts to make all-ceramic restorations, anterior crowns used porcelain with a relatively high concentration of feldspar (a mixture of sodium and potassium aluminosilicates). Although this so-called feldspathic porcelain produced acceptable aesthetic results, the slow propagation of cracks between flaws within the porcelain during function, and also the phenomenon of stress corrosion that arises as a result of hydrolysis of the Si-O groups of the material under favourable alkaline environmental conditions, meant that such crowns could be used only to restore anterior teeth subject to minimal occlusal loading.

Use of this type of crown elsewhere in the mouth simply resulted in premature crown fracture. As a consequence, a considerable amount of research and development has since been undertaken to improve the reliability of dental porcelain to render it suitable for use in anterior and posterior dental restorations. This has centred upon methods of restoration manufacture and the chemical composition of the porcelain. These frequently linked developments are reviewed throughout this chapter and will cover aspects of sintering, casting, hot pressing and injection moulding, and milling.

The addition of alumina to feldspathic porcelain was reported by McLean and Hughes in 1965 and resulted in much stronger dental porcelain which was more resistant to crack propagation. However, aluminous porcelain does not have the same aesthetic qualities as feldspathic porcelain; it does not have the same translucency and cannot reproduce the life-like illusion of a natural tooth crown. Instead, aluminous porcelain can be used to form a coping over the crown preparation (Figure 11.1), which is itself covered with more aesthetic feldspathic porcelain. Using this principle, the first widely used all-ceramic

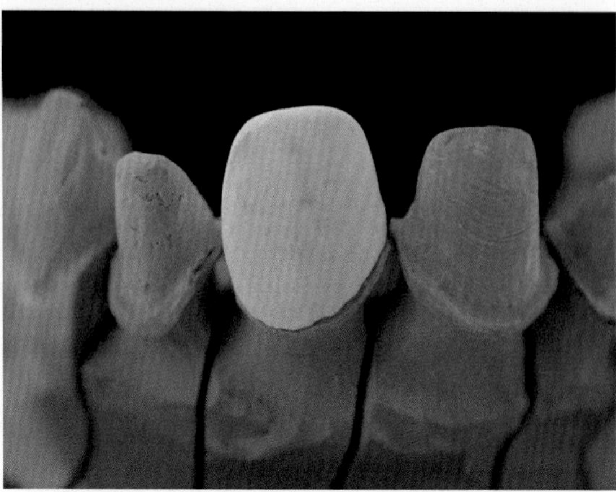

Figure 11.1 Alumina coping to be covered with feldspathic porcelain.

crown was developed and was often referred to as the porcelain jacket crown (PJC). This development increased the strength of the PJC to around 120–150 MPa by reducing the likelihood of crack propagation.

The PJC was widely used to provide an aesthetic restoration for upper anterior teeth. However, it was still not strong enough to resist much occlusal loading without the crown breaking (Figure 11.2). Its use was, therefore, confined mainly to upper incisors, and some premolar teeth in minimal occlusal function. This type of crown is not indicated for molar teeth.

The tooth preparation for and construction of a PJC is described in a stylized diagram in Figure 11.3. The crown preparation requires a shoulder margin all around the gingival aspect of the preparation with an axial reduction of approximately 1.0–1.5 mm. Reduction at the incisal edge is in the order of 1.5–2.0 mm with 1.0–1.5 mm interocclusal clearance required.

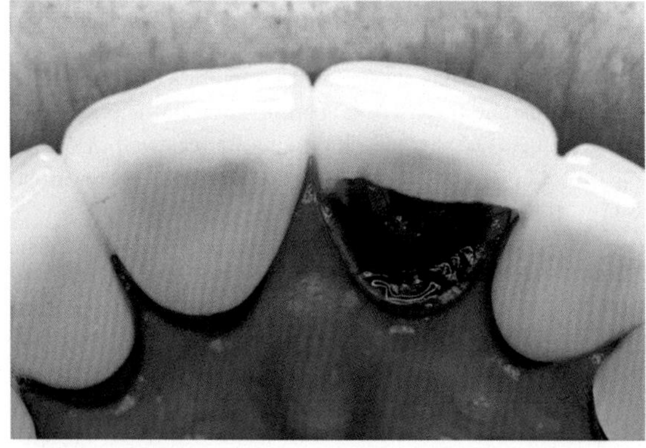

Figure 11.2 Palatal fracture of a porcelain jacket crown (PJC) restoration on the upper left central incisor due to excessive occlusal loading. These teeth were crowned to mask severe tetracycline staining.

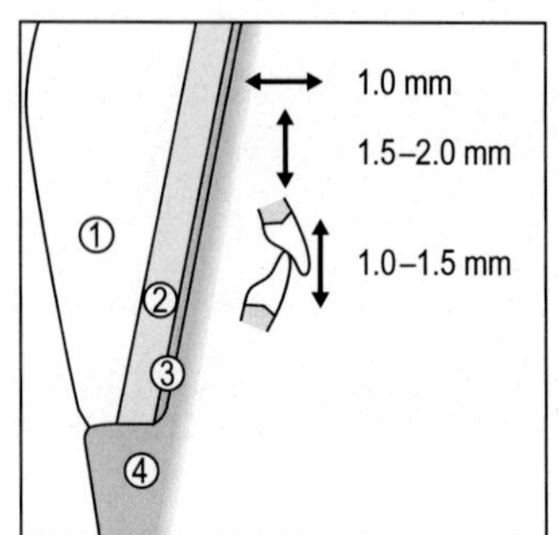

Figure 11.3 Schematic diagram of a porcelain jacket crown: preparation and anatomy.

Fabrication

Traditionally, the impression was cast and a die of the preparation poured using die-stone. A platinum foil matrix was then swaged over the die and an aqueous slurry of aluminous porcelain powder placed over the foil to form the coping. The foil supports the aluminous porcelain slurry in the furnace and may be removed once the crown has been fired and completed. The space left by the platinum foil effectively acts as a die spacer for the luting cement. In order to reduce porosity and shrinkage, firing takes place in a porcelain furnace under vacuum. The process in which the ceramic particles are fused together under heat in this way is called sintering. The aluminous coping is now ready for veneering with feldspathic porcelain which in turn is sintered.

Instead of a stone die model, refractory material may be used which maintains its dimensional stability when subjected to the heat of the porcelain furnace (see Chapter 12 on ceramic veneers). It has been argued that the use of a refractory die results in a more accurate fit of the final restoration to the prepared tooth.

The tooth preparation for the PJC has become a template for modern all-ceramic crowns with one notable exception: the margin has now become a large chamfer or a rounded shoulder. Furthermore, some of the latest all-ceramic crowns now have sufficient strength with an axial tooth reduction of as little as 0.6 mm.

The PJC remained a very popular and widely used restoration for many years. However, there was concern over the bulk of tooth tissue reduction and the inability to withstand occlusal loading. To address these concerns, research concentrated on:

- Decreasing the bulk of tooth tissue reduction required to place an all-ceramic crown
- Development of additional glass ceramic materials and processes by which they can be manipulated
- The use of computer-aided design and computer-aided manufacture (CAD-CAM) and the development of glass ceramic materials with significantly increased strength.

There is now scope to use all-ceramic crowns on any tooth and within increasingly challenging occlusal environments.

DECREASING TOOTH TISSUE REDUCTION FOR AN ALL-CERAMIC CROWN

The dentine-bonded crown

With the advent of adhesively retained porcelain laminate veneers in the 1980s and 1990s, it was a natural progression to extend the preparation to cover the whole surface of the crown, and thus the dentine-bonded crown concept was developed. The strength of this restoration is developed once it is bonded, using a composite resin luting cement, to the underlying tooth structure or composite core. Prior to bonding, the dentine-bonded crown is very fragile and should be treated in the same way as a porcelain laminate veneer.

The use of dentine-bonded crowns is mainly for anterior teeth where occlusal loading is relatively low (Figure 11.4). Such restorations are contraindicated for those patients with an obvious bruxing habit. Application of this type of restoration for premolar and molar teeth, which are normally subject to higher occlusal loading, should be made with caution and after careful examination of the patient's occlusion. Generally, such applications should be avoided. The patient seen in Figure 11.5 has four posterior dentine-bonded crowns chosen for optimum aesthetics as the patient was young. No signs or symptoms of bruxism were noted and canine guidance was achieved; however, despite this, the lower crown fractured and had to be replaced with a metal–ceramic crown.

Tooth preparation for dentine-bonded crowns is kept as minimal as possible and less than that required for metal–ceramic crowns or a traditional PJC. The preparation, in some instances, can be confined to enamel. However, the ceramic should be sufficiently thick to mask discoloured teeth prior to cementation. A minimal shoulder or, more often, a minimal chamfer is the restoration margin of choice. All margins should be supragingival wherever possible to avoid the problems of moisture control at cementation. The axial reduction is in the order of 0.5 mm while the occlusal reduction is between 1.0 and 1.5 mm, with at least 1.0 mm reduction in all excursive movements associated with the preparation (Figure 11.6).

In common with other all-ceramic crown preparations, line and point angles should be rounded to avoid stress concentrations within the porcelain. Figures 11.7–11.9 show the tooth preparation that was carried out for the patients seen in Figures 11.4 and 11.5. Marked palatal erosion (Figure 11.7) has led to exposure of the tertiary (reactionary) dentine that has formed. The only preparation carried out palatally is the cervical chamfer; the tooth wear has removed the rest of the palatal tooth tissue (Figure 11.7). Interocclusal clearance has been created following an

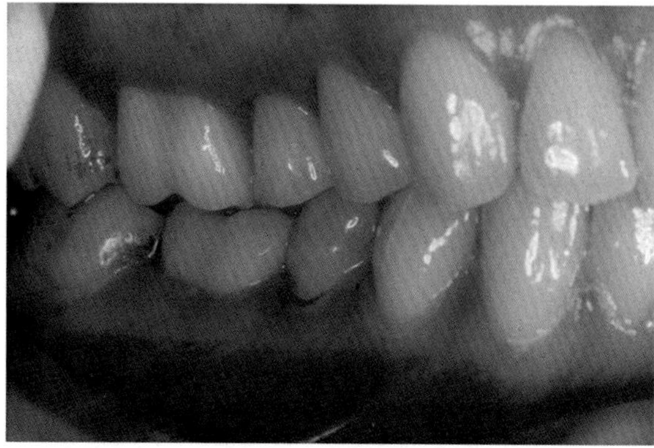

Figure 11.5 Dentine-bonded crowns made from feldspathic porcelain on the upper right premolar and first molar and lower right first molar teeth.

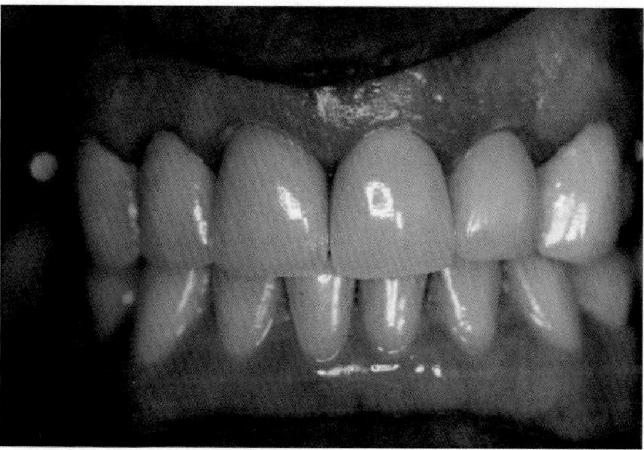

Figure 11.4 Dentine-bonded crowns made from feldspathic porcelain on all six upper anterior teeth.

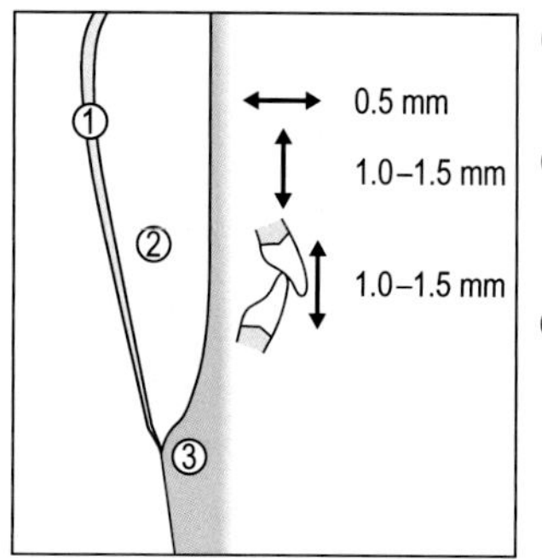

Figure 11.6 Schematic diagram of a dentine-bonded crown: preparation and anatomy.

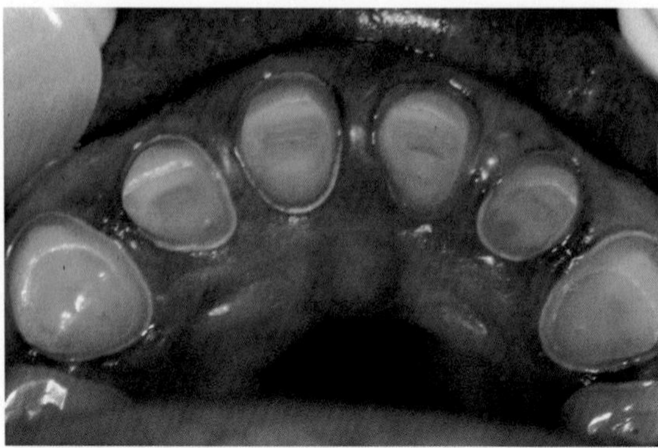

Figure 11.7 Occlusal view of dentine-bonded crown preparations. The majority of palatal tooth removal has been a result of erosion. The completed result is shown in Figure 11.4.

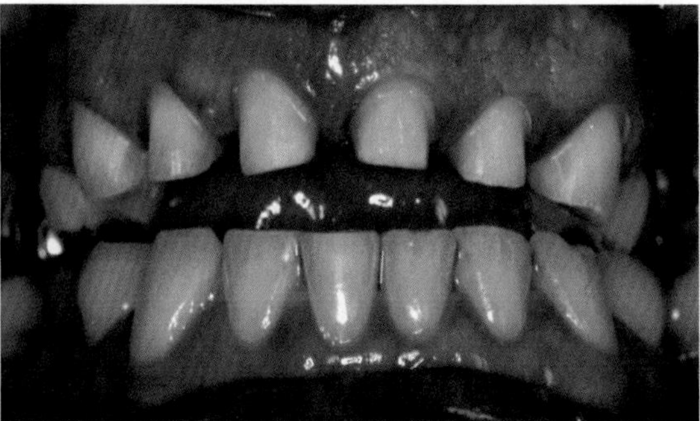

Figure 11.8 Labial view of anterior dentine-bonded crown preparations. The completed case is shown in Figure 11.4.

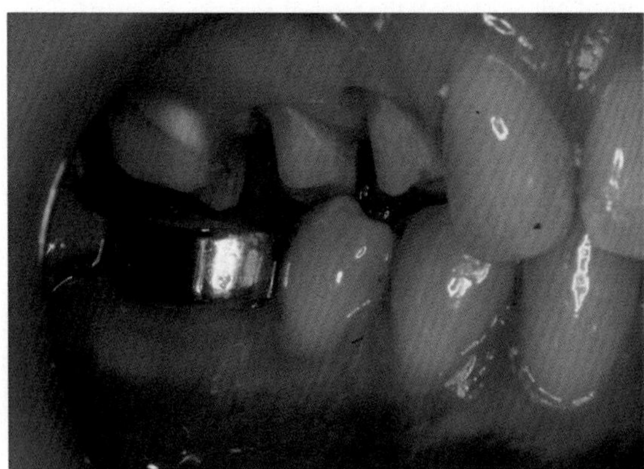

Figure 11.9 Buccal view of dentine-bonded crown preparations for posterior teeth with composite resin core augmentations. The completed restorations are shown in Figure 11.5.

increase in the patient's occlusal vertical dimension by placing gold onlays on some of the posterior teeth (Figure 11.8).

The dentine-bonded crown may be made in a variety of ways using low-fusing feldspathic porcelains, alumina-reinforced porcelains or leucite-reinforced porcelains, all on refractory dies. In addition, castable glass ceramics such as Dicor, as well as hot-press and injection-moulding techniques (e.g. IPS Empress 2), may be used to produce such restorations.

As with a ceramic veneer (see Chapter 12), the fitting surface of a feldspathic porcelain dentine-bonded crown is etched in the laboratory using hydrofluoric acid. Once the fit of the crown has been checked in the mouth, the fitting surface should be cleaned and dried, and a silane coupling agent applied to further enhance adhesion of the resin luting cement. In turn, the tooth preparation is etched, rinsed, dried and bond applied to ensure adhesion of the luting cement to the tooth.

Due to the fragility of this type of restoration when made using feldspathic porcelain, it is recommended that occlusal evaluation and any adjustment be completed once the crown has been cemented. Once cemented, the porcelain is bonded to the tooth structure, each component – crown and core – working synergistically together. The result is a restoration where catastrophic crack propagation and failure is less likely to occur. Because the bonding of this type of restorations is so critical any artificial core material used in conjunction with it must be made of composite (Figure 11.9).

DEVELOPMENT OF ADDITIONAL GLASS CERAMIC MATERIALS AND PROCESSES BY WHICH THEY CAN BE MANIPULATED

The development of glass ceramic materials is summarized in Table 11.1, which has been compiled from manufacturers' data, summarized according to the method of manufacture and the clinical applications of these techniques. Some materials are no longer available (see table for details) but are described here for completeness and because history has a tendency to repeat itself in various guises. Their inclusion also illustrates some of the problems experienced and how they have been overcome.

Castable glass ceramic

The development of a castable glass ceramic meant that the lost wax process could be adapted for use with aesthetic restorations (see Chapter 9 for the lost wax technique). Dicor (Dentsply International) was a 70% tetrasilic fluormica glass within a 30% glass matrix which was cast into the space left after vaporization of a wax

Table 11.1 Clinical applications of porcelain according to manufacturing method of restoration

MANUFACTURING METHOD	AVAILABLE MATERIALS	CLINICAL APPLICATION
Sintering	Feldspathic porcelain, aluminous porcelain	Porcelain jacket crowns, veneers. With appropriate alloy core/framework; dentine-bonded crowns and bridges in both anterior and posterior regions of the mouth
	In-Ceram Alumina (Al_2O_3) (VITA, Zahnfabrik, Germany)	Crowns
	In-Ceram Spinell ($MgAl_2O_4$) (VITA, Zahnfabrik, Germany)	Crowns
	In-Ceram Zirconia (VITA, Zahnfabrik, Germany)	Veneers, crowns and anterior bridges
Casting	Dicor (Dentsply International, USA) (*No longer available*)	Anterior crowns
Hot pressing and injection moulding	IPS Empress (Ivoclar Vivadent, Liechtenstein) (Leucite reinforced glass ceramic)	Anterior onlays and crowns
	IPS Empress 2 (Ivoclar Vivadent, Liechtenstein) (Lithium disilicate glass ceramic)	Anterior and posterior onlays and crowns
	IPS e.max Press (Ivoclar Vivadent, Liechtenstein) (Lithium disilicate glass ceramic)	Anterior to premolar onlays and crowns; anterior 3 unit bridgework
Machining	VITABLOCS Mark II (VITA, Zahnfabrik, Germany) (Feldspathic porcelain)	Crowns, veneers
	VITA TriLuxe Bloc (VITA, Zahnfabrik, Germany) (Feldspathic porcelain)	Anterior crowns, veneers
	In-Ceram Alumina (Al_2O_3) (VITA, Zahnfabrik, Germany)	Crowns
	In-Ceram Spinell ($MgAl_2O_4$) (VITA, Zahnfabrik, Germany)	Crowns
	In-Ceram Zirconia (VITA, Zahnfabrik, Germany)	Posterior crowns
	Lava (3M ESPE, USA) (Partially stabilized zirconia)	Crowns, bridgework
	Procera (Nobel Biocare AB, Sweden) (Partially stabilized zirconia)	Implant abutments
	Procera (Al_2O_3) (Nobel Biocare AB, Sweden)	Implant abutments

pattern invested in a phosphate-bonded investment material. The crown was broken out of the investment and fitted back onto the die. Application of a surface tint and re-firing was used to customize the crown's appearance and ensure the correct shade (Figure 11.10). This type of restoration was made on a conventional all-ceramic crown preparation (see Figure 11.6) but the wearing and chipping of the surface characterization meant that the aesthetics of this restoration could not be assured long term.

Hot-pressed and injection-moulded ceramics

The lost wax technique was also applied to hot-pressed and injection-moulded ceramics. Ivoclar produced a heat-pressed leucite-reinforced glass ceramic to develop the IPS Empress crown (Figure 11.11). Further developments using lithium disilicate glass ceramics gave rise to the IPS Empress 2 and the IPS e.max crowns demonstrating increased strength, thus extending the application of

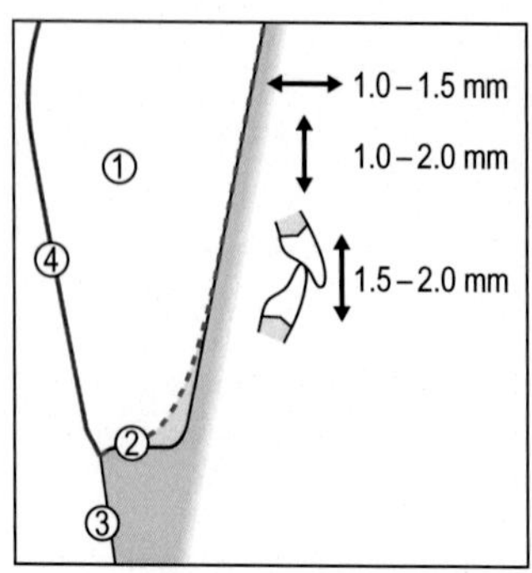

Figure 11.10 Schematic diagram of castable glass, hot-pressed or injection-moulded ceramic crown.

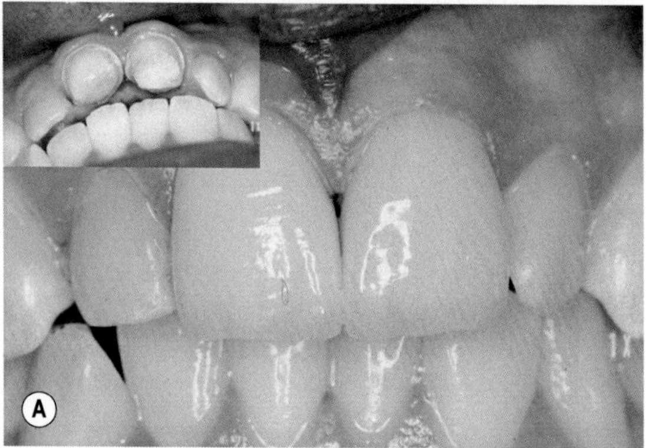

Figure 11.11A Empress crowns placed on upper central incisor teeth. The tooth preparation can be seen inset.

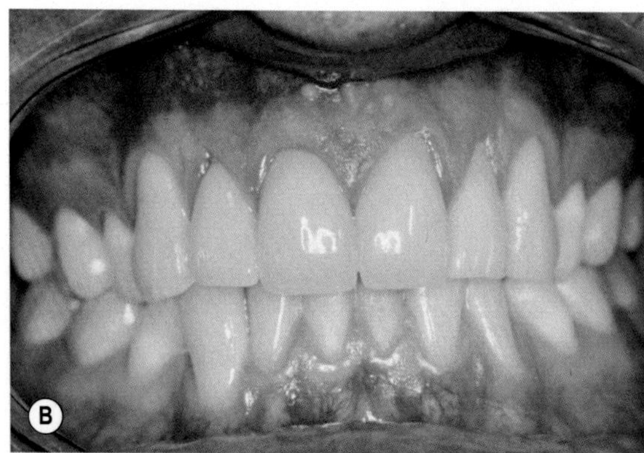

Figure 11.11B Empress crowns placed on the central incisors and upper right lateral incisor. Excellent aesthetic results are possible with such restorations.

such crowns to premolar teeth. In common with cast glass, the surface is characterized with tints although the basic shade has been developed in hot-pressed and injection-moulded glass (see Figure 11.10).

Development of a generic all-ceramic crown preparation

With the further development of alternative materials for all-ceramic crowns, there was increasing demand to develop such restorations for use with posterior teeth. Accordingly, preparations for posterior all-ceramic crowns were developed and generically comprise between 1.0 and 1.5 mm axial reduction, 1.0–2.0 mm incisal edge or occlusal reduction, and between 1.5 and 2.0 mm interocclusal clearance for both anterior and posterior teeth. Such a preparation is outlined diagrammatically in Figure 11.12. Generally, advances in materials have resulted in more minimal tooth reduction and the development of a chamfer margin in preference to a rounded shoulder.

Development of improved coping materials

In order to increase further the strength of all-ceramic crowns, attention focussed on the development of a stronger coping covered with feldspathic porcelain. VITA developed a group of novel coping materials created by building up a coping on a refractory die which shrinks as the coping is fired, thus making it very easy to remove from the die (Figure 11.13). These glass-infused coping materials are:

- Alumina, as the basis for the In-Ceram Alumina crown
- Alumina with added magnesia as the basis for the In-Ceram Spinell crown
- A combination of alumina and zirconia as the basis for the In-Ceram Zirconia crown.

Glass-infused ceramic copings

The basis of many of these is a refractory die of the tooth preparation upon which either an almost pure alumina (Al_2O_3) (In-Ceram Alumina, VITA, Zahnfabrik) or less hard, but of greater translucency, magnesia and alumina

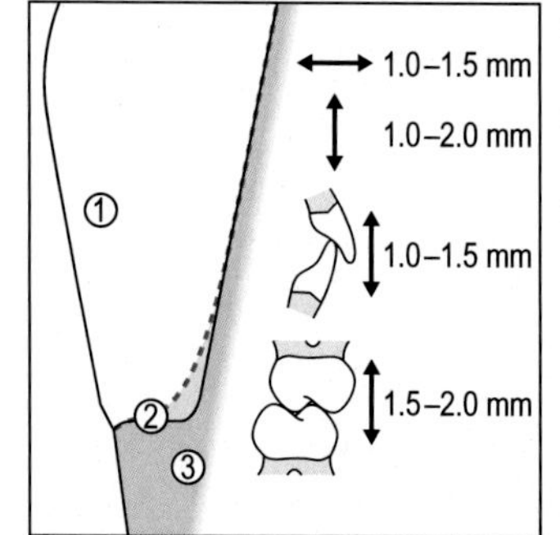

Figure 11.12 The design of a modern all-ceramic crown.

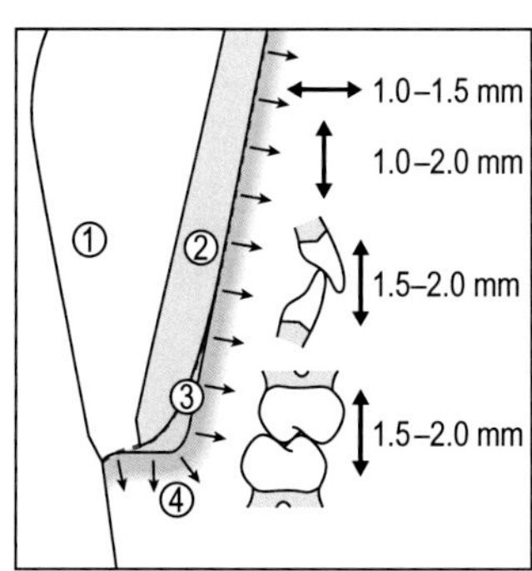

Figure 11.13 Schematic diagram of an In-Ceram all-ceramic crown with a strengthened coping.

$(MgAl_2O_4)$ (In-Ceram Spinell, VITA, Zahnfabrik) coping may be built up. Following sintering (at around 1200°C for 10 hours) the resultant structure is not structurally strong, so a slurry of lanthanum glass is painted on. Upon re-firing (at around 1100°C for 4 hours) the applied glass flows into the voids of the underlying coping, strengthening it.

The completed coping may then be built upon with suitable feldspathic porcelain. With regard to this the coefficient of thermal expansion of the coping and covering porcelain must be the same if cracking of the porcelain is to be avoided during the firing process. It should also be noted that such copings may also be milled from blanks of these glass-infused ceramic core materials using CAD-CAM technology (see later).

THE USE OF CAD-CAM AND DEVELOPMENT OF GLASS CERAMIC MATERIALS WITH SIGNIFICANTLY INCREASED STRENGTH

CAD-CAM has significantly changed all ceramic restorations with respect to:

- The types of material that can be used for the manufacture of all-ceramic crown copings
- The way dies are used and produced
- The way in which crowns can now be made without a master die model.

The advent of computer-aided manufacture to control milling machines has facilitated the use of extremely strong ceramic materials such as pure alumina or zirconium or yttrium-stabilized zirconium to form copings which fit over the prepared die and support more aesthetic feldspathic porcelain.

Nobel Biocare developed a technique whereby a stone die from an impression taken in the clinic is scanned using a laser to produce a digital three-dimensional map. This information can be sent electronically to a milling machine, often many miles away, for computer-aided manufacture of alumina and, more recently, zirconium copings. The copings are returned by post to the laboratory where they are fitted back onto the stone die prior to the addition of aesthetic feldspathic porcelain. This is very important as alumina, and particularly zirconium, is often a dense white colour which can be difficult to disguise with porcelain (Figure 11.14). In this way, Procera crowns are constructed. These crowns have significantly increased strength and have therefore been prescribed for the restoration of molar teeth. The manufacturer claims compressive strength in the region of 500 MPa. The fitting surface of the coping has a similar surface roughness to etched porcelain which assists the bonding process to the underlying core.

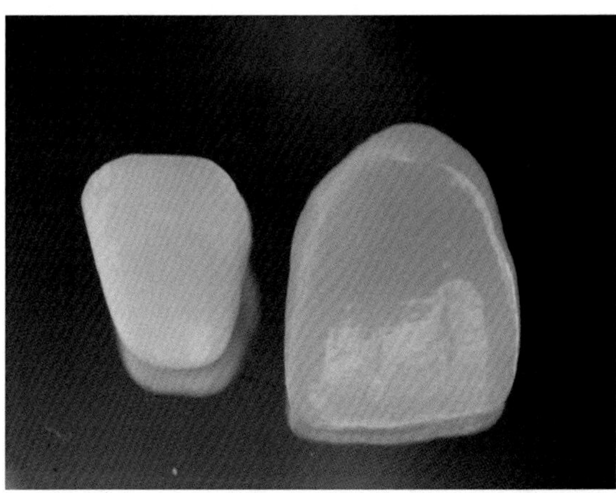

Figure 11.14 Zirconia coping (Lava) and completed anterior crown.

3M ESPE also developed a CAD-CAM method for milling zirconium in its green state followed by a sintering process for which account is taken of the three-dimensional shrinkage of the zirconium (Figure 11.15). This extremely hard and strong coping is then fitted back onto a stone die for the technician to build up the aesthetic feldspathic porcelain superstructure, disguising the relatively unaesthetic zirconium coping. 3M ESPE developed eight basic shades of zirconium for milling which has helped to improve the appearance of what are known as Lava crowns. The manufacturer's claim for the compressive strength of this type of crown is between 700 and 800 MPa.

VITA In-Ceram have used CAD-CAM to develop a set of copings from alumina, zirconium and yttrium-stabilized zirconium with manufacturer-claimed compressive strengths of 500, 600 and 900 MPa, respectively. In common with previously described copings, an aesthetic layer of feldspathic-like porcelain is placed over the coping by the technician.

Long-term studies of all-ceramic crowns manufactured using a CAD-CAM coping covered by a layer of aesthetic porcelain are scarce. However, those that do exist indicate a potential risk of loss of unsupported feldspathic porcelain from the underlying coping, a process called delamination.

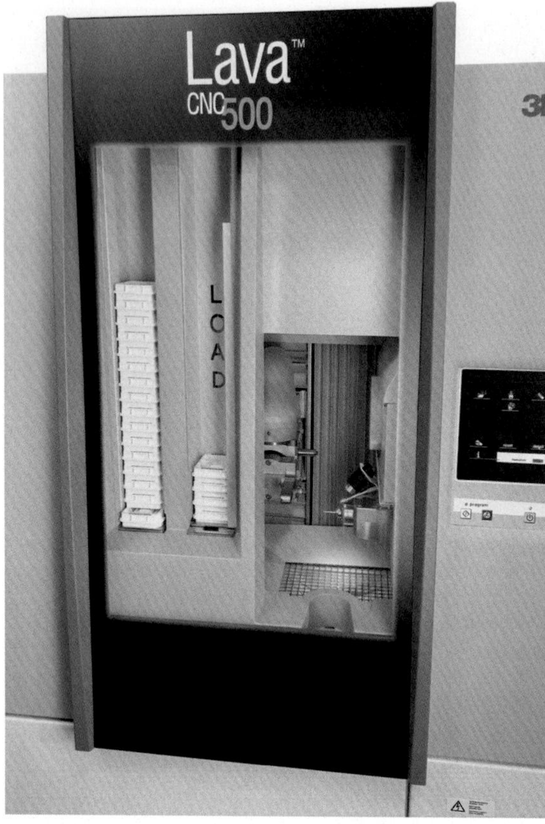

Figure 11.15 The Lava milling machine. The white rectangular zirconia blanks can be seen stacked up to the left, the milling machine is to the right.
(Courtesy of 3M ESPE)

Early copings were designed as 'caps' to cover the prepared tooth. They did not provide support for the overlaid porcelain which is weaker and of uneven thickness. By designing the coping to reflect the shape of what would have been underlying dentine, and using the feldspathic veneering porcelain to represent enamel for the final shape of the completed crown, better support should be provided, thereby reducing the risk of delamination. CAD-CAM technology allows accurate design of these 'biologic' copings.

The use of an intraoral camera to capture a series of images resulting in a three-dimensional composite image has also been developed to produce a so-called optical impression. The cameras require a dry preparation, often best achieved using rubber dam isolation, covered with a non-reflective opaque spray. In this way, the camera and dedicated computer software can identify and build up a dimensionally accurate image which is used for computer-aided design (CAD) of the restoration prior to computer-aided manufacture (CAM) from a single block of material.

Experience suggests quite a steep learning curve to develop this method of optical impression taking and chairside restoration design for all-ceramic restorations. The Sirona Company initially produced the Cerec machine for this purpose but initial results for marginal fit of the restorations were considered to be suboptimal. Development of the process and the advent of Cerec III has resolved this issue and excellent restorations can now be made.

A recent development by 3M ESPE is the Lava chairside oral scanner (COS) whereby a full arch can be scanned by moving a video camera around the arch (Figure 11.16).

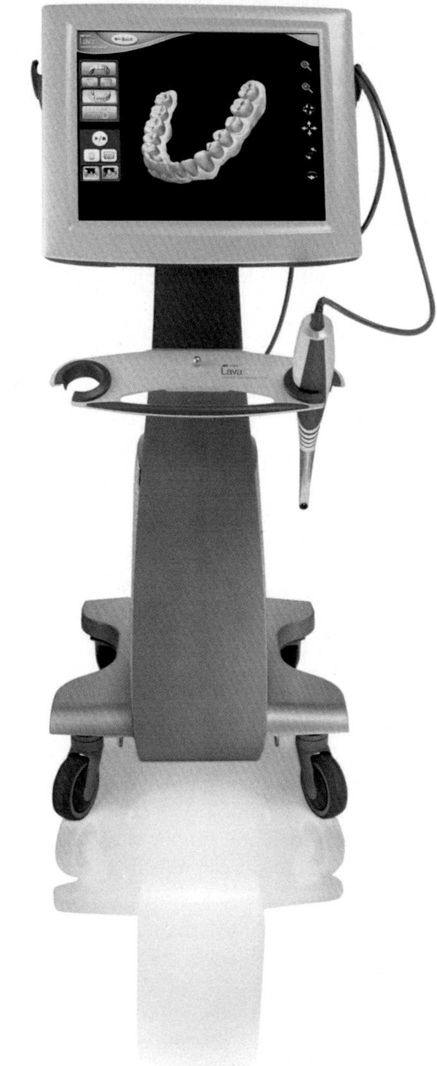

Figure 11.16 The chairside oral scanner (COS). The intraoral scanner is on the right side mount.
(Courtesy of 3M ESPE)

In addition, a three-dimensional image of the opposing dentition ensures restorations can be designed, on virtual dies, without occlusal interferences. Furthermore, the use of a technique called stereolithography (SLA) can be used to produce consistently accurate and durable, resin, occluding models and dies for laboratory construction of conventional extra- and intracoronal restorations such as gold shell crowns and porcelain bonded to metal crowns, in addition to all-ceramic crowns. The SLA model can also be used to ensure the fit of an anatomically accurate milled coping for subsequent addition of porcelain.

Blocks of material from which entire crowns can be milled are manufactured by VITA and include VITA Mark II ceramic blocks where the final shade of the restoration is developed by light scattering from any surrounding tooth structure, thus creating a chameleon effect. Coloured VITA TriLuxe and TriLuxe Forte ceramic blocks reproduce the more intense shading at the gingival margin with the lighter colour of the cusp tip or incisal edge.

Blocks of leucite-reinforced ceramic can also be used (Empress CAD, IPS e.max CAD and Paradigm-C) which come as multichromatic blocks or in five monoshade blocks. In each case, surface tints are added and fired in the laboratory. For the Empress CAD crowns, compressive strengths of 160 MPa are claimed. The IPS e.max CAD crowns are milled in the 'soft' state prior to a short 30-minute crystallization process to produce restorations with a compressive strength of 320 MPa.

3M ESPE have also developed a block based on their Z100 composite (Paradigm MZ100) which comes in five basic shades, claims enamel-like wear characteristics, can be characterized at the chairside with light-cured stains and can be repaired intraorally if required.

CEMENTATION OF PORCELAIN RESTORATIONS

Due to both the aesthetic requirements and brittle nature of some ceramic restorations their cementation poses a challenge. In the case of veneers they must first be tried in, not only to assess their fit but also their appearance. Their aesthetics, by virtue of thinness and translucency, can be markedly affected by the shade of the underlying cement. Resin composite luting agents are used to achieve final cementation and such products are specially formulated for this purpose.

Each manufacturer produces a range of trial pastes that may be applied to the fit surface of the crown or veneer at try in. These are of shades that match the final luting cements. Once this has been carried out the veneer is readily removed and both the tooth preparation and veneers must be debrided of residual paste prior to final cementation of the restoration. This is readily accomplished by a prophylaxis of the tooth and steam cleaning of the veneer. Cementation of ceramic veneers will be discussed in further in Chapter 12.

In relation to final cementation of all porcelain restorations it is important to note that the materials used for this should exhibit shear thinning (a reduction in viscosity with applied pressure) to minimize fracture of the restoration upon seating. The cementing medium should also provide a firm foundation for the restoration to maximize resistance to fracture. Acid-based conventional cements (e.g. zinc oxyphosphate, zinc polycarboxylate and conventional glass polyalkenoate) should be avoided as they may interact with porcelain, exacerbating any flaws and enhancing crack propagation in function. As a consequence, resin composite luting agents are recommended. Such materials are not acid based and exhibit superior flexural strength. Those that are dual cured are considered best, since lone chemical curing lacks operator control and satisfactory light curing alone may not be accomplished if the restoration is either deep in dimension or dark in colour.

The exception to this choice of cement type is zirconia oxide-based crowns that may, if desired, be cemented with conventional cements. Their high fracture resistance diminishes the need for support and their underlying tooth preparation requires no adhesive interface for retention.

The fit surface of all feldspathic porcelain restorations, to be cemented with resin composite luting agents, must be etched prior to cementation with hydrofluoric acid (5–9.5%). This is best accomplished in the dental laboratory. As an alternative, air abrasion is to be avoided as this will induce and exacerbate any flaws in the porcelain. The fit surface of the restoration should then be silanated just prior to the application of the resin composite luting agent. It is important to realize that silane is a chemical coupling agent that will bond the porcelain to the luting agent. This chemical exhibits good wetting but degrades in the presence of both moisture and air. Its application should therefore be as near as possible to the cementation of the restoration. Bonding of the resin luting agent to tooth substance is achieved by acid etching the preparation, rinsing, drying and applying a bonding agent prior to seating the resin composite loaded restoration.

Glass infiltrated alumina-based ceramics are resistant to hydrofluoric acid etching and, in the case of restorations fabricated from this material, one manufacturer (3M ESPE) advocates a tribochemical silica coating process instead. This roughens the fit surface to facilitate bonding of the resin composite luting agent. This is accomplished by laboratory cleaning of the restoration by application of 100 μm high purity aluminium oxide under a pressure of 250 kPa for 14 seconds. A similar process pertains for sintered aluminium oxide crown copings.

SUMMARY

The long history of all-ceramic crowns has utilized advances in ceramic materials and production methods to create functional and aesthetic restorations which require increasingly less tooth reduction to achieve an adequate result. On-going clinical studies will inform greater understanding about the modes of failure of these restorations and help to further develop materials and techniques, thus extending the range of clinical circumstances in which this type of restoration may be used.

Many of the clinical studies reporting the results of all-ceramic crowns indicate that they are successful for anterior teeth. The situation on posterior teeth, either single crowns or bridges, is more complex. Small fractures or chips are commonly found and whilst these may not result in failure of the restoration, they are unwanted complications. As such, these restorations should be carefully considered for patients using high occlusal loading, particularly bruxists. The balance between the need to achieve a good aesthetic result and a long-term successful restoration means that these restorations need careful planning and prescription.

FURTHER READING

Burke, F.J., 2007. Four year performance of dentine-bonded all-ceramic crowns. Br. Dent. J. 202, 269–273.

Conrad, H.J., Seong, W.J., Pesun, I.J., 2007. Current ceramic materials and systems with clinical recommendations: a systematic review. J. Prosthet. Dent. 98, 389–404.

Donovan, T.E., 2008. Factors essential for successful all-ceramic restorations. J. Am. Dent. Assoc. 139 (Suppl.), 14S–18S.

McLean, J.W., Hughes, T.H., 1965. The reinforcement of dental porcelain with ceramic oxides. Br. Dent. J. 119, 251–267.

Miyazaki, T., Hotta, Y., Kunii, J., Kuriyama, S., Tamaki, Y., 2009. A review of dental CAD/CAM: current status and future perspectives from 20 years of experience. Dent. Mater. J. 28, 44–56.

Sadowsky, S.J., 2006. An overview of treatment considerations for esthetic restorations: a review of the literature. J. Prosthet. Dent. 96, 433–442.

Spear, F., Holloway, J., 2008. Which all-ceramic system is optimal for anterior esthetics? J. Am. Dent. Assoc. 139 (Suppl.), 19S–24S.

Sutton, A.F., McCord, J.F., 2001. Variations in tooth preparations for resin-bonded all-ceramic crowns in general dental practice. Br. Dent. J. 191, 677–681.

Chapter 12

Inlays, onlays and veneers

David Bartlett, David Ricketts

CHAPTER CONTENTS

INTRODUCTION

Historically, gold was the material of choice for inlays and onlays. The accuracy and malleability of gold made it an ideal material to restore lost tooth structure and protect weakened cusps destroyed by caries and trauma. Although gold is versatile, its use has declined over recent years but is still used by those clinicians who recognize its unique qualities in areas of the mouth where appearance is not important. Modern attitudes to appearance and colour have seen a preference for tooth-coloured materials.

Modern materials utilize the properties of adhesive cements to reduce the necessity for extensive tooth preparation and restoration, so conserving tooth tissue. Both ceramic and composite-based materials are regularly used as an alternative to gold in restoring broken down teeth, and veneers have been designed to improve the appearance of minimally restored teeth.

INLAYS AND ONLAYS

The most common indication for inlays or onlays is extensively restored and weakened teeth. The distinction between the two designs is unclear but simply those restorations without cuspal coverage that remain within the body of the tooth would be considered inlays (Figure 12.1) whereas onlays replace tooth tissue including cusps (Figure 12.2).

Inlays

Inlays are usually used when difficulty is anticipated or experienced in obtaining an acceptable contour, contact point and occlusion on a directly placed restoration. Repeated fracture of a directly placed restoration may also indicate the placement of an inlay, and in this situation a gold inlay may be advocated for its strength. Composite and ceramic inlays may also be chosen for their aesthetics in situations where strength is not a major requisite. This can be particularly relevant for the mesial surfaces of upper premolar teeth and the occlusal surfaces of lower teeth when appearance is important to the patient. Increasingly, patients are concerned about the placement of amalgam and request an alternative when the restorations need replacement and in rare situations amalgam replacement is necessary because of lichenoid reactions.

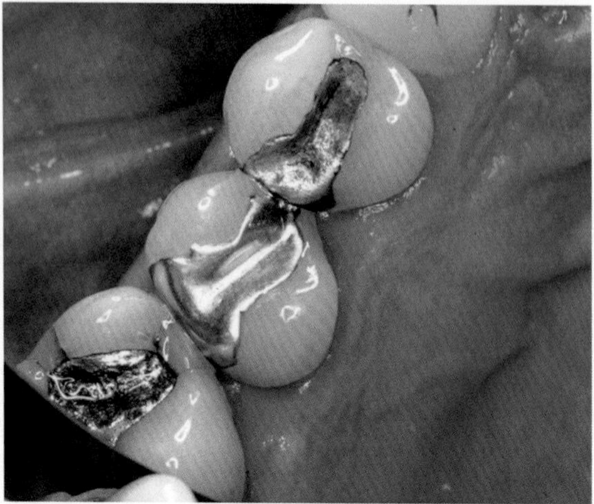

Figure 12.1 Gold inlay placed due to repeated fracture of the previous amalgam restorations. Aesthetics is not a problem in this upper premolar tooth.

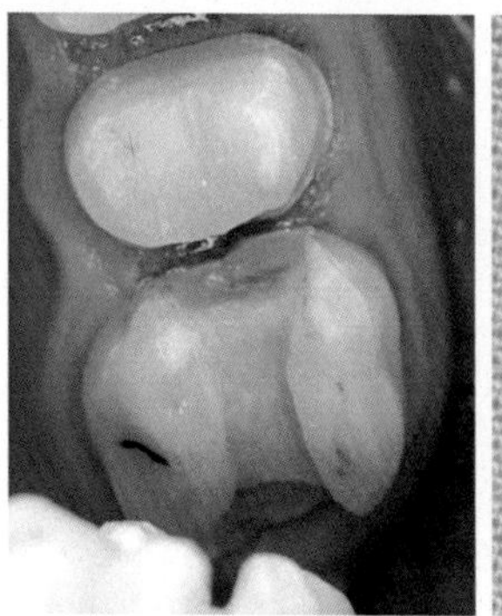

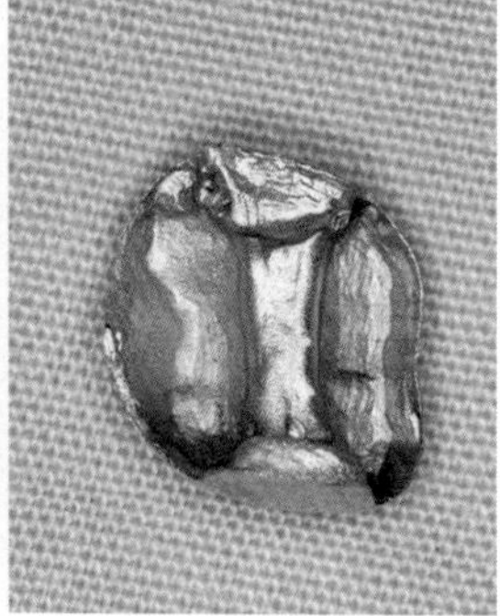

Figure 12.2 Gold mesial occlusal distal (MOD) with cuspal overlay; the tooth preparation can be seen on the left with the fit surface of the restoration to the right.

In these situations, directly placed composites must be considered the most appropriate material to restore minimal cavities. The necessity of using an indirect material with associated elimination of undercuts and laboratory costs means their indications are limited to more extensive cavities.

Onlays

The most commonly placed partial coverage extracoronal restoration would be an onlay where weakened tooth structure can be protected without further extensive tooth removal. A common indication for an onlay would be a root-filled posterior tooth where cuspal protection is required. Root canal treatment in posterior teeth is usually the result of caries and restorative procedures and, as such, these teeth are extensively broken down and have weakened cusps. The coronal access cavity needed for a root treatment removes the roof of the pulp chamber, weakening the tooth further, and can leave a limited amount of buccal and lingual tooth tissue which might be completely removed if prepared for a crown (Figure 12.3). Preservation of some part of the buccal and lingual tooth helps to retain the core and reduces the need to consider a post, especially in premolar teeth (Figure 12.4). The three-quarter gold crown preparation on a premolar tooth, particularly when only the buccal cusp remains, will preserve tooth tissue but the colour and appearance of gold within the smile line is considered by some to be a disadvantage (see Chapter 8 and Figure 12.5).

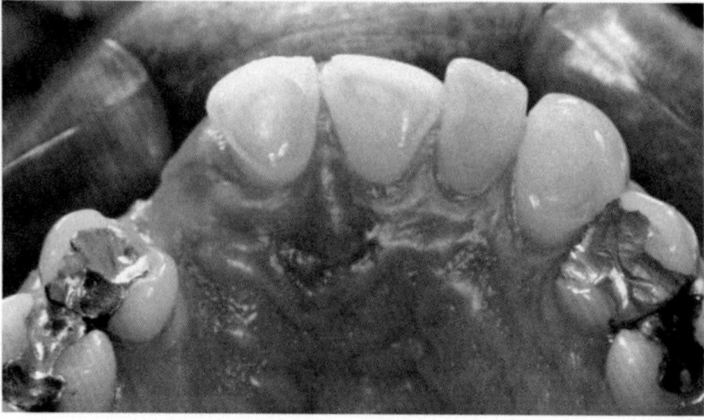

Figure 12.3 The upper left first premolar tooth has an extensive mesial-occlusal-distal (MOD) amalgam restoration; preparation of this tooth for a metal–ceramic crown might result in the loss of the entire buccal cusp, leaving the amalgam unsupported or poorly retained, with potential loss of the restoration. An onlay or inlay preparation would preserve the buccal tissue.

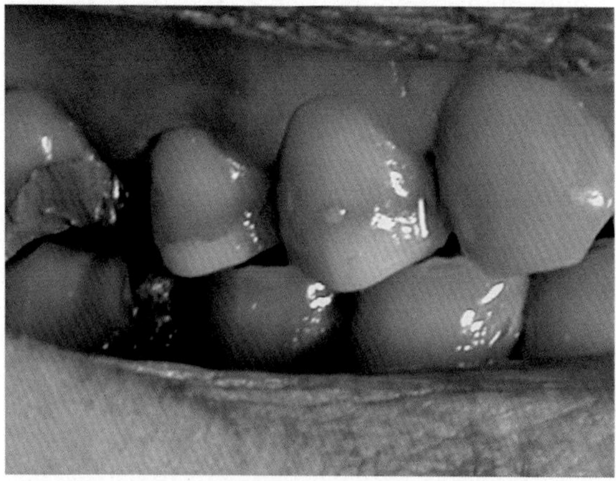

Figure 12.4 Onlays cemented to both premolars restoring teeth which were extensively destroyed by caries. By using an onlay rather than a crown the buccal tooth tissue is preserved, avoiding the need for a full coverage restoration.

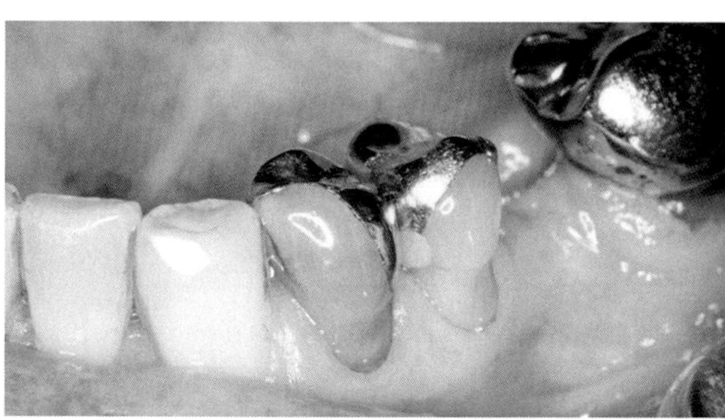

Figure 12.5 Three-quarter crown preparation on the lower left second premolar tooth has preserved buccal tooth tissue, but may be regarded by some patients as having an unacceptable appearance.

Bonding materials (including gold) to a tooth, using adhesive cements, reduces some of the need for conventional principles of retention. Onlays can be considered when there is no or little intracoronal shape to the preparation and where retention is poor. Despite the retention provided by adhesive cement, conventional concepts of tooth preparation for retention should not be ignored and, where possible, should be incorporated into the design of the preparation (Figures 12.2 and 12.6); routine use of adhesive cements to achieve retention poses problems if retrieval is ever necessary.

Dental materials

Gold

Whilst gold is gradually being superseded by tooth-coloured materials for the provision of indirect restorations, its use should not be ignored as gold has some advantages over indirect composites and ceramics when used for inlays and onlays. It has high strength, ductility and has the ability to be cast accurately, especially into thin sections. A dentist would be unable to obtain full consent from a patient if gold (with its advantages and disadvantages) was not discussed as a treatment option.

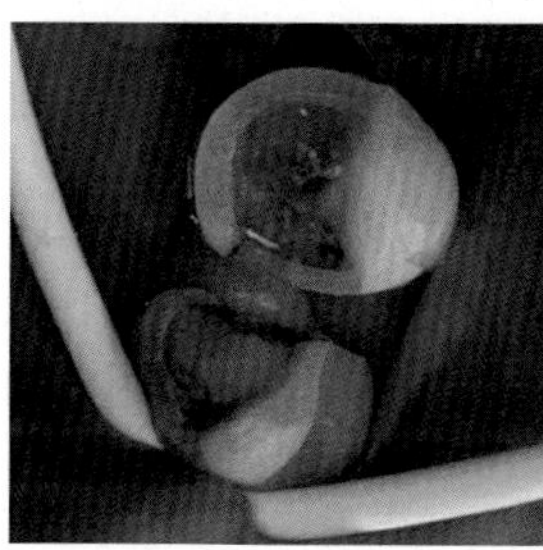

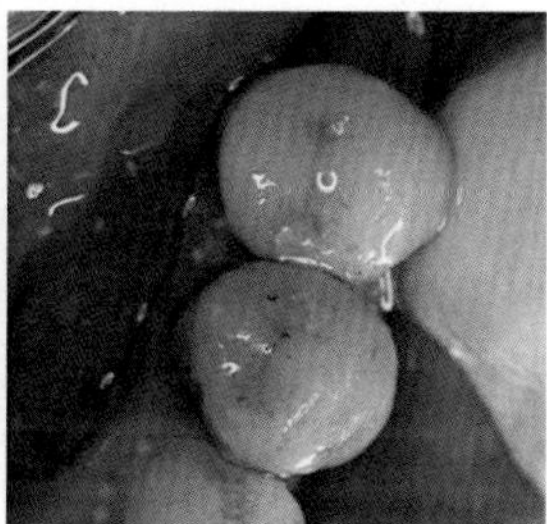

Figure 12.6 The intracoronal preparation for an onlay. The sharp line angles on the buccal and lingual surfaces allow the porcelain or indirect composite an ideal margin. Internal line angles can be rounded.

Gold onlays need less occlusal and axial reduction than that needed for tooth-coloured materials, as the latter tend to be more brittle and require greater bulk for strength. The ductility of gold and its ability to be highly polished means that it is not as abrasive to the opposing dentition, especially for those patients with tooth wear. All intra- and extra-coronal restorations made from gold need tooth preparation with near parallel walls and an absence of undercuts (Figure 12.7).

Composite

The need for tooth-coloured inlays competes with directly placed composites for aesthetically pleasing tooth-coloured restorations. Laboratory-made indirect composites have a theoretical reduction in polymerization shrinkage as the curing is completed in the laboratory. The curing occurs by subjecting the composite to heat, pressure or intense light, and this higher degree of cure improves strength and reduces wear; the indirect composite inlays/onlays are often referred to as 'super cured'. This super curing does, however, leave fewer reactive resin groups to bond to the resin luting cement. The accuracy of fit is significantly less than restorations made in either ceramic or gold and they can absorb dietary stains after a few years which significantly affects their appearance.

Ceramic

Ceramic restorations are indicated where the aesthetic demands of the patient are high. The colour matching of modern porcelains allows the margin between the tooth and material to be almost imperceptible. Where there is a slight difference in colour, the margin of a ceramic inlay/onlay will be obvious (see Figure 12.4) as there is a sudden transition from ceramic to tooth. Ceramic materials, unlike directly placed composite, cannot be placed into progressively thinner layers to blend and merge the

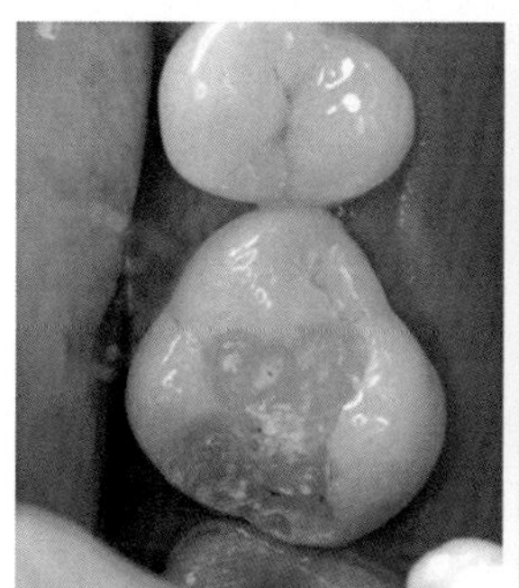

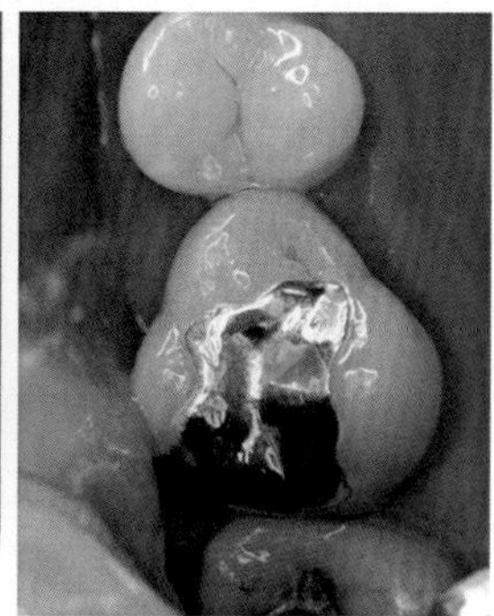

Figure 12.7 Disto-occlusal inlay preparation and cemented inlay. The retentive features in the inlay preparation, i.e. near parallel walls and occlusal key, are adequate and adhesive resin luting cements are not necessary.

colour to that of the tooth, due to their brittleness. This progressive transition with direct composite can camouflage the restoration. Ceramic is a hard material and has high wear resistance; however, it can be abrasive to the opposing dentition when used on the occlusal surfaces, especially if the glaze is lost and the restoration has been adjusted.

The manufacturing techniques used for porcelain and indirect composites generally cannot tolerate such parallel preparations as those produced for a gold inlay, and more tapered walls are needed. Undercuts in the tooth preparation can either be eliminated by further tooth preparation or be blocked out with an adhesive tooth-coloured material. All variants of the preparations should avoid sharp line angles, particularly intracoronally (Figure 12.8).

The traditional method of manufacture of onlays and inlays was the lost wax technique for gold-based materials and the use of refractory dies for all-ceramic restorations (see manufacture of veneer later in this chapter). More recently, computer-aided design and computer-aided manufacture (CAD-CAM) technology has allowed laboratory and chairside production of indirect restorations. Most systems utilize scanners to record the tooth preparation or its model digitally and then send the data to an automated milling machine. The milled crown, inlay or onlay has a fit accuracy of a few microns and is adjusted to fit the occlusion with the opposing tooth. There are a variety of commercial systems on the market and all use the same basic principles (see Chapter 11).

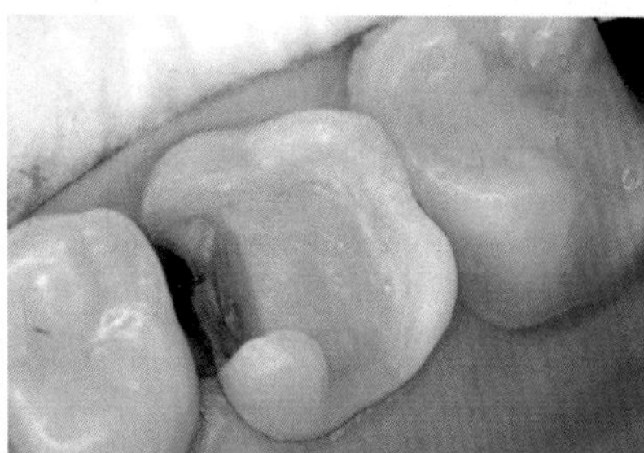

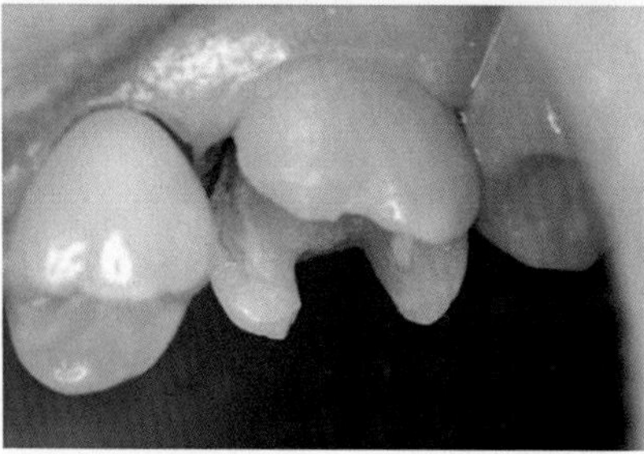

Figure 12.8 Tooth prepared for ceramic inlay. Note that undercuts are blocked out with bonded composite, avoiding further tooth removal to eliminate undercuts. The preparation is slightly more tapered and has rounded internal line angles. *(Courtesy of Dr Suzanne Blacker)*

Ceramic inlays and onlays are cemented with a resin-based luting cement and are handled in the same way as described for ceramic veneers below.

TOOTH PREPARATION FOR INLAYS AND ONLAYS

Tooth preparation for intra- and extra-coronal restorations follows the same basic concepts as used for all indirect restorations. The preparation should avoid undercuts between opposing walls within the cavity; however, the more complex the shape, the harder it is to avoid them. Multiple surface intracoronal restorations, particularly those including proximal boxes, are particularly demanding and, as a result, cavities tend to be over-tapered. Since all-ceramic restorations rely upon the cement lute for most of the retention, provided there are no undercuts a slightly over-tapered cavity is acceptable. However, gold restorations gain most of their retention from the cavity shape and are therefore more reliant upon near parallel preparations.

The major advantage for inlay and onlay restorations is the preservation of some tooth tissue to retain the core. If existing cavities contain undercuts they can be blocked out with composite or glass ionomer cements to provide the necessary cavity shape (Figures 12.9 and 12.10). Tapered burs provide the most convenient shape to prepare inlays and onlays and reduce the chance of creating undercuts. If an onlay preparation is to be cut, occlusal clearance/reduction will be required consistent with the material chosen. Similarly, the marginal configuration (shoulder, chamfer or deep chamfer) will also be dictated by the material planned.

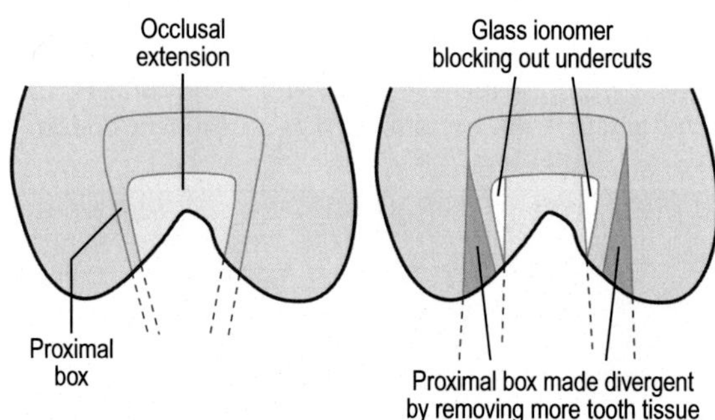

Figure 12.9 Diagrammatic representation of an undercut Class II cavity which has been prepared for an amalgam restoration (left). To convert this to an inlay preparation, the undercuts have to be eliminated. This can be achieved either by blocking out the undercuts with an adhesive restorative material or by removing more tooth tissue to produce a divergent cavity (right).

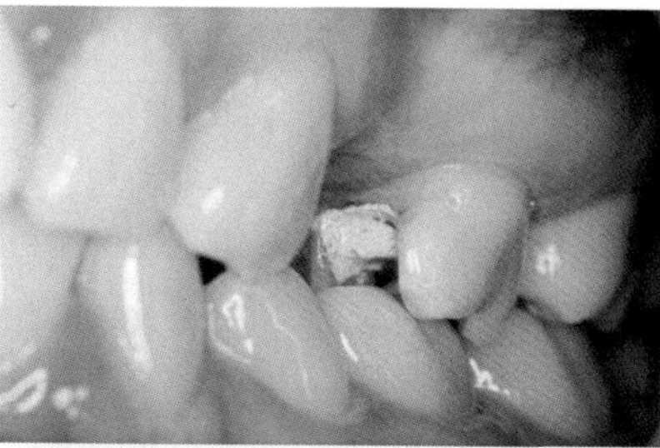

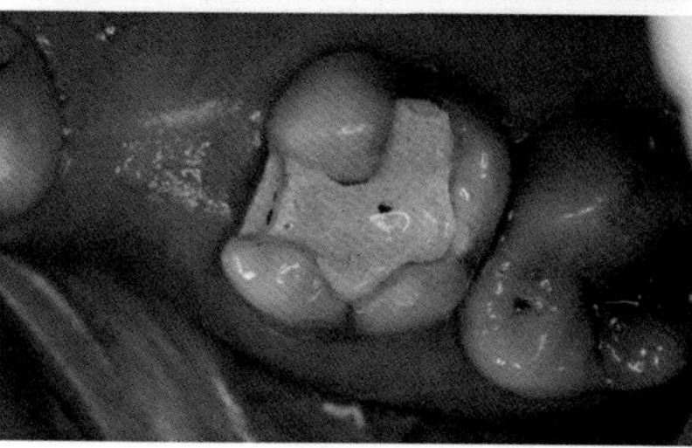

Figure 12.10 The upper left first molar tooth has been prepared for an inlay which is to act as a retainer for a cantilever bridge. A silver reinforced glass ionomer has been used to block out the undercut and all margins should be on tooth tissue. *Note*: Further removal of the material is required at the floor of the box to allow the margin of the inlay to be placed on tooth tissue.

CERAMIC VENEERS

Ceramic veneers are thin layers of ceramic (Figure 12.11) used to mask discoloured teeth and to alter the shape and alignment of minimally restored teeth. It is important to understand that whilst tooth preparation for veneers is relatively conservative of tooth tissue compared to full coverage crowns, some tooth preparation is required and the procedure is irreversible. Adequate tooth preparation should allow for a veneer 0.5–0.75 mm thick.

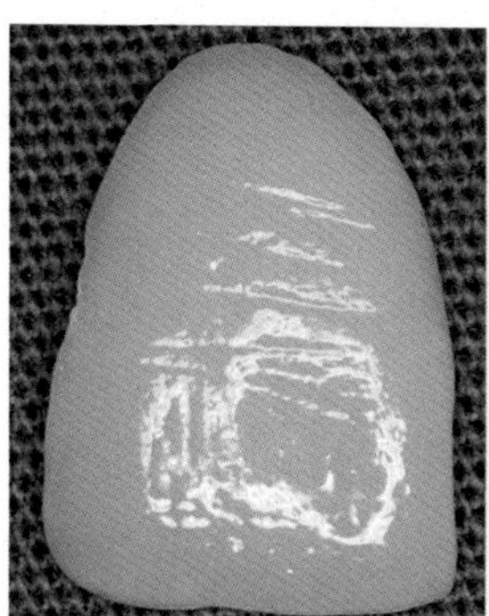

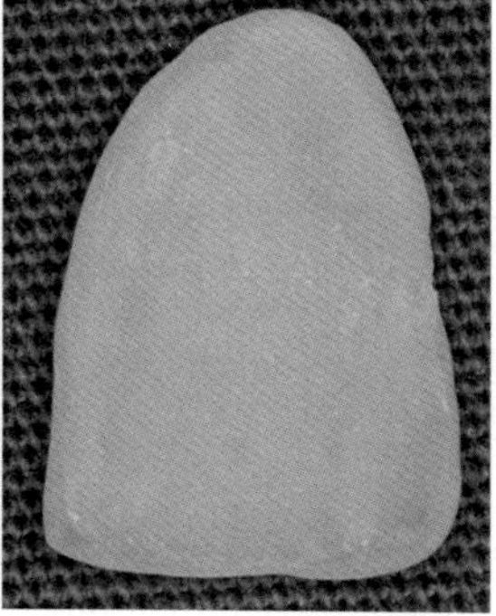

Figure 12.11 Labial (left) and fit (right) surfaces of a ceramic veneer.

Specific considerations

If poorly aligned in-standing teeth are veneered, they may not need as much reduction, as the veneer thickness can be used to align the teeth (Figure 12.12). However, the outer, aprismatic, surface of mature enamel should always be removed as it provides an inferior bond compared to that of etched subsurface prismatic enamel. When using ceramic veneers to improve the appearance of restored teeth, small cavities containing old discoloured composite restorations should be replaced to minimize the appearance of any shine-through and to ensure a superior bond from the veneer to the newly placed composite. Water sorption and limited reactive chemical groups found in old polymerized composites lead to an inferior bond with the luting resin, leakage, staining and increased failure (Figure 12.13). When treatment planning for veneers, careful attention to the occlusion between the restoration and the opposing tooth is needed as those placed under heavy occlusal loads are more likely to debond or fracture. In the upper anterior region, for example, caution is needed when veneers are planned for teeth with incisal edge-to-edge contacts, cross bites and signs of parafunctional habits such as wear facets (Figure 12.14).

Tooth preparation for veneers

When discoloured teeth are well aligned, a uniform reduction in the labial enamel should be carried out (Figure 12.15). Inadequate tooth reduction leads to the veneer appearing too bulky or a veneer too thin to mask the discolouration. Uniform reduction of tooth tissue can be difficult when done 'freehand and eyeballed'. Multiple dimples cut with a round diamond bur of radius ~0.5 mm and held at 45° to the tooth surface may help as a depth guide. The angulation

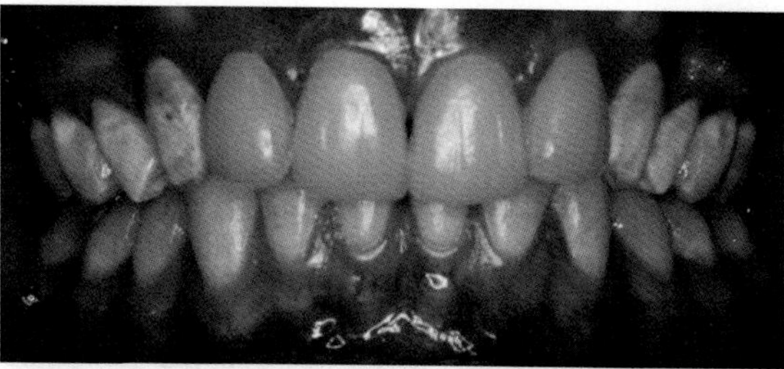

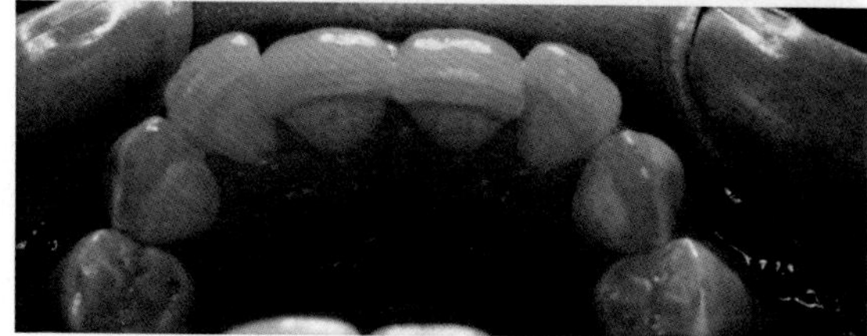

Figure 12.12 Ceramic veneers have been used to align the incisors in a patient with a Class II Division II incisor relationship, with retroclined central incisors. Note the contact points are broad bucco-lingually.

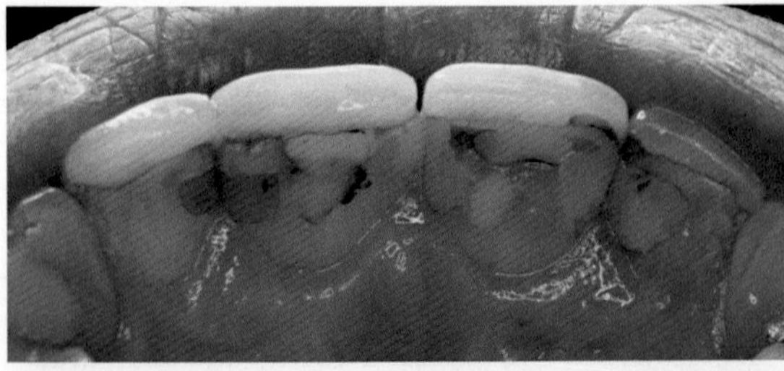

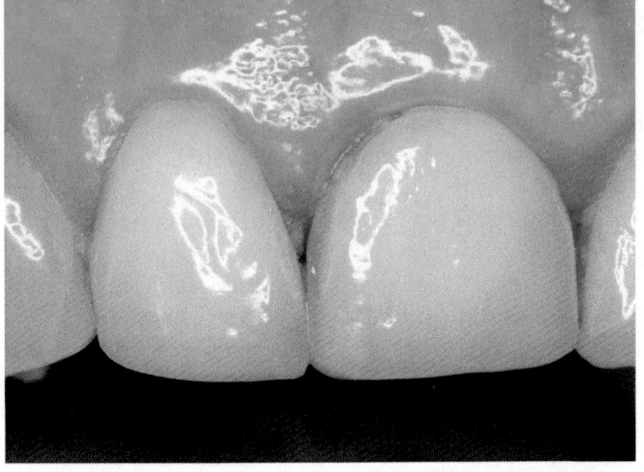

Figure 12.13 The ceramic veneer on the upper right central incisor has been placed on an old distal composite. An inferior bond has led to leakage and staining.

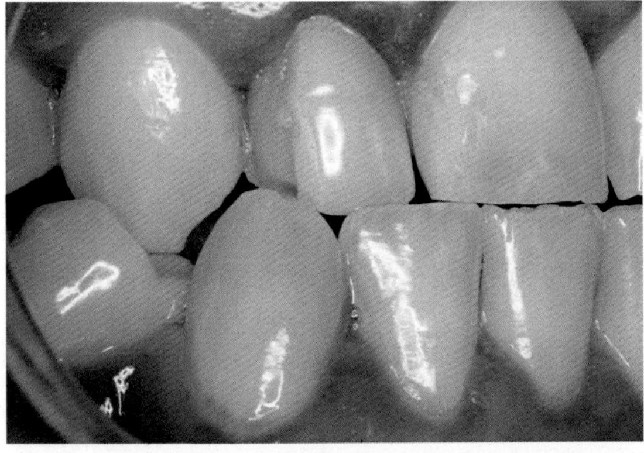

Figure 12.14 Inappropriate placement of a ceramic veneer on the upper right lateral incisor tooth, which is in cross bite with the lower canine, has led to fracture and partial debond of the veneer.

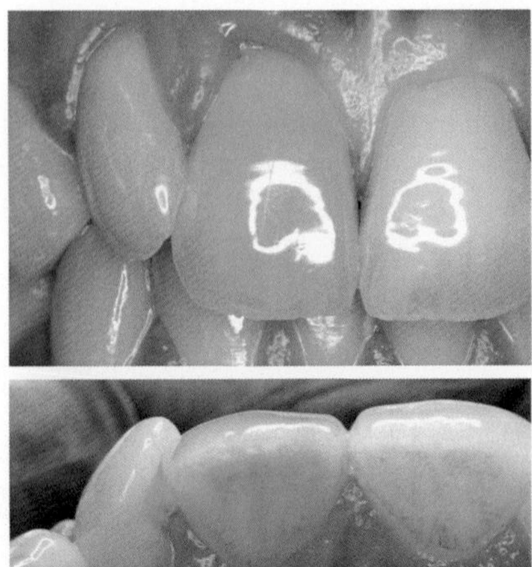

Figure 12.15 Discoloured upper right central incisor where a ceramic veneer is planned. It is in alignment with the upper left central incisor and the labial face will have to be reduced to create space for the veneer.

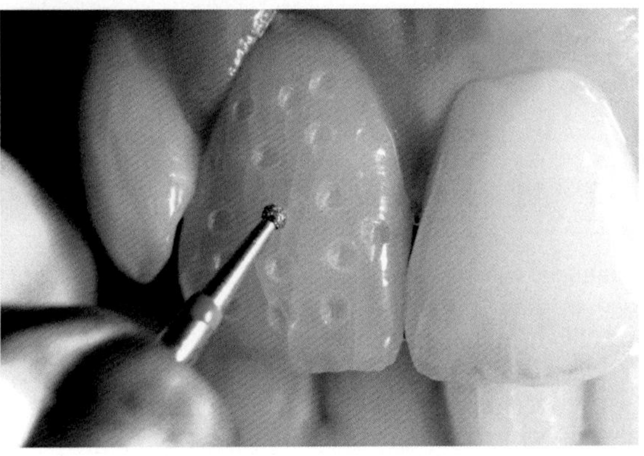

Figure 12.16 Dimples cut into the labial face with the bur at 45° to the tooth ensures the dimples do not become too deep. The dimples act as depth cuts, guiding uniform labial reduction for the veneer.

that the bur is held ensures that the dimples do not become too deep as the shank of the bur engages the tooth surface (Figure 12.16). A specially made bur with a blank shank and diamond wheels (Figure 12.17) can also be used in a similar manner to make horizontal depth cuts in the enamel. A tapered bur can then be used to reduce the remaining labial tooth tissue until the dimples or horizontal grooves just disappear. With all burs it is important to remember that the labial face of a tooth is curved and the reduction needs to conform to this (Figure 12.18) as with any crown preparation.

At the cervical margin a chamfer finish should be created with a round-ended tapered bur. Some burs have a finer diamond grit at the tip to ensure better adaptation and fit of the ceramic veneer at the margin (Figure 12.19). The veneer preparation should be extended proximally, sufficient to completely mask the tooth tissue and prevent a dark line being seen at the margins (Figure 12.20). However, the contact point between teeth must be preserved, if temporary veneers are not placed, as proximal space closure will prevent the veneer from seating fully.

Incisally, a number of preparations have been described, each with their advantages and disadvantages (Figure 12.21). The feather edge finish is easy to prepare

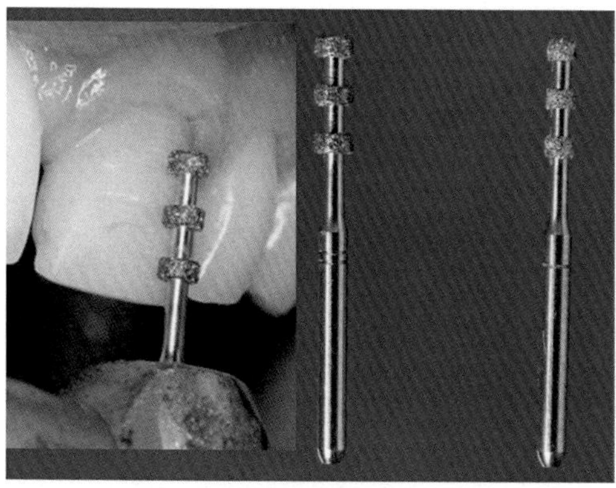

Figure 12.17 Bur with smooth shank and diamond wheels used for producing horizontal depth cut grooves to aid veneer preparation.

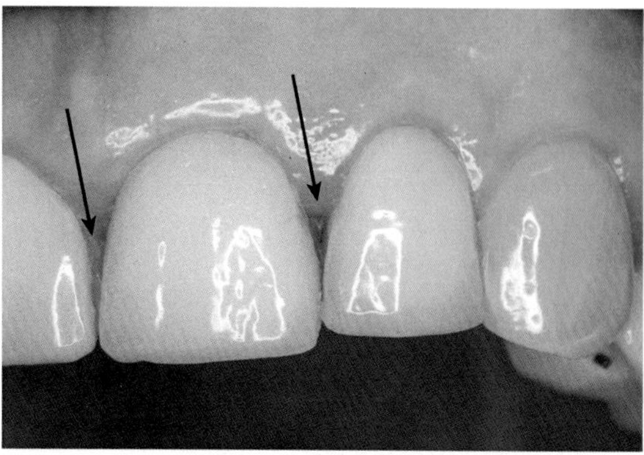

Figure 12.20 Inadequate extension of the veneer preparations proximally has led to the appearance of dark proximal lines.

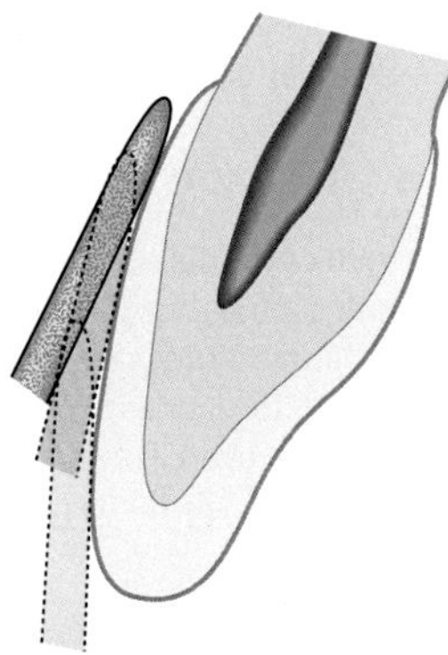

Figure 12.18 The tapered diamond bur should be held in at least three different planes to ensure the labial curvature of the preparation conforms to that of the tooth, giving an even 0.5 mm reduction.

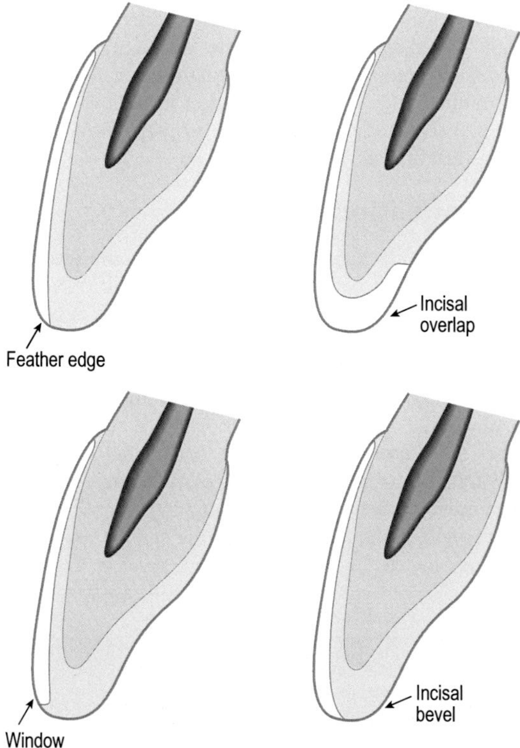

Figure 12.21 Various types of incisal preparation that have been described for veneers.

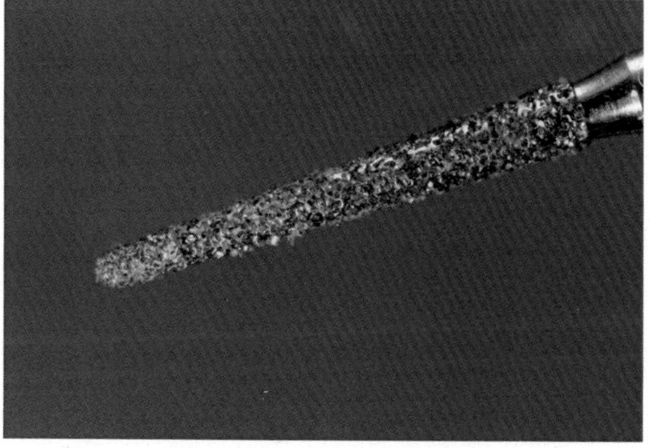

Figure 12.19 Tapered bur with finer diamond grit tip to produce a chamfer margin with fewer irregularities.

and there is little risk of damage to the ceramic in most occlusal schemes; however, it does not allow a translucent incisal tip on the ceramic (Figure 12.22). The incisal overlap overcomes this but the preparation is more destructive and the palatal finish line is in a position where occlusal contacts could lead to damage. The window preparation is difficult to prepare and is not normally recommended; however, the incisal margin of the veneer is protected from occlusal

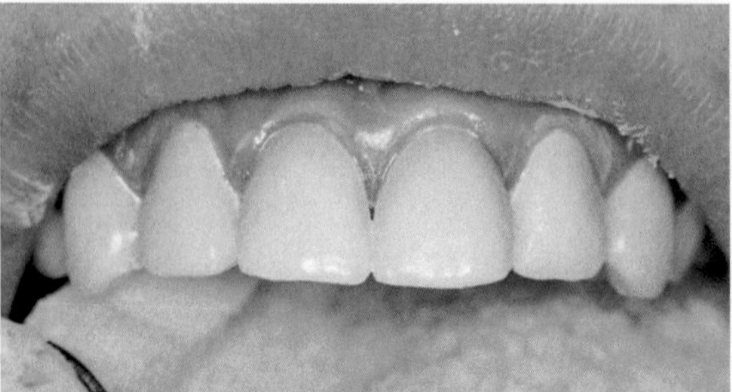

Figure 12.22 Feather edge finish to the incisal aspect of the veneer preparation has led to no incisal translucency and a monotone finish. Excess luting cement still has to be removed.

forces. Unfortunately, the incisal edge of the tooth may be visible, compromising the result (Figure 12.23). The incisal bevel overcomes this but the ceramic margin becomes thin and fragile and is more suited for restorations using a directly placed composite veneer. The choice of preparation will depend upon each clinical situation, but those most commonly used are the feather edge or incisal overlap. Figure 12.24 shows the completed veneer preparation for the patient seen in Figures 12.15 and 12.16.

Temporization

Once the tooth preparation has been completed, an impression is taken and consideration can be given to temporization. Placement of temporary veneers is usually unnecessary, particularly if a conservative intra-enamel preparation has been carried out. Preparing teeth for a veneer reduces the thickness of enamel and if the teeth are markedly discoloured the appearance may become worse. If temporary veneers are considered necessary, these are best made out of directly placed composite resin and bonded to the tooth by acid etching a small spot of the enamel, leaving the majority of the enamel unaffected and ready for etching for the definitive veneers. Composite veneers 'spot welded' in such a way are easy to remove.

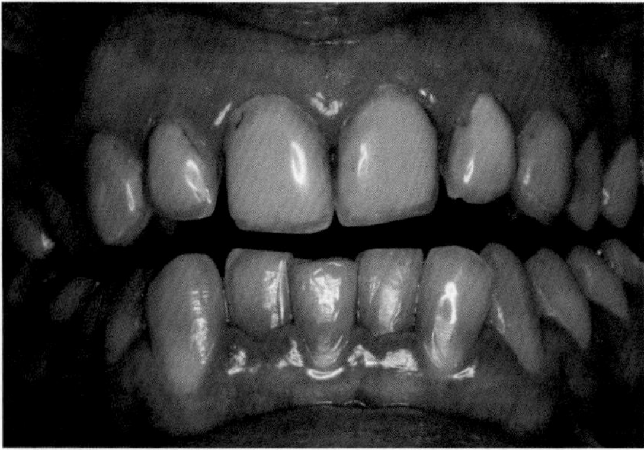

Figure 12.23 Window type preparation for these composite veneers has led to a darker incisal line.

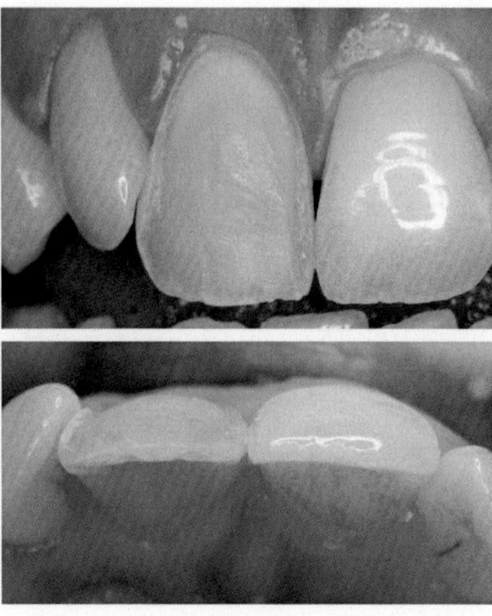

Figure 12.24 Veneer preparation for the patient seen in Figures 12.15 and 12.16 completed until no signs of dimples remain. The margins are prepared to a chamfer finish cervically and proximally, and a feather edge incisally.

Manufacture of ceramic veneers

Two models are required when making ceramic veneers. The first model is made from a refractory die material onto which the ceramic can be built and which can withstand the temperature needed within the furnace when the ceramic is fired (Figure 12.25). A glaze porcelain is usually applied to the refractory die before building up the ceramic. The ceramic

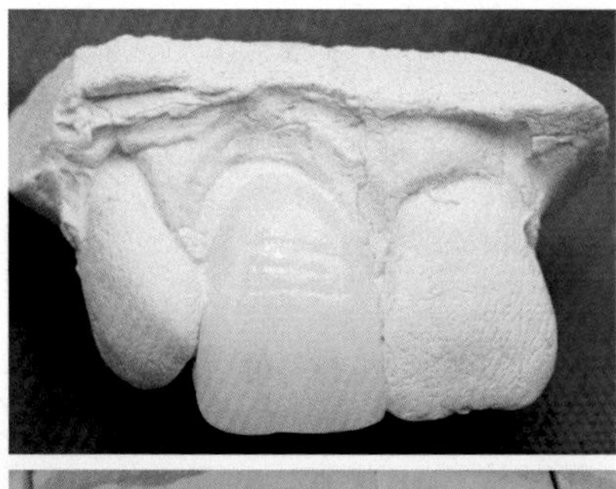

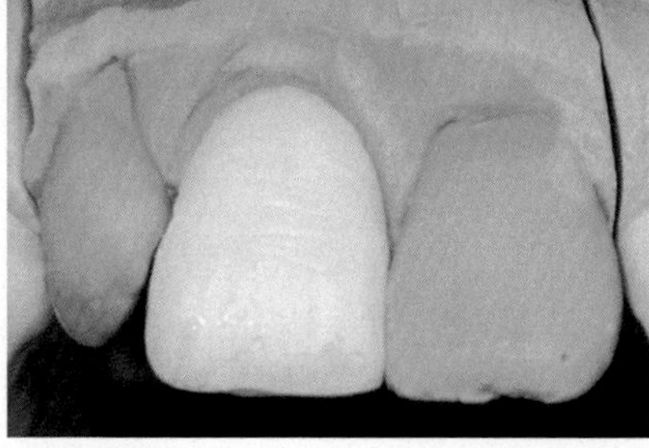

Figure 12.25 Refractory die (above) onto which the ceramic is built and fired. Once the refractory die has been sandblasted from the fit surface of the ceramic it can be tried on the stone master die (below).

powder is usually made from feldspar (80%), quartz (15%) and kaolin (5%) which is mixed with an aqueous medium to produce a paste. This is built up on the refractory die and the particles are condensed by vibration and water absorption using a tissue paper. The refractory die and ceramic are then put through a firing cycle which fuses the porcelain particles together. Once removed from the furnace and cooled, the refractory die material is sandblasted from the veneer, taking care not to damage the thin laminate. This also roughens the fit surface of the veneer, improving the bond with the luting cement. The fit surface may be roughened further by etching with hydrofluoric acid gel. This is extremely caustic and should not come into contact with patients; its use is confined to the laboratory. The second model made by the dental technician is a conventional die stone model onto which the veneer is seated to assess fit and shape.

As with all-ceramic crowns, ceramic veneers can also be produced using CAD-CAM technology (see Chapter 11).

Try-in and cementation

To try-in and cement a veneer, an appropriate resin luting cement system should be used. These usually have water soluble try-in pastes of various shades which correspond to the definitive resin luting cement and can modify the overall shade of the veneer. Try-in pastes are generally composed of either glycerine or polyethylene glycol resin to which has been added a variety of additives and pigments. They exhibit the phenomenon of shear thinning which allows the controlled loading of the fit surface of the veneer, with no running off of the material. The subsequent reduction in viscosity that occurs upon seating the restoration upon the tooth both facilitates positioning and minimizes the chances of porcelain fracture occurring in this procedure. Thereafter the viscosity increases, minimizing the chances of displacement of the veneer by the patient's circumoral musculature whilst the appearance is assessed. Even if the ceramic appears to be a good colour match, a neutral or clear try-in paste should be used as this can alter the light transmission and reflection at the veneer–tooth interface which can affect the appearance (Figure 12.26).

When operator and patient are happy with the appearance of the veneer at try-in, cementation can take place. The water soluble try-in paste should be thoroughly rinsed off and the veneer dried. A silane coupling agent is then applied to the fit surface of the veneer and gently air dried. This chemical exhibits good wetting but degrades in the presence of both moisture and air. Its application should therefore be as near as possible to the cementation of the restoration. The silane is a chemical coupling agent that will bond the porcelain to the luting agent.

For cementation the tooth should ideally be isolated under a rubber dam and a split-dam technique may avoid interference with the seating of the veneer cervically (Figure 12.27). A cellulose strip should be placed between

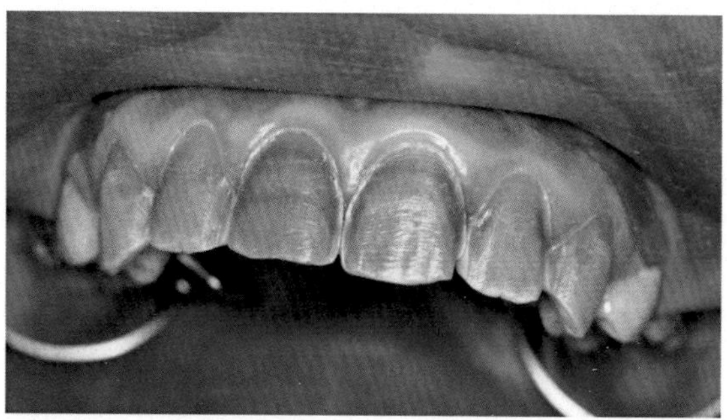

Figure 12.27 Teeth isolated using a split rubber dam technique, in preparation for cementation of veneers.

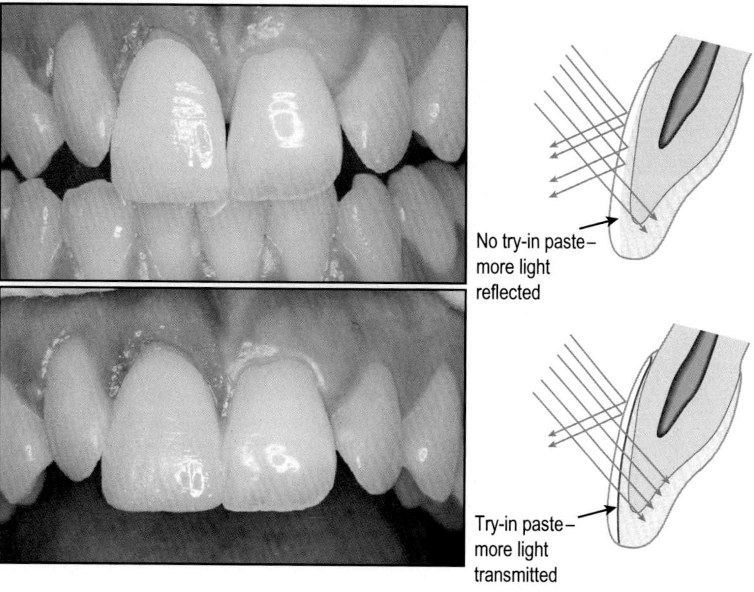

Figure 12.26 Ceramic veneer try-in; with no try-in paste above and with a neutral try-in paste below. Note that the veneer looks lighter when no try-in paste is used due to greater reflection of light from the veneer surface and the veneer tooth interface – placement of a try-in paste and the definitive luting cement lead to more light transmission.

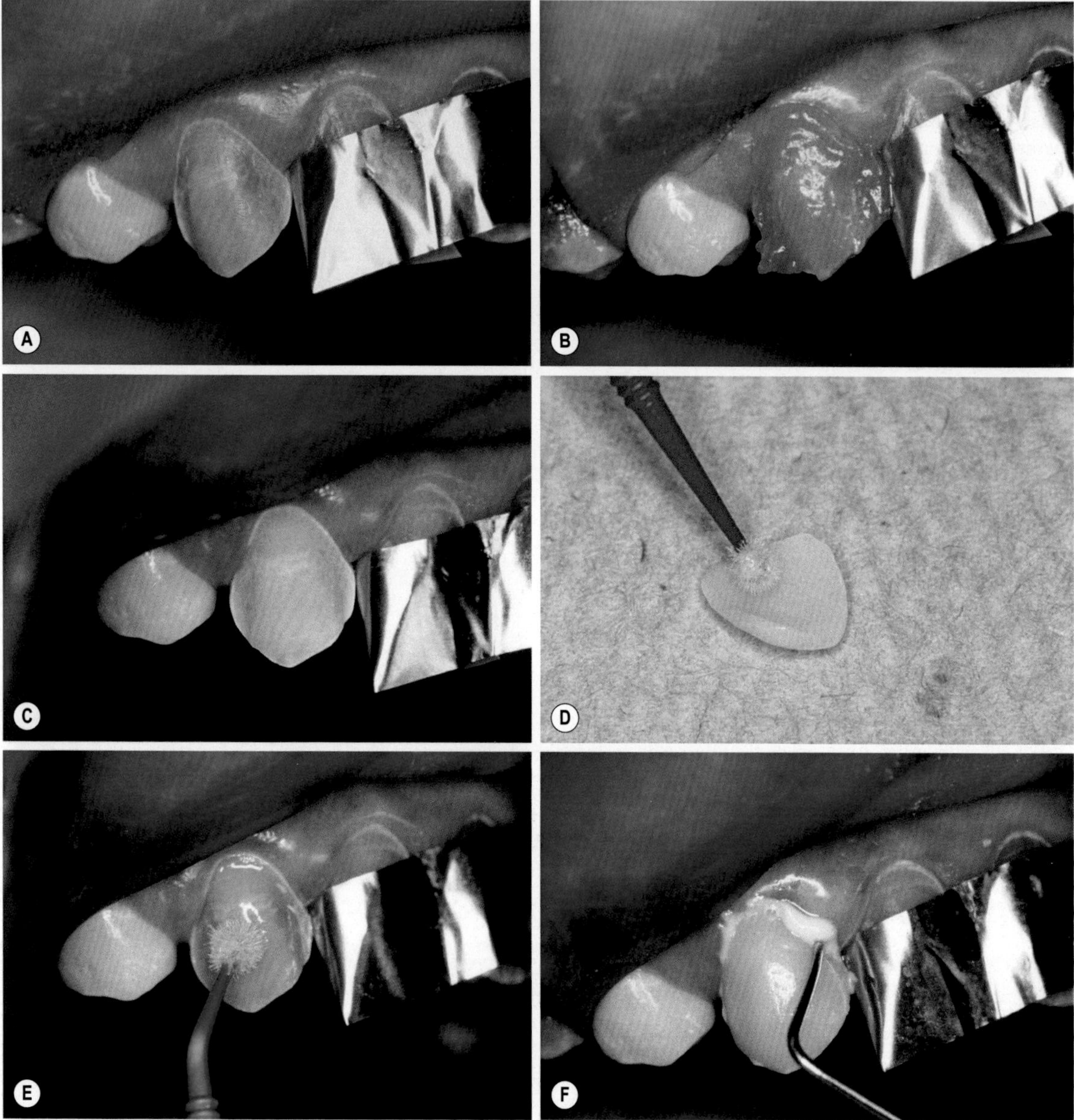

Figure 12.28 Stages in cementing a ceramic veneer. Tooth isolation (**A**), acid etch tooth (**B**), rinse and dry thoroughly (**C**), apply silane coupling agent to veneer (**D**), apply bond to tooth (**E**), load the veneer with resin luting cement and seat, removing excess before light curing (**F**).

the teeth to avoid bonding adjacent teeth together. If difficulty is experienced with access to the tooth due to the cellulose strip, a soft, thin, malleable metal strip can be used instead which can be moulded around the contact point of the adjacent teeth, giving better access (Figure 12.28).

Once the prepared tooth has been acid etched, rinsed, dried, bond applied and cured, the resin luting cement can be loaded onto the fit surface of the veneer and seated (Figure 12.28). Excess cement can be removed with a microbrush dipped in resin and the cement light cured, as most resin luting cements used for cementing veneers are dual cured. It is better to leave a little excess luting cement which can be trimmed away and polished, rather than overzealously trying to remove all excess which can lead to cement lute being dragged out from the veneer–tooth interface.

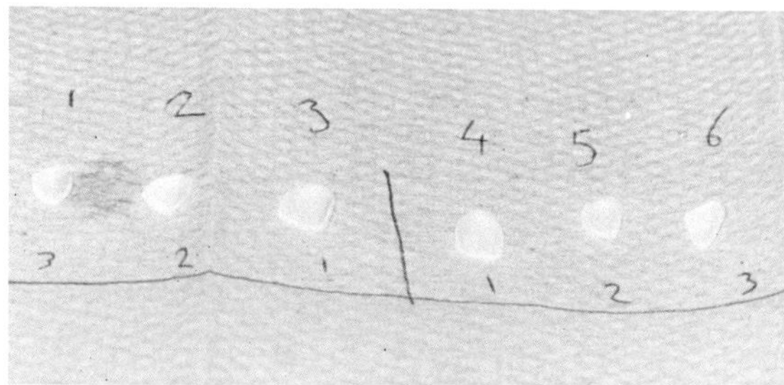

Figure 12.29 Veneers for patient seen in Figure 12.27. The order in which the veneers were tried-in was from right to left. It is important to repeat the same order when cementing so as not to alter the paths of insertion.

When cementing multiple veneers, each veneer should be tried-in individually to assess fit and appearance. The veneers then need to be tried-in *en masse* and the order in which they are seated should be recorded (Figure 12.29). This order should be repeated when they are finally cemented to avoid problems that can arise with different paths of insertion when a different order of cementation is used.

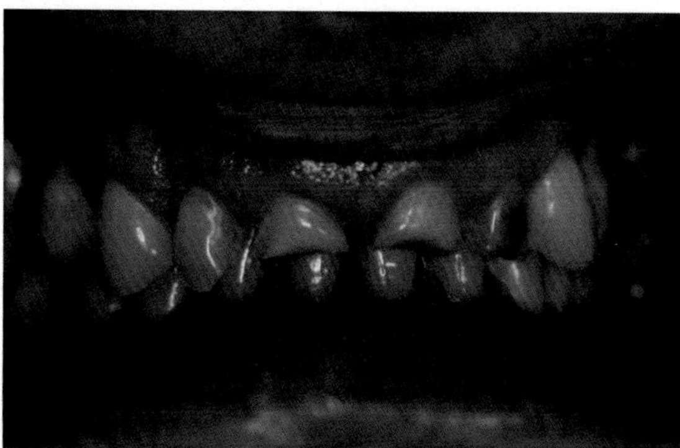

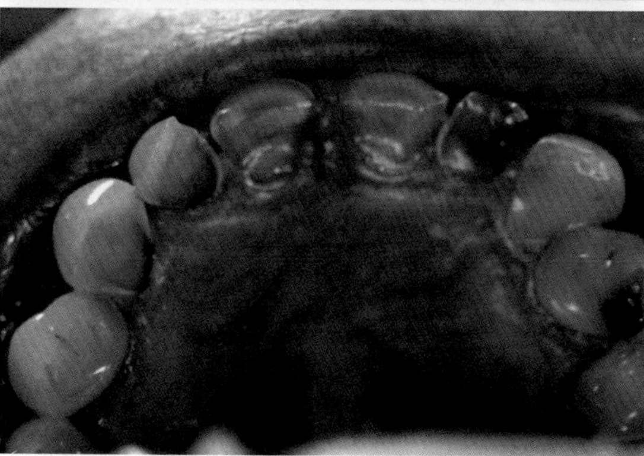

Figure 12.30 This patient has tooth wear affecting the palatal surfaces of the upper anterior teeth. The incisors are short and require crowns; the canines are only affected palatally and require gold palatal veneers.

GOLD VENEERS

Tooth wear can either affect the entire dentition or can be localized, typically to the upper anterior teeth (see Chapter 4). The pattern of tooth tissue loss can also vary. Consider the patient in Figure 12.30: all of the upper anterior teeth are worn palatally, but only the incisors have lost crown height and require crowns. The palatal wear on the canine teeth can simply be restored with gold alloy veneers, the tooth wear having effectively prepared the teeth so that no further preparation is required (Figure 12.31). Originally high copper gold alloys were oxidized or tin plated to achieve improved bond strengths with adhesive resin luting cements such as Panavia (Kuraray Dental). However, recent data (Chana et al., 2000) have shown that sandblasting gold veneers with alumina and cementation with Panavia 21 leads to clinically acceptable survival rates.

Where tooth wear occurs labially as well as palatally, some clinicians have suggested 'double veneers', that is, gold palatal veneers and ceramic labial veneers. Although this might be modestly more conservative of tooth tissue, the multiple interfaces between veneers and tooth tissue make these restorations less predictable than metal–ceramic crowns and the latter are usually favoured in such a clinical scenario.

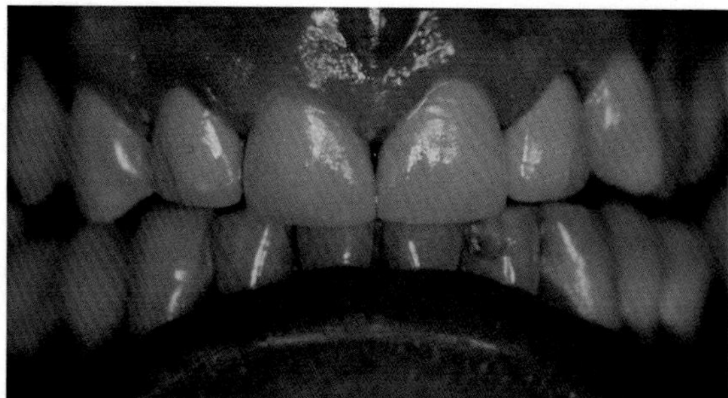

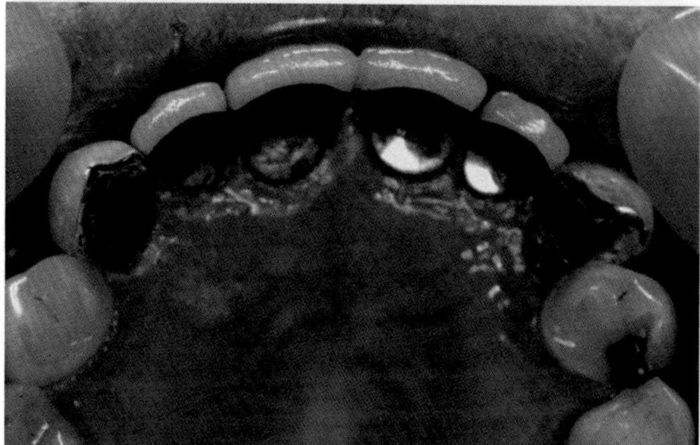

Figure 12.31 Patient seen in Figure 12.30, with metal–ceramic crowns placed on the incisor teeth and palatal gold veneers on the canine teeth.

SUMMARY

Inlays and onlays often provide a conservative alternative to full coverage crown preparations for the restoration of heavily restored teeth which are either not suitable for direct restorations or where direct restorations have failed. Similarly, ceramic veneers can alter the appearance of teeth, avoiding the need for more destructive all-ceramic or metal–ceramic crowns. However, the merits of directly placed composites should not be overlooked.

FURTHER READING

Chana, H., Kelleher, M., Briggs, P., Hooper, R., 2000. Clinical evaluation of resin-bonded gold alloy veneers. J. Prosthet. Dent. 83, 294–300.

Della Bona, A., Kelly, J.R., 2008. The clinical success of all-ceramic restorations. J. Am. Dent. Assoc. 139 (Suppl), 8S–13S.

Manhart, J., Chen, H., Hamm, G., Hickel, R., 2004. Buonocore Memorial Lecture. Review of the clinical survival of direct and indirect restorations in posterior teeth of the permanent dentition. Oper. Dent. 29, 481–508.

Mjör, I.A., Davis, M.E., Abu-Hanna, A., 2008. CAD/CAM restorations and secondary caries: a literature review with illustrations. Dent. Update 35, 118–120.

Peumans, M., Van Meerbeek, B., Lambrechts, P., Vanherle, G., 2000. Porcelain veneers: a review of the literature. J. Dent. 28, 163–177.

Sadowsky, S.J., 2006. An overview of treatment considerations for esthetic restorations: a review of the literature. J. Prosthet. Dent. 96, 433–442.

Chapter 13

Impression materials and techniques

David Ricketts

CHAPTER CONTENTS

INTRODUCTION

Impressions of teeth and related structures are taken for making implants, crowns, bridges and dentures, and the material selected will partly depend on the personal choice of the clinician and the use. The choice of impression tray used will also be dictated by the impression material and its viscosity. Impression materials used for advanced operative procedures such as crown and bridgework must have elastic properties to allow the removal from undercut areas in the mouth without creating permanent distortion; these can be either water based (hydrocolloids) or synthetic elastomers.

THE MATERIALS

Hydrocolloid impression materials

Agar is an example of a *reversible hydrocolloid* impression material. It consists of long chain polysaccharide molecules and water. When cool, the polysaccharide chains are linked together by hydrogen bonds between hydroxyl groups on the polysaccharide chains, resulting in the characteristic gel. When the temperature is raised, the hydrogen bonds are broken and the gel liquefies; on cooling again the gel state reforms, hence the name 'reversible hydrocolloid'. Whilst it is a hydrophilic material and gives an accurate impression, it suffers from a number of disadvantages, namely it is dimensionally unstable and needs to be cast up within 1 hour, it has low tear resistance, is hot and uncomfortable on insertion and requires additional equipment such as

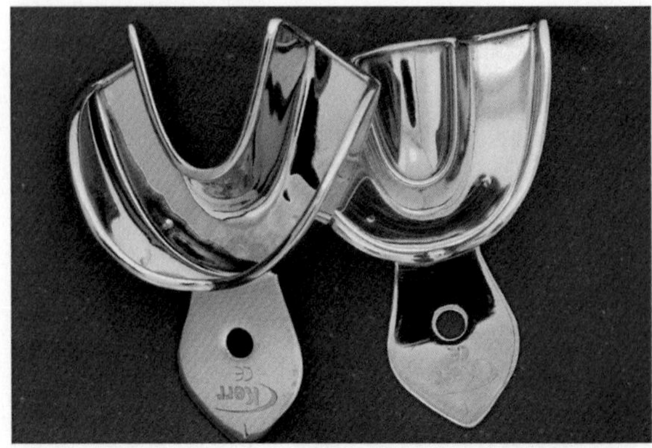

Figure 13.2 Metal non-perforated impression stock trays. The rolled metal rim affords some degree of retention to the set impression material; however, an adhesive is also required.

specially designed water baths, impression trays and tubing (for the water coolant). The use of a water bath is a major drawback in relation to contamination and problems with cross infection control; as such, the material is rarely used in contemporary practice.

Alginate is an *irreversible hydrocolloid* material whose main ingredients are sodium alginate, calcium sulphate dihydrate and inert filler particles. Alginates are long polysaccharide chains derived from a marine plant (seaweed). It is presented as a powder which is mixed with water. When this is done a setting reaction takes place which involves the calcium ions irreversibly cross-linking the polysaccharide chains, so converting the sol into a gel. This would be a rapid reaction if a retardant was not added. Sodium phosphate is therefore added which preferentially reacts with the released calcium ions forming calcium phosphate; the calcium ions initially are therefore not available to cross-link the polymer chains. Once all of the sodium phosphate has been used up in this reaction, the remaining calcium released is used in forming the cross-linkages and the gel. The filler particles give the set material its rigidity.

Alginate is a commonly used material but suffers from the same disadvantages of the reversible hydrocolloids, that is, they have poor tear resistance and are dimensional unstable. If alginate impressions are stored dry, they dry and shrink; if stored under water, they imbibe water (imbibition) and swell. In addition, the impression is not as detailed as that taken with a synthetic elastomer and therefore not suitable for impressions of crown and bridge preparations; its main use is for study casts and opposing models.

Before taking the impression an appropriately sized impression tray should be selected (Figure 13.1). A perforated plastic stock tray is ideal for this as the material is not too viscous and should not distort the tray on seating. Such trays are for single use only and would distort if heated during a decontamination process. Although a metal tray could be used as an alternative (Figure 13.2), thorough cleaning and decontamination of the trays between patients is time consuming and, as such, disposable single-use plastic trays are more popular and cost effective. A tray should be selected that seats fully over the dentate arch with its flanges not bedding into the soft tissues of the buccal, labial and lingual sulci. Occasionally, the stock tray needs modifying with impression compound to increase its extension to completely cover the dentition and areas of interest.

Despite the fact that stock trays have perforations and ridges to retain the set impression material in the tray, a tray adhesive should also be used. Alginate adhesive is supplied either in a bottle for use with a brush or in an aerosol can (Figure 13.3). Brushing the adhesive on the fit surface of the tray and just over its flanges ensures an

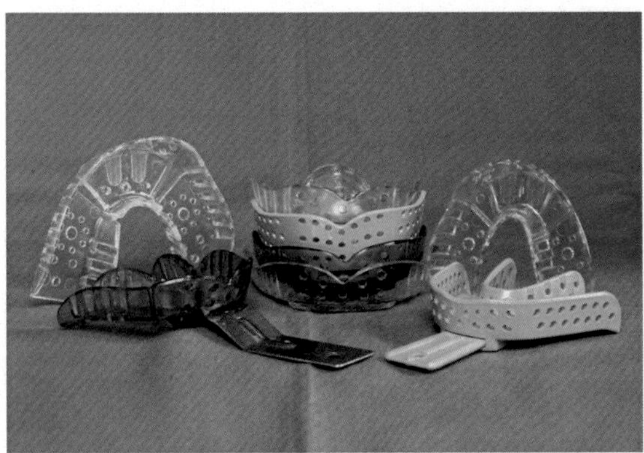

Figure 13.1 Selection of impression stock trays. Light blue plastic (opaque) trays are suitable for alginate impressions. Clear coloured polycarbonate trays are more rigid and are suitable for more viscous elastomeric impression materials. Three colour-coded sizes are seen.

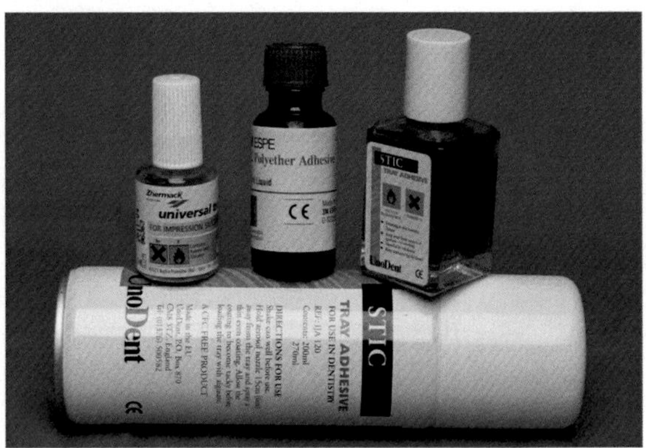

Figure 13.3 Selection of tray adhesives. The alginate adhesive is provided as either paint on (top right) or aerosol (bottom). A universal adhesive can be used for silicone impression materials (top left) and a specific polyether adhesive (top centre) should be used for polyethers such as Impregum (3M ESPE).

even thin layer of adhesive; however, the adhesive needs to be dispensed into a disposable dappens pot first and applied with a single-use brush to prevent contamination of the adhesive in the bottle. To simplify matters and avoid problems with cross-infection control, aerosol adhesives can be used. The work surface should be covered with a paper napkin and the fit surface sprayed with an even thin application of adhesive. Before use the adhesive should be dry and tacky; if the adhesive is applied too thickly it will not dry and will act as a lubricant, with the risk of the impression material pulling away from the tray on withdrawal from the mouth.

When mixing alginate it is important to use the correct proportion of powder to water. To achieve this, manufacturers provide a measuring scoop for the powder and a measuring cylinder for the water. Before use the powder should be stirred in its container to thoroughly mix the ingredients and to ensure the material has not become compacted during storage. The number of scoops of powder will be dictated by the size of the impression tray and the patient's mouth. The powder is mixed with the correct amount of water and evenly combined in a mixing bowl. Most alginate materials have a mixing time of about 1 minute. The mixed alginate is then loaded into the impression tray to the level of the flanges and posterior extremity using a spatula. Overloading the tray should be avoided as this will lead to difficulty in seating the impression in the mouth and will be unpleasant for the patient, with a risk of obstructing the airway.

When taking alginate impressions the patient should be seated upright in the dental chair with their head at about the elbow height of the operator. Once the tray has been loaded with alginate, a portion of alginate can be scooped up on the operator's finger and smeared over the occlusal surfaces of the teeth and any areas of importance. Rubbing the material into fine recesses such as pits and fissures reduces the risk of incorporating any air bubbles. The loaded impression tray is then seated before the smeared alginate starts to set (single-stage technique). For the lower impression, if right handed, the operator should stand on the patient's right-hand side facing the patient. The impression tray is then rotated into the mouth, with that part of the tray on the patient's left entering first. Once the tray is over the dentate arch the lips should be retracted before seating the tray, allowing the alginate material to flow into the sulci. The patient should then be asked to raise the tongue over the tray to mould the lingual sulcus and the material in the buccal and labial sulci can be moulded with external light pressure on cheeks and lips. If the operator is left handed they should stand on the patient's left-hand side and carry out the procedure in a similar mirror fashion.

The upper impression is taken in a similar way, with the exception that the operator now stands behind the patient's right shoulder (if right handed) and the tray is rotated into the mouth with the patient's right side of tray first. Once positioned over the dental arch, the tray should be seated posteriorly first, lifting the lip up and out when seating the tray anteriorly. This ensures that the impression material flows forwards and not backwards towards the patient's throat. If the patient retches it is important not to remove the tray when the material is unset, but ask the patient to lean forwards and breathe deeply through their nose. This should effectively close the oral cavity from the oropharynx and prevent material flowing posteriorly.

The speed with which the material sets can be altered by the manufacturer, and regular and rapid-set materials are available with working and setting times ranging from 1 to 4 minutes depending on the material chosen. The setting time can also be influenced by the temperature of the water; using warmer water will speed up the setting reaction. Alginate when initially mixed is alkaline (pH $\approx$11) but when set is near neutral. Some manufacturers have taken advantage of this and include a pH indicator which changes colour with the pH. Once set, the tray should be removed from the mouth with a rapid technique. This is because the material is viscoelastic and if removed rapidly elastic recovery should take place; slow removal from undercuts would lead to distortion of the material.

Once removed from the mouth any saliva should be rinsed off the surface and the impression should be decontaminated; prolonged immersion in a disinfectant solution leads to distortion of irreversible hydrocolloid impression materials. Ideally, if there is a laboratory facility, the impression should be cast within 30–60 minutes. If not, the impression should be stored at 100% humidity by wrapping the impression in wet gauze or a napkin and placing it in a sealable plastic bag during transit to the laboratory.

The impression provides the technician with a negative mould into which stone can be poured. This is done by holding the impression over a vibrator so that air bubbles in the stone rise to the surface as the material flows into all recesses. Once the impression is filled to the level of the sulcus, it is inverted and based onto stone mounded up on the bench top. Once the stone has set the impression can be removed and the excess stone trimmed. The alginate impression should not be left on the cast for any period after the stone has set as it dries out and becomes difficult to remove.

Elastomeric impression materials

Impressions for indirect restorations need to be accurate to record fine detail of tooth preparations and they need to be dimensionally stable with time. Usually there is a delay in taking the impressions and casting them up as most practices do not have a laboratory on site and have to send impressions through the post. An ideal impression material should also have good elastic recovery when it is used in undercut situations and should have good tear resistance. The synthetic elastomeric materials in general meet these high demands. The elastomeric impression materials available are silicones (addition and condensation cured) and polyethers. Historically, *polysulphide* impression materials were included in the list of elastomeric impression materials and favoured by some for their long setting time; however, they are rarely used in contemporary practice due to a list of disadvantages which include an unpleasant smell, shrinkage on storage resulting in distorted dies, and the need to use it in conjunction with a laboratory-made special tray.

Silicones

Addition cured silicones

The most commonly used elastomeric impression material is the *addition cured silicone*. These materials consist of polyvinyl siloxane polymer chains which have terminal vinyl groups that are cross-linked by a silanol (present in the base paste) in the presence of a platinum catalyst (present in the catalyst paste). No by-products are produced during the setting reaction and, as such, the material is dimensionally stable.

Manufacturers usually produce addition cured silicone base and catalyst in putty, heavy bodied, medium bodied and light bodied forms dependent on the amount of filler content. Base and catalyst with the same viscosities are mixed together. Usually addition cured silicones are used in a two-phase, single-stage technique using a stock tray.

A two-phase, single-stage technique

The *two-phase* (or twin mix) refers to the fact that two viscosity materials are used to take a single impression, with a light body wash being syringed around the tooth preparation to record the fine detail and either a heavy body or putty material loaded into the tray to take up the bulk of space between the preparation and the tray. The wash is syringed around the tooth preparation whilst the dental nurse is mixing the heavy body or putty and loading it into the stock tray (Figure 13.4); the heavier bodied materials have the benefit that they do not flow from the tray. Before the wash begins to set, the loaded tray is seated over the teeth, with the heavier bodied material forcing the low viscosity wash into the intricate recesses around the tooth preparation (Figure 13.5). Both wash and heavier bodied materials set at the same time, hence the term *single-stage technique*.

Most light bodied materials are now supplied in dual cartridges (base and catalyst) which are loaded into guns onto which double helix mixer tips are attached (Figure 13.6). As the gun is activated, the plungers express the base and catalyst through the mixer tip which ensures a perfectly proportioned, bubble-free mix of base and catalyst. A small amount of material should be syringed onto a pad or bracket table to allow its setting to be monitored. Occasionally, especially with new cartridges, air inclusions at the end of either the base or catalyst cartridge mean that only one or other of the materials exits the mixer tip in an unmixed state which will obviously not set. Syringing the material onto the bracket table first ensures only mixed material is syringed around the teeth.

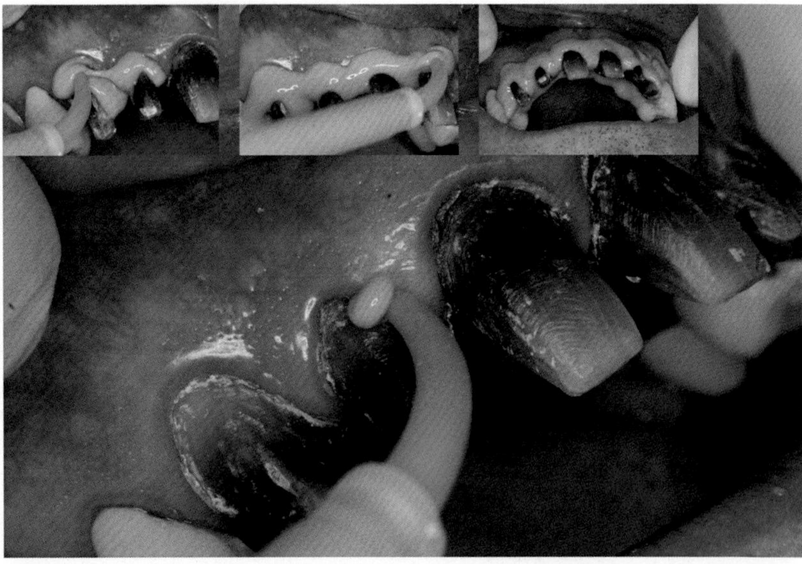

Figure 13.4 Light bodied wash being syringed around upper anterior tooth preparations.

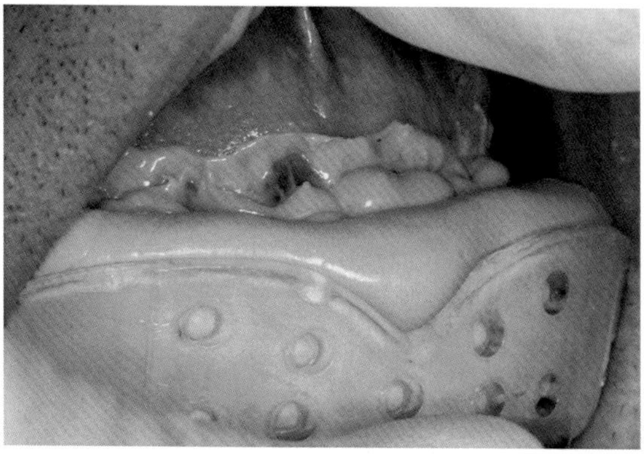

Figure 13.5 Putty in stock tray being seated over wash before it starts to set.

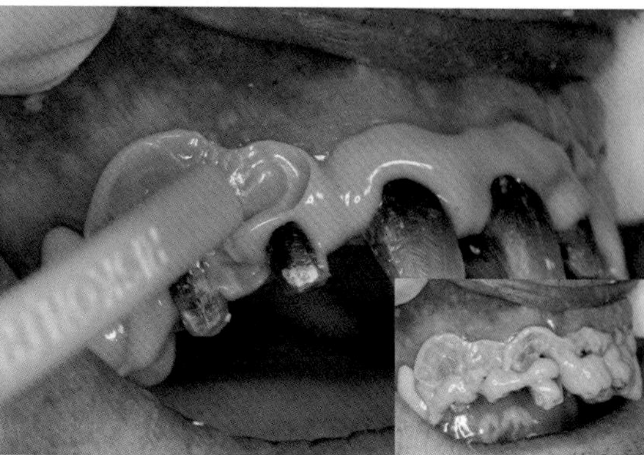

Figure 13.7 Air blown onto light bodied wash, dispersing it into recesses of the preparation.

The fine tips that attach to the double helix mixers allow the mixed material to be deposited at the preparation margins and internal recesses such as slots and grooves (see Figure 13.4). Some clinicians advocate gently blowing air through the three-in-one syringe to disperse the wash and to blow it into areas such as the gingival sulcus (Figure 13.7). Care should be taken if this is done as too strong an air pressure could lead to air being incorporated into the wash with resultant bubbles in the set impression or the wash could be simply blown off the prepared tooth. The latter is more likely if there is moisture contamination on the tooth surface.

Putty materials are usually provided in tubs with colour-coded scoops for colour-coded base and catalysts, respectively; cross contamination of scoops should be avoided. Equal proportions of the base and catalyst are mixed by hand until an even, streak-free mix is obtained. As the set of some addition cured silicone materials is inhibited by residues from latex gloves, the materials should be mixed with vinyl or nitrile gloves donned; most manufacturers are overcoming this problem but if in doubt avoid latex gloves. Some putty and heavy bodied materials are provided in cartridges for use in an electrically driven Pentamix automatic mixing unit (3M ESPE) with a double helix mixer tip, giving all of the advantages that the corresponding tips have for mixing the light bodied materials (Figure 13.8).

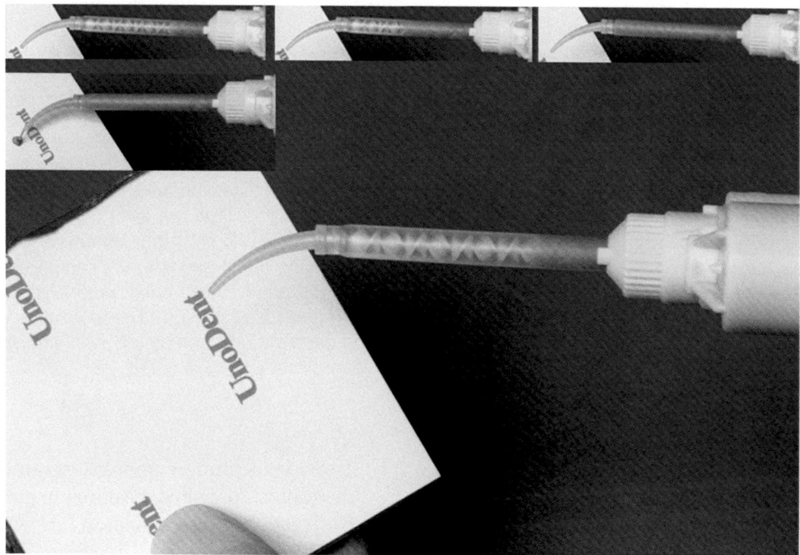

Figure 13.6 Light bodied wash cartridge containing separate base and catalyst loaded into a mixing gun to which is attached a double helix mixer tip.

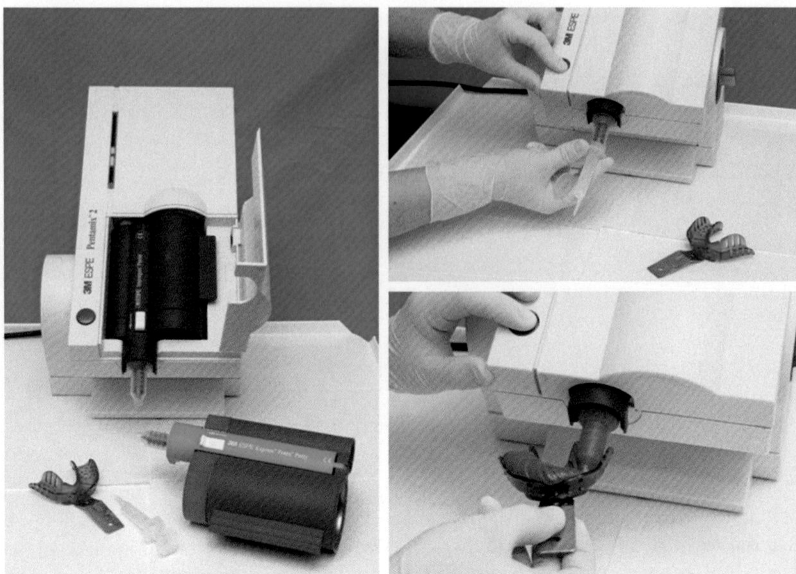

Figure 13.8 Pentamix for automated mixing of polyethers and heavy bodied impression materials (left). Polyether being loaded into a syringe (top right) and the impression tray (bottom right).

A rigid plastic or polycarbonate tray is required for such an impression technique as the heavier bodied materials could distort less rigid trays on seating (see Figure 13.1). Metal trays could be used but with caution; if the materials set into deep undercuts, removal might be difficult and in this situation sectioning the tray to salvage the situation would be almost impossible. Despite the fact that most trays have perforations and ridges to retain the impression material, an appropriate adhesive for addition cured silicones must be used (see Figure 13.3).

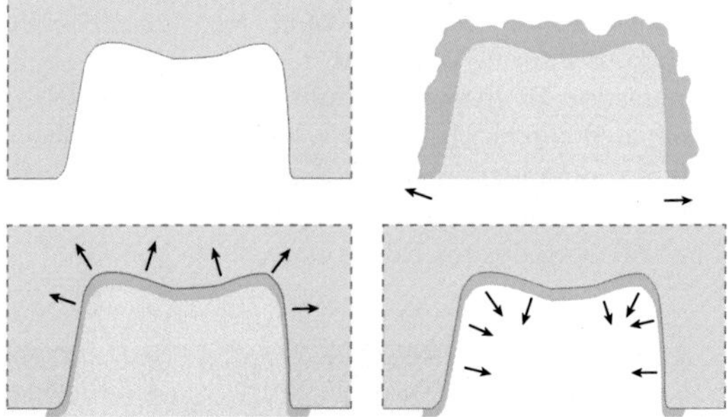

Figure 13.9 Diagrammatic representation of a two-phase, two-stage impression technique. First the putty or heavy bodied impression is taken and allowed to set (top left). Wash is syringed around the tooth preparation (top right) and before it is set the first stage impression is reseated. As this is a good 'fit' there is little space for the wash to escape and compression of the first stage impression occurs (bottom left). On removing the impression, the compressed impression recoils and provides an imprint (impression) of the prepared tooth which is smaller (bottom right). A crown made on this model will be too small and will not fit the prepared tooth.

Two-phase, two-stage technique

As previously described, the two-phase technique refers to the fact that two viscosity materials are used, usually putty or heavy body and wash. However, the two-stage aspect refers to the fact that, in the first stage, the putty or heavy bodied material is seated in the mouth, allowed to set and then removed. The second stage to the impression involves syringing the wash around the tooth preparation(s) and, before it sets, reseating the putty or heavy bodied impression over it. This forces the wash into all the recesses of the preparation. The wash, however, takes up space and on reseating the putty impression, compression of the putty occurs (Figure 13.9). When the impression is removed the putty recoils and the distorted impression will result in a smaller die of a full coverage crown preparation, for example. The risk of distortion using this technique can be reduced in two ways which provide space for the wash between the tooth preparation and primary impression:

- The first or primary impression can be taken before the tooth is prepared, resulting in greater space for the wash once tooth preparation has been carried out. However, gauging how much wash to use to completely fill this space without leaving voids is difficult.

- Use of a cellophane spacer over the tooth preparation provides a small space but distortion of the primary impression is still a high risk.

To reduce the risk of distortion further, V-shaped grooves can be cut into the primary impression that corresponds to the area between the tooth preparation and the buccal (and where possible lingual) sulcus. This effectively allows venting of the wash without excessive build-up of pressure and distortion of the putty.

Wherever possible the two-stage technique should be avoided with addition cured silicones. In addition to the problems associated with distortion of the impression, reseating rigid putty materials may be difficult, especially where there are deep undercuts.

Condensation cured silicones

Condensation cured silicones also consist of polyvinyl siloxane polymer chains and filler particles in a base paste; however, in these materials, the polymer chains end with hydroxyl terminal groups. The catalyst or activator paste contains tetraethyl silicate molecules which can cross-link up to three polyvinyl siloxane polymer chains at a time. This cross-linkage setting reaction is accompanied by the release of alcohol groups as a by-product. The release of alcohol during the setting reaction also makes the material less dimensionally stable, with the greatest shrinkage with time of all the elastomeric materials. As with addition cured materials, manufacturers produce various viscosity base pastes, but the activator paste is often of a different viscosity from the heavier bodied materials, making mixing more difficult.

Condensation cured silicones can be used in either a single-stage impression technique or a two-stage technique. In the two-stage technique any compression of the primary putty impression on reseating over the wash during the secondary impression will be compensated for to some degree by the shrinkage of the material. Compression and shrinkage cannot, however, be accurately predicted and the condensation cured materials are therefore not as accurate as the addition cured materials.

Polyethers

Polyethers are presented as a base and activator paste of the same viscosity. Unlike the silicone impression materials, polyethers are only available in one viscosity and are therefore an example of a monophase impression material; the same viscosity material is syringed around the tooth preparation(s) as is loaded into the impression tray. It is therefore a monophase material that should always be used in a single-stage technique. Polyethers have good elastic properties and are particularly suited for implant prosthodontics.

The base paste of a polyether contains inert fillers and polyether polymer chains which terminate in an amine group. These polymer chains are cross-linked by an aromatic sulphonate ester in the activator paste, which also contains inert filler particles. There are no by-products to this setting reaction and, as such, the material is dimensionally stable; however, since the materials will take up water, the set impression should be stored dry. Polyethers which are presented in tubes for manual mixing on a pad are messy and difficult to mix and it is for this impression material that the Pentamix was originally designed (see Figure 13.8). Polyether impressions should be cast within a few days as prolonged storage leads to deterioration of the material.

GENERAL CONSIDERATIONS FOR ELASTOMERIC IMPRESSION MATERIALS

Blocking out undercuts

The most commonly used elastomeric impression materials are the addition cured silicones and polyethers and these materials are the most rigid once set. It is therefore important prior to taking any impression in these materials to check intraorally for undercuts into which the materials may flow and become lodged once set. Common undercuts to look out for are buccal undercuts in the sulcus, periodontal bone loss and large interdental spaces and recesses beneath bridge pontics (Figure 13.10).

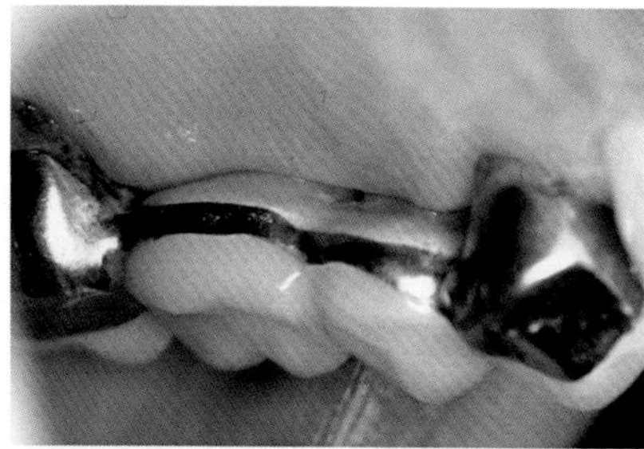

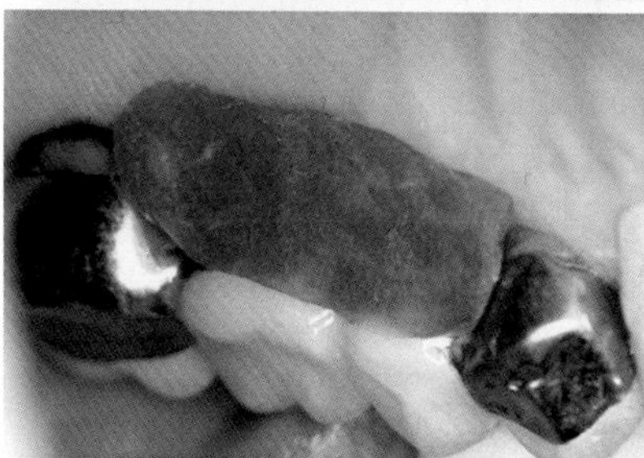

Figure 13.10 An elastomeric impression material could flow into the recess beneath the bridge pontics and make removal of the impression difficult once set as they are relatively rigid and have a high tear resistance. Such recesses (undercuts) can be blocked out with soft wax.

Undercuts can simply be blocked out intraorally by placing soft wax, ensuring the wax does not interfere with the occlusion and appearance in the aesthetic zone.

Protecting the dentine

Preparation of teeth for indirect ceramic or composite restorations, in particular full coverage crowns, leads to freshly cut dentinal tubules. These tooth-coloured restorations should be cemented with resin luting cements and a systematic review of the literature has suggested that the dentine could be sealed with a dentine bonding agent prior to taking an impression. This so-called immediate dentine seal (IDS) protects the pulp during the drying and impression taking, leads to improved bond strengths when the indirect restoration is cemented, and reduced microleakage and postoperative dentine hypersensitivity (Magne, 2005). Whether these findings can be extrapolated to metal-based restorations will depend on the subsequent luting cement used; if it is resin based, similar findings might be expected.

Keeping a dry environment

All elastomeric materials suffer from the major drawback of being hydrophobic. The degree to which a material is hydrophobic or hydrophilic is reflected in its ability to wet a surface; this is measured by the contact angle of water on the material's surface. Polyethers are less hydrophobic (contact angle 49°) than addition cured silicones (contact angle 98°). Some manufacturers have tried to overcome the problem of the highly hydrophobic silicones by adding surfactants to their materials; however, no elastomeric material can be regarded as hydrophilic and impression-taking techniques demand that the teeth are perfectly dry.

Whilst it is important to take alginate impressions (especially the upper) with the patient sitting in the upright position, most elastomeric materials are viscous or do not flow unless placed under pressure. This, together with the fact that the teeth need to be dry, necessitates that the impressions are taken with the patient lying back. It is only then that the teeth in question can be adequately dried with a three-in-one syringe and isolated with cotton wool rolls or absorbent pads and a saliva ejector placed to remove excess saliva. Once the wash has been syringed around the preparation, the cotton wool pads and saliva ejector have to be removed quickly prior to seating the loaded impression tray. Cotton wool embedded into the impression prevents appropriate decontamination prior to sending to the laboratory.

Checking the impression

When using the two-phase, single-stage impression technique, speed is of the essence. The wash should be in an unset state when the putty is seated. Once the impression material has set it is important to evaluate the impression for accuracy and any potential faults in relation to the prepared teeth:

- The wash should have merged imperceptibly with the putty (Figure 13.11). If there is a demarcated line between the wash and the putty, this indicates that the wash had started to set before the putty was seated (Figure 13.12).The impression must be retaken as the set wash is likely to have distorted under the pressure of seating the putty.
- All preparation margins should be clearly visible (Figure 13.11), with no drags or air bubbles. Taking an impression of subgingival margins can be difficult.
- No drags or defects between the putty and wash should be found corresponding to the axial walls of the preparation, internal line angles or recesses such as slots, grooves and boxes.

Focus has been placed on taking an impression of the tooth or teeth that have been prepared for indirect restorations; however, it is important to ensure that an adequate impression of the entire arch is made to ensure that the occlusion and shape of the remaining teeth can be recorded. Once the wash has been syringed around the prepared teeth, it can then be syringed into the pits and fissures of posterior teeth or areas of particular interest. Alternatively, where two-phase, single-stage impressions are concerned, wash can be syringed into the loaded impression tray corresponding to the arch form.

The impression should also be checked for errors elsewhere and areas remote from the site of the prepared tooth. This is important to confirm that a model can be produced, not only to ensure that a restoration can be made on the master die, but also to ensure that the occlusion can be formed correctly. For example, an impression might be taken of a lower molar tooth for a gold crown. Although the impression might be satisfactory for construction of the crown margins, a drag labial to the lower incisors might prevent upper and lower models seating together in a Class I incisor relationship and hence inability to check the occlusion. Occasionally the impression will pull away from the impression tray, distorting the occlusal plane. In these situations the impression should be retaken.

GINGIVAL MANAGEMENT – RETRACTION

Chapter 2 emphasized the importance of establishing periodontal health prior to the placement of indirect restorations. If this is achieved and careful tooth preparation is carried out with appropriate placement of cervical margins, there is little need for gingival management or retraction prior to taking an impression. Wherever possible preparation margins should be placed supragingivally;

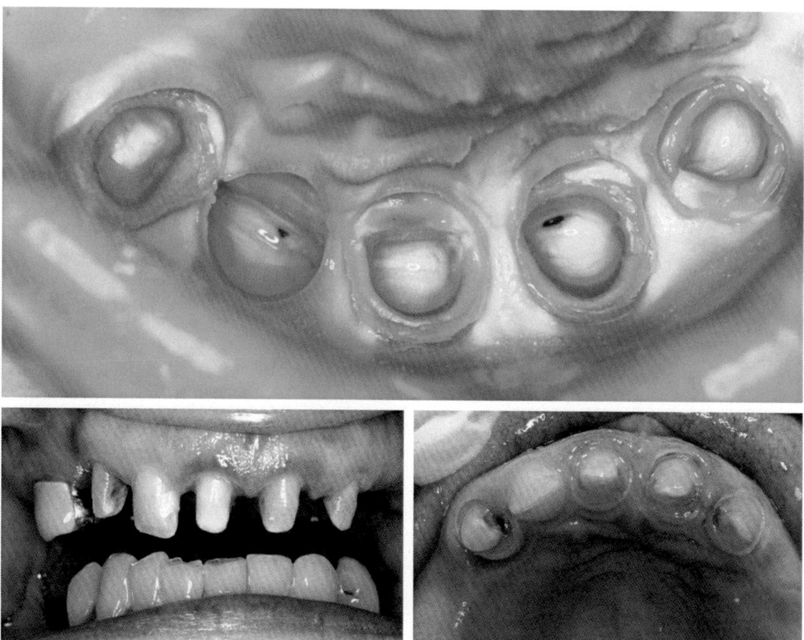

Figure 13.11 An addition cured silicone putty (light blue) and wash (dark blue) impression of five upper anterior teeth. Failed porcelain jacket crowns have been removed from four of the teeth, hence the shoulder preparations. The upper right lateral incisor has a minimal veneer preparation. All margins are visible in the impression, the wash has merged with the putty and no bubbles, drags or defects are visible. The impression tray is visible in two areas, but this is unlikely to have any impact on the model cast.

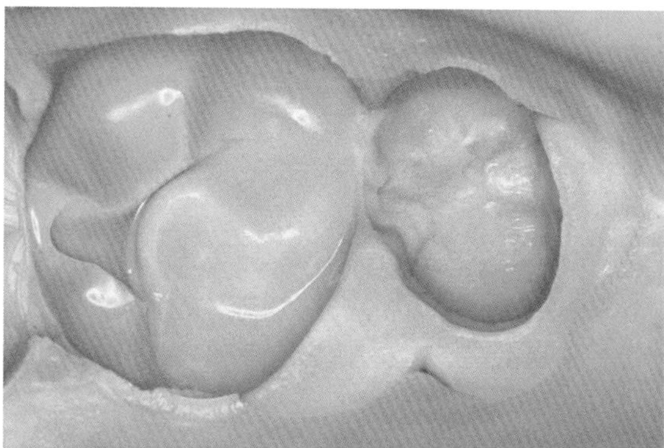

Figure 13.12 An impression for a resin retained cantilever bridge using the premolar tooth as an abutment. The impression of the mesial and distal rest seats are clear; however, the wash (orange) is demarcated from the putty (green), indicating that the wash had set before the putty was seated. The impression should be retaken.

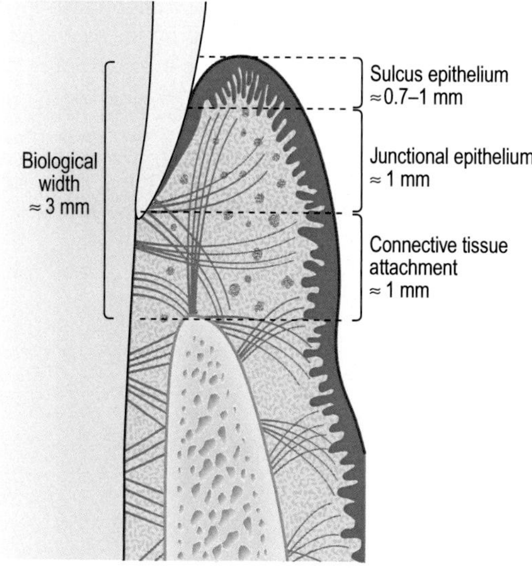

Figure 13.13 Diagrammatic representation of the biological width.

the closer the margins are to the gingivae, the greater will be the potential adverse effect on gingival health.

When considering indirect restoration margins in relation to gingival health it is important to reconsider the biological width. The supra-alveolar gingival apparatus consists of the gingival sulcus (0.7–1 mm), the junctional epithelium (≈1 mm) and the connective tissue attachment (≈1 mm), making up approximately 2.7–3 mm of biological width (Figure 13.13). The biological width makes up the body's natural defence mechanism and when

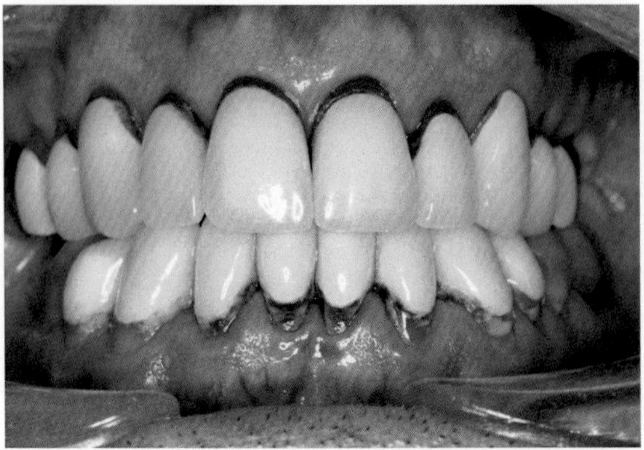

Figure 13.14 This patient has severe tetracycline staining. Original placement of the crown margins subgingivally to mask the discolouration encroached upon the biological width and led to attachment loss and recession. Poor oral hygiene has probably exacerbated the situation. Following successful basic periodontal treatment, further crowns will be required due to the patient's high lip line.

this is encroached upon, for example by a subgingival restoration, the body's reaction is to re-establish the biological width. This takes the form of alveolar bone loss, new connective tissue attachment, apical migration of the junctional epithelium and gingival recession, the crown margins now becoming supragingival (Figure 13.14).

Where appearance is of paramount importance in the aesthetic zone in patients with a high lip line, subgingival margins may have to be accepted as a compromise, but these should not extend deeper than 0.5 mm from the free gingival margin. If deep extensive restorations or short clinical crowns dictate that the margins should be more apically placed than this, surgical crown lengthening should be considered.

Occasionally a pragmatic approach has to be taken when a restoration margin extends subgingivally beyond the ideal 0.5 mm and crown lengthening is neither desirable nor appropriate. In these situations retraction of the gingiva has to be achieved in order to obtain an accurate impression of the tooth preparation margin and occasionally arrest haemorrhage. This can be achieved by mechanical retraction, chemomechanical retraction or surgical retraction. In any case a sulcus width of 0.2 mm or more is required to record the preparation margin accurately and have an adequate thickness of impression material for durability.

Mechanical retraction

Retraction cord

The most time-honoured method of mechanically retracting the gingival tissue is the use of retraction cord. Retraction cords can be twisted like a rope, braided or knitted, and are provided in different diameters (Figure 13.15). Plain retraction cord is placed into the gingival sulcus with a gentle packing technique using either a flat plastic instrument or a specially designed instrument which has a rounded, serrated head. A single length of retraction cord is usually packed into the sulcus for the full circumference of the tooth. Care must be taken not to use excessive pressure on packing retraction cord so as not to cause

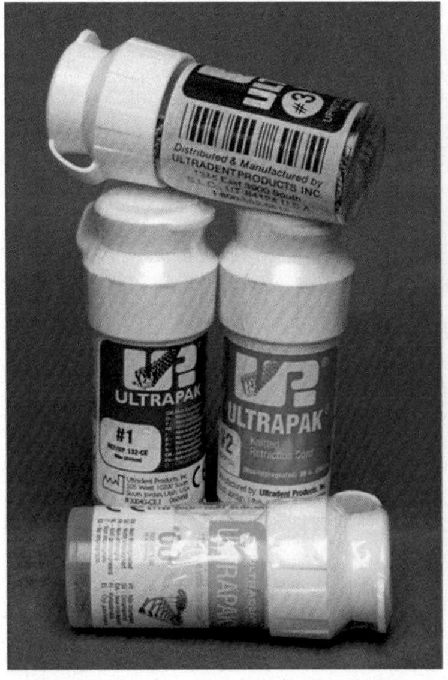

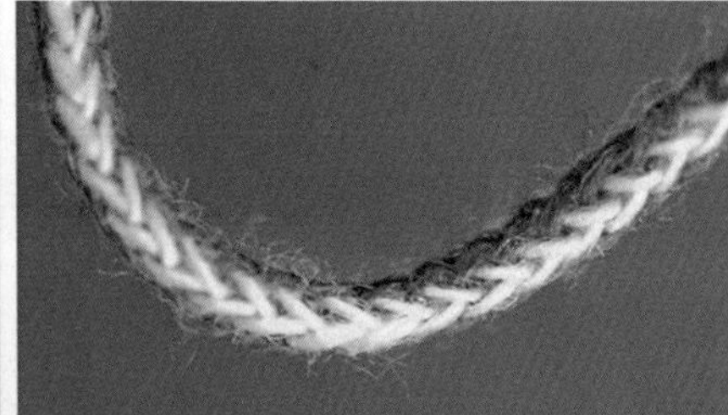

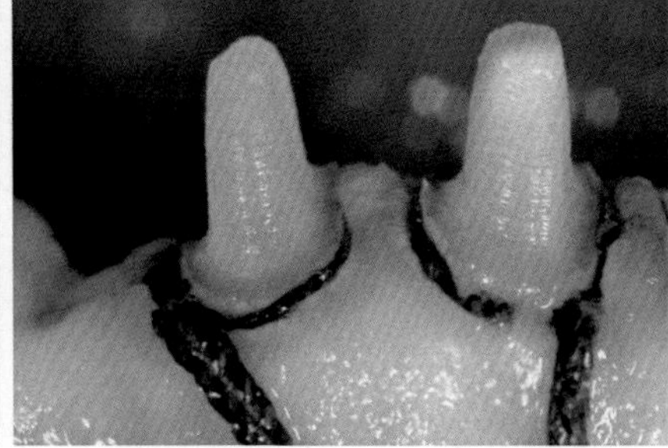

Figure 13.15 Knitted retraction cord in pots of various sizes (left). Magnified image of cord (top right) and placed in situ (bottom right).

trauma to the soft tissues, minimizing subsequent recession on healing.

Twisted retraction cord tends to unwind on packing and for this reason braided cords are easier to use. When retraction cord is used in its plain, untreated form to physically push the tissues away from the tooth, gingival crevicular fluid and/or blood becomes absorbed into it. Subsequent removal of the cord can cause trauma of the sulcus epithelium or can remove any blood clot, leading to haemorrhage and problems with impression taking. Wetting the retraction cord prior to removal and re-drying the preparation may reduce the risk of this happening.

Some clinicians may argue that the retraction cord should remain in situ whilst the impression is being taken, and some even advocate a double cord technique. In the latter, a narrow first cord is packed into the gingival sulcus and a second wider cord packed on top. Only the second cord is removed prior to taking the impression, leaving the first in situ during the impression to maintain the gingival retraction. If retraction cord is left in situ it is important to ensure that it lies beyond the preparation margin so that the impression material records the entire margin and just beyond. Retraction cord lying level with the preparation margin makes it impossible to record and see the margin on the subsequent model (Figure 13.16).

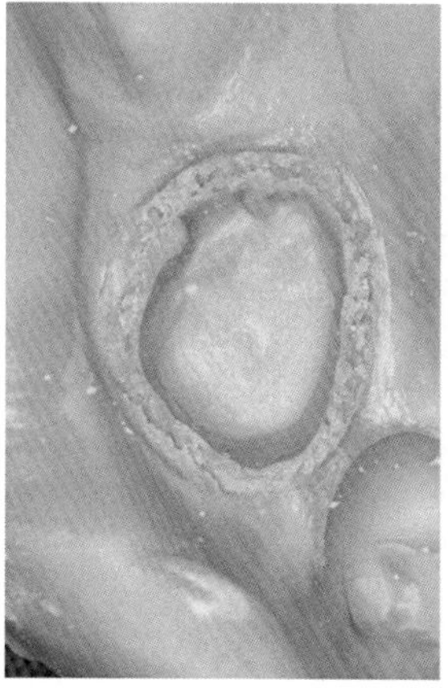
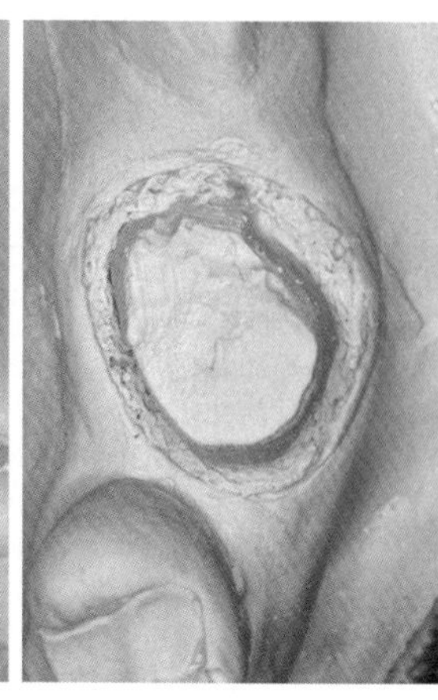

Figure 13.16 Retraction cord left in situ for impression taking (left) has led to an inaccurate impression and subsequent model (right). The retraction cord sat at the level of the crown preparation margin and, as a result, the crown preparation margins cannot be seen on impression or model.

Magic Foam Cord (Coltène Whaledent)

Possibly a less traumatic method to retract gingival tissues mechanically is with the use of Magic Foam Cord (Coltène Whaledent Ltd, Sussex, UK). This material is an expanding polyvinyl siloxane which is syringed around the cervical margin of the tooth (Figure 13.17). A Comprecap, similar to a contoured cotton roll, is then held in place over the silicone. As the silicone begins to set it starts to effervesce, and it is the production of air bubbles that causes the material to expand and mechanically push the gingivae away from the tooth. The material should be left in place for up to 5 minutes and removed prior to taking the impression. It is therefore time consuming to use and does not have a haemostatic agent which limits its use.

Chemomechanical retraction

Retraction cords revisited

Astringents or vasoconstrictor-impregnated retraction cords can overcome some of the problems associated with impression taking. Plain cords can also be dipped in these

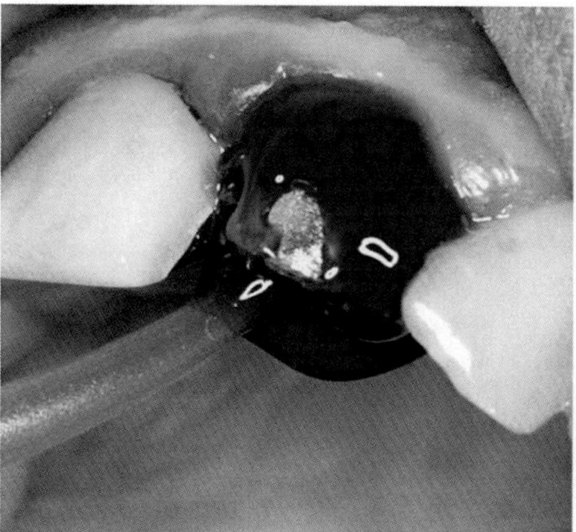
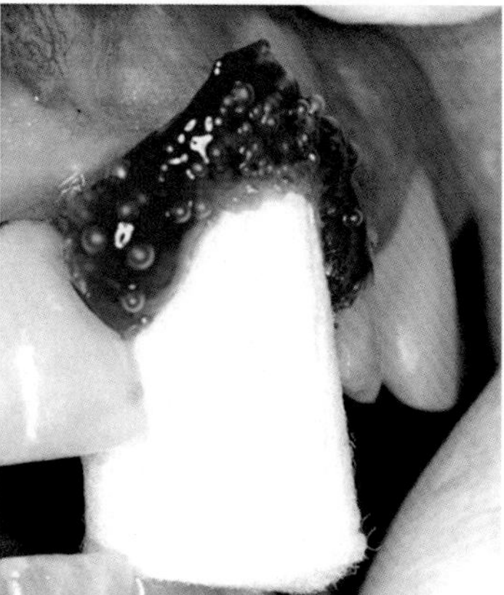

Figure 13.17 Magic Foam Cord (Coltène Whaledent) is a polyvinyl siloxane which is syringed around the tooth preparation (left). A Comprecap is then seated over the tooth (right) and on setting the silicone effervesces and expands, leading to less traumatic mechanical retraction of the gingiva.

chemicals. The cord mechanically retracts the gingivae and the chemicals help to arrest haemorrhage. Astringents such as aluminium chloride, ferric sulphate, potassium aluminium sulphate and zinc chloride help to reduce moisture, improving the impression result. The least damaging to the soft tissues and the astringent of choice is aluminium chloride.

Adrenaline has also been impregnated into retraction cords to produce vasoconstriction and arrest of haemorrhage. However, concerns have been raised over the absorption of adrenaline into the bloodstream and the concomitant systemic effects such as tachycardia, increased blood pressure and heightened anxiety, and interactions with drugs such as tricyclic antidepressants. The amount of adrenaline absorbed is unpredictable and will depend on gingival health, dilution from saliva or gingival crevicular fluid, and concentration of adrenaline used. The use of adrenaline-impregnated cord should therefore be avoided or used with caution, taking the patient's medical history into consideration.

Expasyl (Kerr Dental)

Expasyl is a relatively new method of chemomechanically retracting gingival tissues. It consists of a kaolin-based paste which is injected, using a unique gun, into the gingival sulcus (Figure 13.18). The material is very viscous and maintains its rigidity, effectively displacing the gingivae away from the tooth without the trauma that can be caused when packing retraction cord. Expasyl also contains aluminium chloride to arrest bleeding. The paste is left in place for up to 2 minutes and is then removed atraumatically by rinsing it away with a three-in-one syringe. The preparation then needs to be dried thoroughly prior to taking the impression.

Surgical retraction

Electrosurgery

Occasionally surgical removal of tissue and arrest of haemorrhage is required prior to taking an impression. For example, when a subgingival core is placed with a poor contour and surface finish, the gingivae can become hyperplastic, hindering impression taking following tooth preparation. Electrosurgery units utilize high-frequency electrical currents which can cut and/or coagulate soft tissue and have interchangeable active electrode tips of different configurations; probably the most commonly used are the loop and straight tip (Figure 13.19). The cutting tips are inserted into a handpiece connected to a current generator and the electrical circuit is completed to a passive electrode which is usually a plate placed beneath the patient's shoulder blade whilst lying in the dental chair (Figure 13.20). The passive electrode plate should not make direct contact with the patient's skin.

When using electrosurgery the working field should be dry and metal-free instruments should be used to reduce the risk of conduction burns. Electrosurgery around metal restorations should also be done with care so as not to

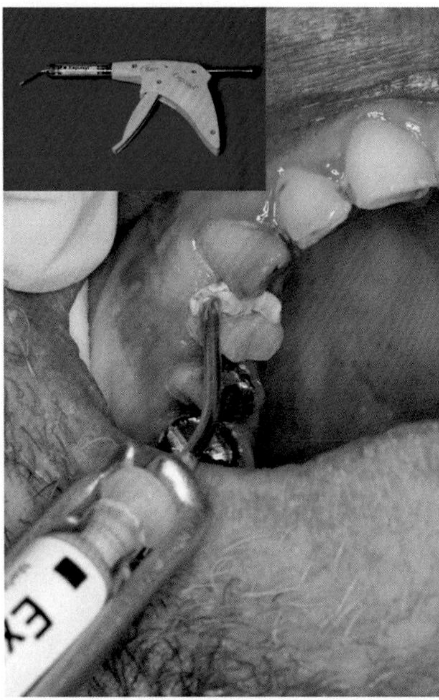

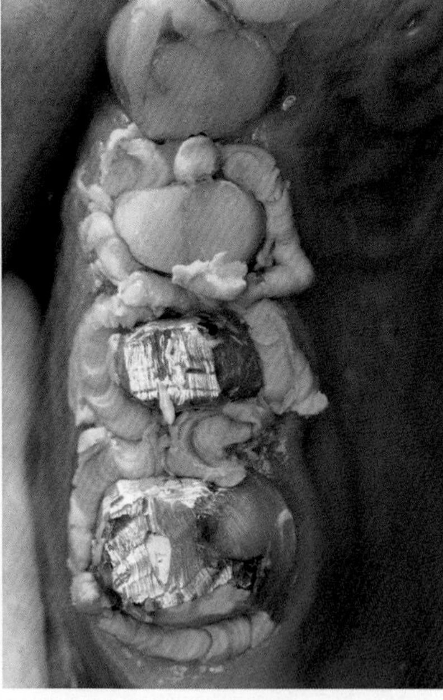

Figure 13.18 Expasyl being syringed into the gingival sulcus (left); slight blanching of the tissues can be seen as the tissues are retracted. The Expasyl is left in situ for up to 2 minutes and then rinsed off with a three-in-one syringe until completely removed.

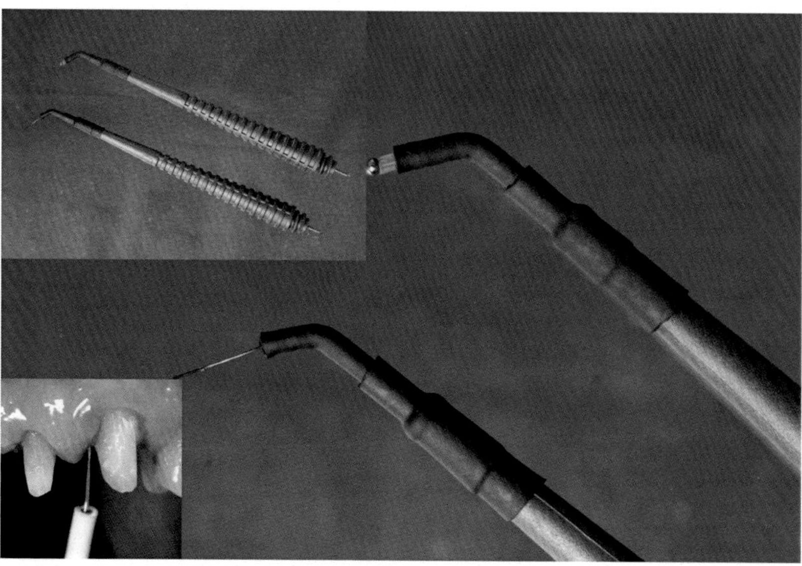

Figure 13.19 Two electrosurgery tips: a straight (left) and ball end (right). The straight tip or loop (not shown) is probably the best for gingival tissue management.

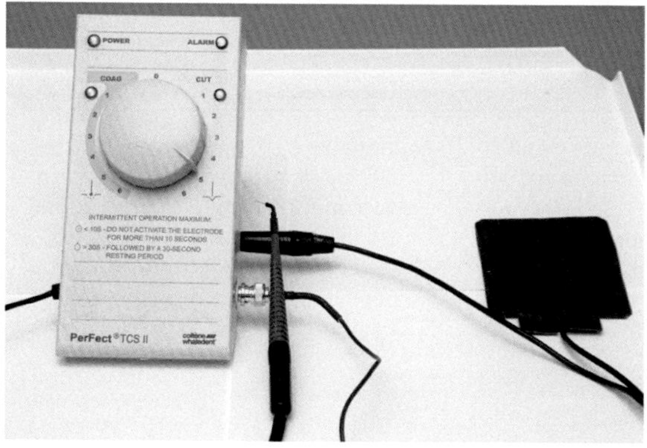

Figure 13.20 Electrosurgery unit with main box with setting dial, the electrosurgery straight tip to its right and the passive electrode plate to the far right which is placed beneath the patient's shoulder.

contact the restoration. Considerable heat is generated at the active electrode cutting tip and can cause necrosis of soft tissues and bone if used incorrectly. To reduce the heat generated, smooth sweeping movements are required; the tip should not stay stationary at any point. Cutting should not be repeated in the same area until the tissues have had time to cool which can take 5 seconds or more. Cutting movements should therefore be rehearsed prior to actual surgery. Once happy with the cut planned, the power can be applied to the unit and surgery commenced. The power may need to be increased to achieve adequate cutting of the soft tissue.

High-speed cutting burs

High-speed cutting burs have also been used to remove soft tissues surgically (Figure 13.21). Whilst quick, such 'curettage' is traumatic and associated with considerable bleeding; as such, they are rarely used.

Lasers

Lasers have also been used to cut soft tissue effectively and arrest haemorrhage; however, their use in the management of gingival tissues is uncommon. They lack tactile feedback and the equipment required is expensive. There are also health and safety issues with the use of lasers which preclude their use in the vast majority of surgeries.

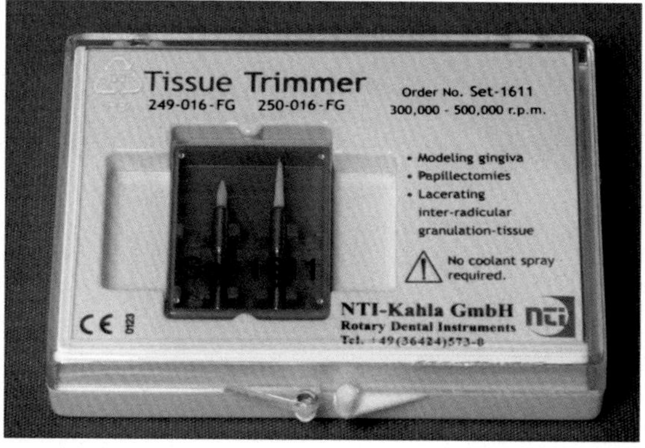

Figure 13.21 An example of tissue trimming burs.

It must be remembered that some forms of gingival retraction are particularly traumatic: the greater the trauma, the greater the risk of gingival recession once the tissues have healed. The least traumatic technique should therefore be chosen in each clinical situation to bring about the desired result.

DISINFECTION OF THE IMPRESSION

It is essential for infection control that all impressions are disinfected prior to sending them to the laboratory. Impressions can be sprayed or immersed in a disinfectant. A number of disinfectants have been used previously for dental impressions and include chlorine, aldehyde, iodine or phenol-based solutions. The most commonly used are sodium hypochlorite and glutaraldehyde. Polyether and alginate can expand if soaked in a disinfectant solution for longer than 10 and 15 minutes, respectively. These materials should therefore be sprayed with an appropriate disinfectant and placed in a sealed bag or immersed for less than 10 minutes in a disinfectant solution. Addition cured silicones are dimensionally stable and can be soaked in most disinfectant solutions for the desired duration.

It is important for each material being used (impression and disinfectant) that the manufacturer's instructions are followed. It has been recommended that the minimum disinfection procedure should include immersion of the impression in a 1% sodium hypochlorite solution for at least 10 minutes.

SUMMARY

Good atraumatic tooth preparations and periodontal health make impression taking easier and reduce the need for any additional soft tissue gingival management. In general, a two-phase, single-stage impression technique in a disposable rigid stock tray and a polyether monophase impression (also in a disposable stock tray) are the most commonly used materials and techniques suitable for most fixed prosthodontics procedures. Where soft tissue gingival management is required prior to taking an impression, various options are available which are outlined in this chapter; the least traumatic should be chosen for each clinical situation. Following these guidelines will ensure good impressions, models and restorations.

FURTHER READING

Blair, F.M., Wassell, R.W., 1996. A survey of the methods of disinfection of dental impressions used in dental hospitals in the United Kingdom. Br. Dent. J. 180, 369–375.

Goldberg, P.V., Higginbottom, F.L., Wilson, T.G., 2001. Periodontal considerations in restorative and implant therapy. Periodontol. 2000 25, 100–109.

Magne, P., 2005. Immediate dentin sealing: a fundamental procedure for indirect bonded restorations. J. Esthet. Restor. Dent. 17, 144–154.

Padbury Jr., A., Eber, R., Wang, H.L., 2003. Interactions between the gingiva and the margin of restorations. J. Clin. Periodontol. 30, 379–385.

van Noort, R., 2007. Introduction to dental materials, third ed. Mosby, Edinburgh.

Chapter | **14** |

Provisional restorations

John Radford, David Ricketts

CHAPTER CONTENTS

INTRODUCTION

During the time period between tooth preparation and fit of an indirect restoration it is important in most situations to provide a patient with a high-quality provisional restoration. Failure to do so could lead to the early demise of the definitive restoration for reasons which will be outlined in this chapter. This comes at great expense to both patient and dentist, in terms of both monetary and biological cost, and professional relationship and trust.

Some may argue, why waste precious time crafting a bespoke provisional restoration only for it to be replaced within weeks? Moreover, the cynic would argue that acceptance of the definitive restoration can be problematic if the dental aesthetic and function of the provisional restoration is comparable to that of the final restoration. To the contrary, when the dentist appreciates the relationship between form and function of a provisional restoration and its relationship to the immediate and long-term health of the teeth, supporting structures and the definitive restoration, its importance is unquestioning; the dentist/health care professional now only has to acquire the knowledge and skills to construct one.

Oral health care and treatment planning for advanced operative procedures follows a logical sequence as outlined in the earlier chapters of this textbook: initially stabilizing (including preventing further) dental diseases, evidence of oral health and then the possible reconstruction of teeth. The success of each stage of management depends upon the success of the preceding stage. The same is true when providing laboratory-fabricated indirect restorations. It is unacceptable to provide a laboratory-fabricated restoration without the prior placement of a provisional restoration. Whilst it is true that a less than ideal provisional restoration might not always influence long-term outcome of the definitive restoration, it may result in a lengthy 'fit appointment'. A health care professional would not be discharging their responsibility if any aspect of their treatment is substandard, including the placement of provisional restorations. The synergy between an empowered patient, dentist and dental technician can and should provide a seamless continuum of dental care and provisional restorations are a part of this.

With respect to terminology, there is a facile debate as to whether or not such restorations should be called provisional or temporary. The debate is perhaps academic and in this section they will be referred to as provisional restorations.

CHARACTERISTICS OF A PROVISIONAL RESTORATION

When considering provisional restorations it is most logical to consider features that must be achieved and then other 'value-added' functions of the restoration. Before exploring these, at the centre of every carer's ethic is '*Primum nil nocere*' (First, do no harm). Preparing a tooth for a laboratory-fabricated restoration will, however, by necessity:

- Compromise its dental aesthetic if in the smile line
- Degrade the tooth's function as a result of occlusal reduction
- Result in an unstable occlusion due to occlusal and approximal reduction
- Render a vital tooth sensitive due to unprotected freshly cut dentine
- Compromise the coronal seal to root-filled teeth.

A provisional restoration should therefore restore the characteristics that have been lost and additionally allow optimum home care. 'First, do no harm' also applies to something seemingly as trivial as providing a provisional restoration. Consider the provisional crowns provided in Figures 14.1 and 14.2. The provisional restoration in Figure 14.1 demonstrates an adequate fit cervically and home care should therefore not be compromised. In contrast, the provisional restoration that has been placed on the molar tooth in Figure 14.2 had overhanging margins and during the short time in situ adequate oral hygiene has not been possible and gingival inflammation has ensued.

Specifically, therefore, a provisional restoration must:

- *Establish and/or maintain the dental aesthetic.* A 'value-added' function of a provisional restoration would be to evaluate a patient's satisfaction with the dental aesthetics if this is to be changed in the definitive restorations. A diagnostic wax-up can be made of the ideal aesthetics for the tooth/teeth. This can then be duplicated in stone to allow a vacuum-formed splint to be made which can then be used to make a custom-formed temporary crown(s) (see later).
- *Confirm that the tooth preparation is adequate.* This includes sufficient occlusal reduction and intra- and extracoronal design characteristics, including maintaining occlusal stability (the prepared tooth must not be allowed to drift or overerupt in an uncontrolled fashion). A 'value-added' function of a provisional restoration is as a tool to help the dentist maintain a conformative approach to the occlusion.

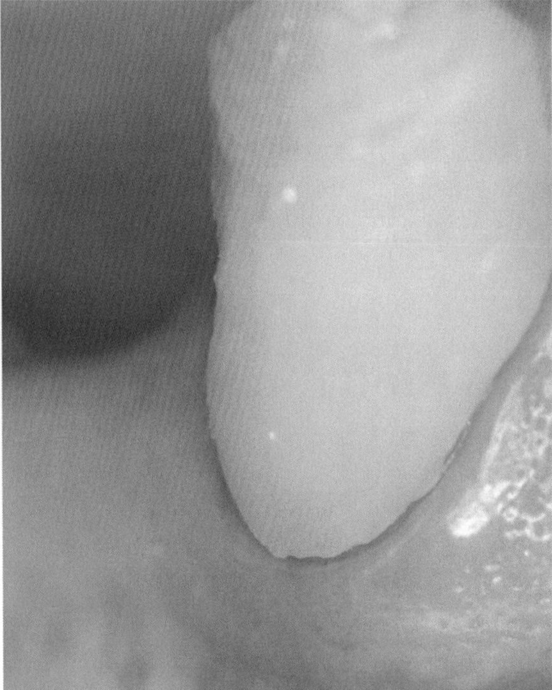

Figure 14.1 This provisional restoration demonstrates an adequate fit, cervically. Home care should therefore not be compromised and periodontal health maintained.

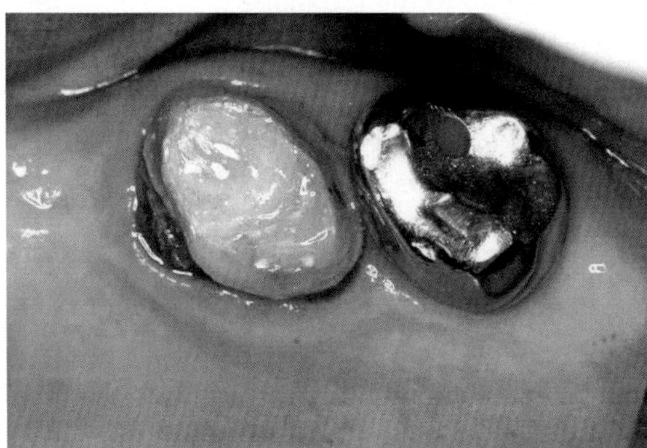

Figure 14.2 A poorly fitting provisional crown has been removed from the upper left first molar tooth. The overhanging margins mesially and palatally have prevented adequate home care with resultant plaque accumulation and gingival inflammation.

- *Prevent tooth sensitivity* by covering all exposed, freshly cut dentinal tubules in vital teeth and preventing fluid movement in the dentinal tubules.
- *Prevent bacterial leakage* at the provisional/tooth tissue interface in vital teeth and non-vital, root-filled teeth. The former reduces pulpal inflammation and

the latter maintains a good coronal seal to the root canal filling.
- *Allow optimum home care.* Ledges are unacceptable, but anecdote would suggest it is preferable to have a negative (tooth) ledge when compared with a positive (restoration) ledge (Figure 14.2).

Provisional restorations can be either custom-formed to each individual situation or preformed by manufacturers in standard shapes and sizes and adjusted to fit at the chairside. The custom-formed temporaries are preferred, but are perhaps a more demanding technique to master.

CUSTOM-FORMED RESIN REPLICA PROVISIONAL CROWNS

The most appropriate material to be used for a custom-formed resin replica provisional restoration is a chemically cured bis-acrylic composite resin, for example Protemp Plus Temporisation Material (3M ESPE) or Integrity Temp-Grip Temporary Crown and Bridge Material (Dentsply). The merit of using this as a provisional restorative material is that it can be customized so that its internal aspect custom fits the preparation and its external surface reproduces accurate contact points and occlusion with the opposing arch.

It is important that the provisional restoration is made before the impression is taken. This is because the provisional restoration can be used to affirm that the tooth preparation characteristics are satisfactory. These include whether sufficient tooth/core has been prepared to accommodate the definitive restoration (Figure 14.3) and other preparation characteristics such as whether the preparation is undercut or not (Figures 14.4 and 14.5). If deficiencies in the preparation are found these can be remedied and the temporary can be relined or remade. An impression of the preparation can now be made with reassurance that the preparation is satisfactory.

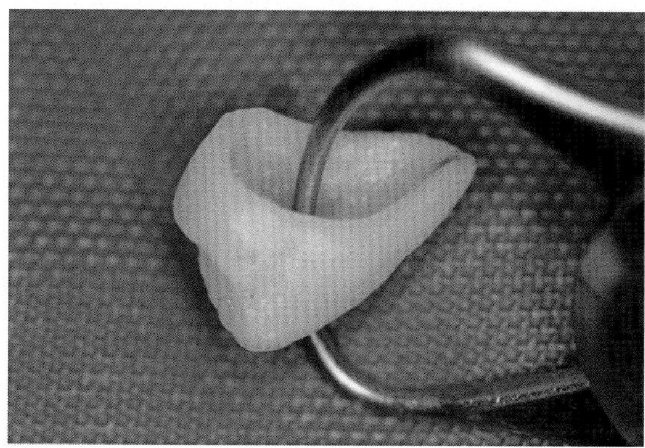

Figure 14.3 An Iwanson gauge can be used to measure the thickness of the provisional restoration in relation to the buccal cusp occlusal reduction, for example. If it is shown that there is insufficient tooth reduction, further preparation is carried out and the provisional restoration is relined.

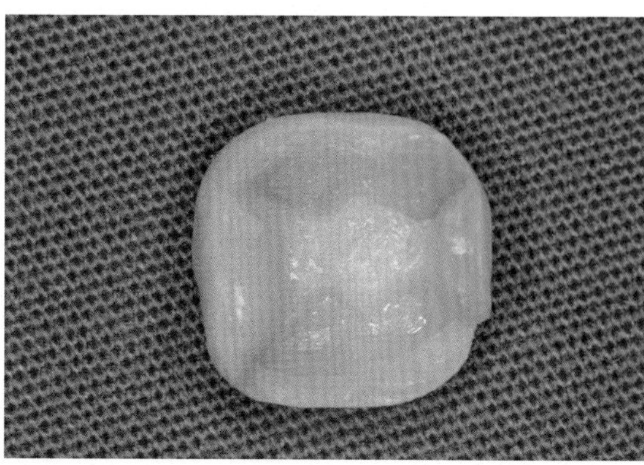

Figure 14.4 Bis-acrylic composite provisional restoration, affirming a satisfactory preparation for a gold overlay. This provisional restoration shows mesial and distal gingival bevels to the proximal box preparation.

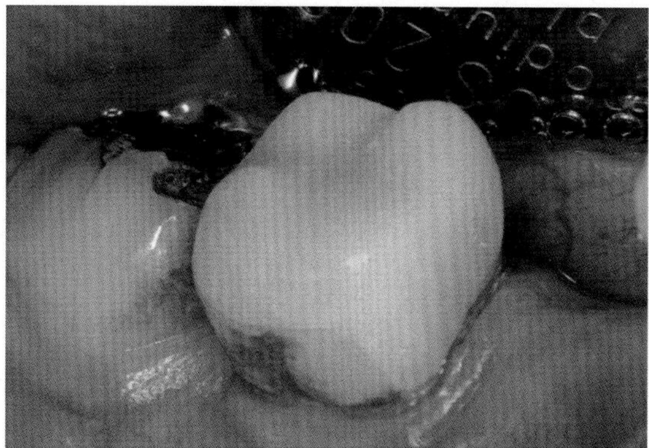

Figure 14.5 The provisional restoration shown in Figure 14.4 in situ.

How to make a custom-formed provisional restoration (Figure 14.6)

Firstly a sectional impression of the tooth to be prepared is made. A full arch impression is unnecessary for this and would make it more difficult to relocate on the teeth. This can be done in a number of materials:

- An addition cured silicone putty is preferred as this can be disinfected and given to the patient (Figure 14.6). If the temporary is lost or breaks in function in the ensuing weeks whilst the crown is being made, the impression can be reused (as it is dimensionally stable) to make a new custom-formed

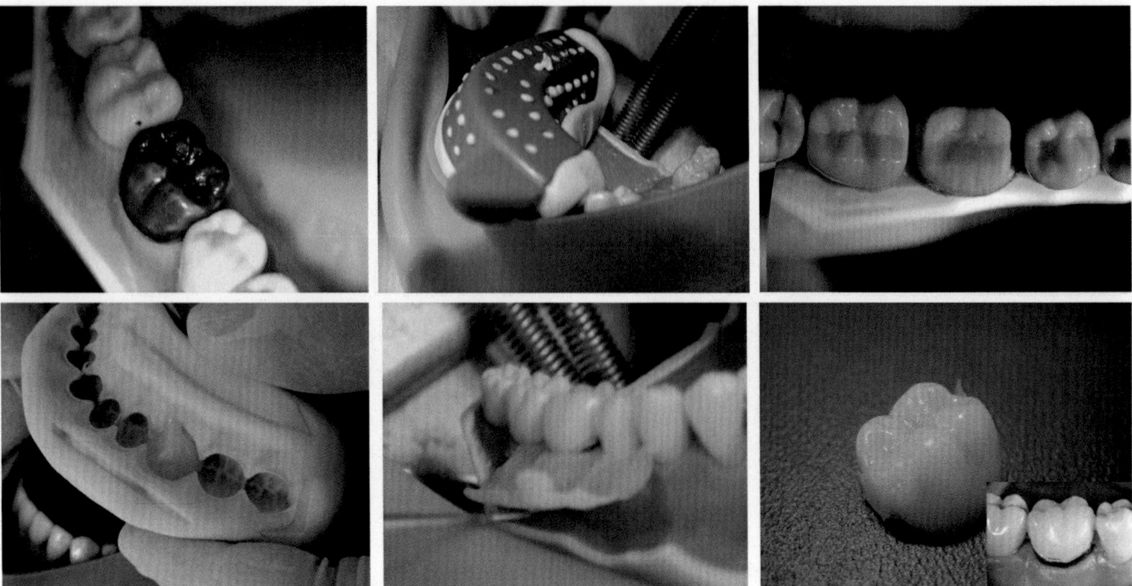

Figure 14.6 The stages involved in making a custom-formed resin replica provisional crown. From left to right and top to bottom: an impression is taken of the tooth prior to preparing it for a crown. The tooth is then prepared, the impression of the tooth is filled with a bis-acryl resin and reseated fully in the mouth. Once the bis-acryl resin has almost set (rubbery stage) the impression is removed. The provisional restoration is removed from the tooth and trimmed.

provisional restoration. Such a material has the advantage over alginate, in that it can be used repeatedly without tearing.

- Alginate is cheaper, but cannot easily be reused or kept by the patient should the provisional restoration fail in function.
- Some clinicians use softened modelling wax. This has the advantage that it can easily be adjusted and smoothed with a hot instrument (see later) but is not suitable where there are deep undercuts as it would easily distort. Whilst cost effective and convenient to make, it cannot be stored and used again, unlike the silicone matrices. For this reason the technique is suitable for simple and single restorations that copy the original shape of the tooth.
- A custom vacuum-formed plastic mould can be made from a study model or a model made from a diagnostic wax-up (see later).

The tooth is prepared for the chosen design of restoration, which in Figure 14.6 is a full coverage gold crown. A thin layer of petroleum jelly can be smeared onto the preparation to facilitate the removal of the provisional restoration from the tooth once set; this is not always necessary. The bis-acrylic composite resins used are supplied in cartridges which fit into dispensing guns onto which double helix mixer tips are attached. Before syringing the material into the impression, some of the material should be dispensed onto the bracket table or a mixing pad to ensure it is completely mixed (occasionally, base or catalyst moves into the double helix mixer tip ahead of the other and hence emerges in an unmixed state) and to monitor its set. The bis-acrylic composite resin is then syringed into the sectional impression of the tooth that has been prepared and the impression is relocated in the mouth, ensuring it is fully seated over the teeth; an obvious click is often felt as the impression passes over the bulbosity of the remaining teeth.

Before complete polymerization of the bis-acryl resin, remove the impression. At this stage the resin on the pad or bracket table will feel rubbery. This is an important step as waiting for the final set may result in difficulty in removing the temporary restoration as it can set into existing undercuts. For this reason at the rubbery stage carefully move the matrix up and down with a small amplitude so as to ensure no setting occurs into such undercuts. The provisional restoration that has formed may either stay on the tooth or will be removed in the impression. In the former situation, gently ease it off the preparation as soon as possible using an instrument beneath the contact points. If this is not done, the bis-acrylic composite will completely polymerize into the interdental undercuts, making it impossible to remove without destroying the provisional restoration. If the provisional is removed in the impression, let it set completely as trying to remove it in a partially polymerized stage could lead to distortion and damage.

Once removed from the mouth or impression, any material flash and ledges can be removed with a high speed diamond bur or abrasive polishing discs, paying particular attention to the interdental areas where the material goes into the undercut areas beneath the bulbosity of the adjacent teeth. Following this, confirmation of an adequate tooth preparation can be carried out as described earlier and in Figures 14.3 and 14.4, comparing the fit surface of the provisional restoration with that of the prepared tooth. The marginal fit and occlusion are checked with the provisional restoration in situ and adjusted if necessary; ideally, the provisional restoration should be removed and adjusted outside of the mouth. Finally, the patient should be shown the restoration to confirm that the dental aesthetic is satisfactory. The provisional restoration can then be cemented with a temporary luting cement such as a non-eugenol temporary cement (TempBond NE, Kerr Dental). It is argued that eugenol-containing cement would inhibit the polymerization of a permanent resin luting cement. Excess temporary cement is then meticulously removed from the margins, carefully using dental floss interdentally. To avoid dislodging the provisional restoration by pulling the floss back through the contact point, the floss can be pulled out buccally/labially.

Modifications to the technique

Occasionally it is necessary, before preparing the tooth, to modify its shape with soft wax or resin composite (placed and cured but not etched and bonded to the tooth or core) to achieve a better contour for the provisional restoration. This is necessary in situations where the core or shape of the tooth is inadequate. For example, the amalgam core seen in Figure 14.7 has no disto-buccal cusp created in the core and it is not in occlusal contact in this area with the opposing teeth. Minimal or no occlusal reduction is needed in this area but using the custom-formed technique for making provisionals as described above would lead to a very thin layer or no provisional material in the unprepared area and a corresponding perforation in the provisional restoration would result. To address this, wax or composite can be placed to build up the cusp to form and function before the preoperative impression is taken, ensuring the provisional restoration is intact and correctly contoured.

An alternative method to overcome such problems is that the impression itself can be adjusted in the relevant areas using a scalpel blade or instrument such as an excavator. The amount of impression material removed is arbitrary and the provisional restoration often needs more adjustment. Advocates of using softened wax as an 'impression material' claim that the wax is easier to remove and can be smoothed with a hot instrument.

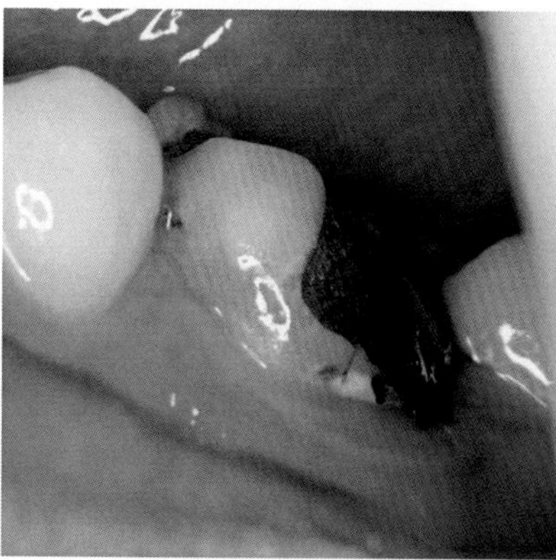

Figure 14.7 Poorly contoured amalgam restoration which is to act as a core for a full coverage crown. The occlusal surface can be modified using composite or wax to create the ideal occlusal form, prior to taking an impression for a custom-formed resin replica provisional restoration.

Establishing the occlusion and aesthetics with custom-formed provisional restorations

When placing crowns and/or bridges on anterior teeth which have lost their original form, for example through tooth wear or repeated restoration over many years, the shape of the teeth needs to be re-established; the occlusion and aesthetics can be piloted on provisional restorations. Ideally, guidance (anterior/incisal) should be produced on the crowns and this can be created in a diagnostic wax-up on articulated study models. Once this and the appearance are satisfactory, the wax-up can be duplicated in stone and a vacuum-formed mould (template/splint) made. At the patient's subsequent visit, the anterior teeth can be prepared and the mould used to make custom-formed provisional restorations to the new occlusal scheme and appearance created in the diagnostic wax-up. The patient can then wear the provisional restorations for some time until happy with the form and function (Figure 14.8). During this time the occlusion and appearance (shape of the teeth) can be altered by removing provisional material with a bur or the addition of a colour-matched composite, if necessary.

The guidance created in such provisional restorations can be transferred to the definitive restorations using a technique such as a customized formed incisal guidance table (Figure 14.9). In this technique, impressions of the upper (including the provisional restorations) and lower arches are made and the resultant models mounted on a semi-adjustable articulator as described in Chapter 6. Lateral and protrusive movements are reproduced on the articulated models. As this is done the incisal pin raises up off the incisal guidance table according to the steepness of the guidance created on the provisional restorations. The technician then places cold cure acrylic on the incisal guidance table and repeats the excursive movements, the

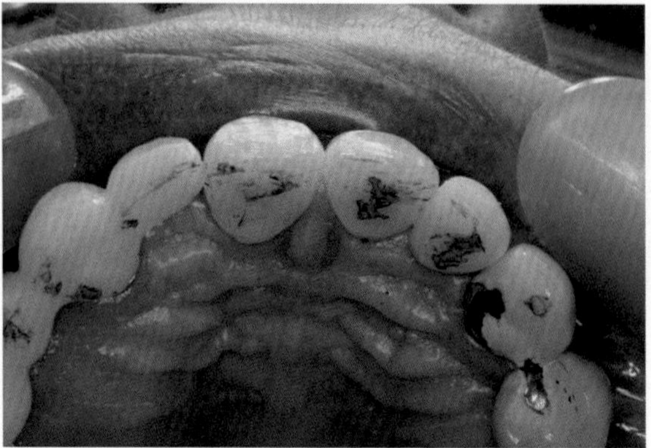

Figure 14.8 Establishing incisal/anterior guidance on the provisional restorations. Note 'light' if any contact on pontic upper right lateral incisor to minimize unfavourable forces during protrusion and excursion.

incisal guidance pin moulding (scoring) the setting acrylic. The so-called customized incisal guidance table is therefore formed.

Impressions of the tooth preparations are then made and the resultant master model mounted on the articulator to the lower model. As the definitive restorations are being made, the technician repeatedly makes the excursive movements, now guided by the custom-formed incisal guidance table. The palatal contours of the crowns are adjusted to have simultaneous contact with the incisal pin on the guidance table, so reproducing the guidance of the provisional restorations in the definitive crowns.

Fortunately for most circumstances a diagnostic wax-up produced by a technician can satisfy the aesthetic demands of a patient. Using the guides described in Chapter 15, the form and shape of restorations can be made to complement the mouth. However, on occasion, some patients can have a high aesthetic demand. In these situations the initial provisional crown may be altered or replaced to achieve the demands of the patient. Chairside alterations, provided they are minor, can be undertaken by removing and reshaping with burs or adding small amounts of provisional material. More extensive changes may need a replacement provisional restoration; this is more likely on upper anterior teeth where the aesthetic demands of most people are higher. After agreement on the restoration shape, an alginate impression can be recorded to help the technician reproduce the result in the final restoration.

Establishing gingival contours with custom-formed provisional restorations

In certain situations custom-formed provisional crowns can allow shaping of the gingival tissues in order to achieve a satisfactory emergence profile of the definitive restoration. This is indicated particularly when restoring bone-level dental implants. For details on this the reader should refer to a text on implantology.

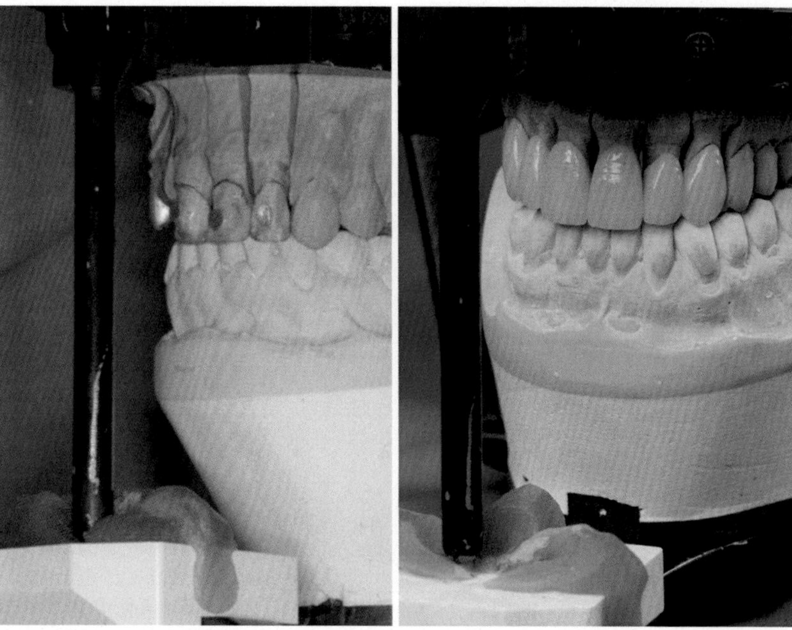

Figure 14.9 Customized incisal table replicating the palatal contours of those established in the provisional restorations made in Figure 14.8 (left), and for another patient whose guidance is being replicated in replacement crowns (right).

PREFORMED PROVISIONAL CROWNS

A number of preformed provisional crowns are available. These can be tooth coloured (polycarbonate crowns) or clear plastic crown forms which can be filled with bis-acryl composite resin (for use within the smile line), or they can be metal based. Each type of crown is provided as a series with different tooth morphologies and sizes. This poses two problems: (1) it is unlikely that a preformed crown will fit cervically, occlusally and interdentally with any degree of accuracy and, as such, will require chairside adjustment; and (2) a large bank of crowns (at a monetary cost) is required to fit any eventuality. This having been said, they are particularly useful in situations where an impression of the tooth prior to crown preparation does not exist, for example when a patient presents following trauma and significant loss of coronal tooth tissue.

Provisional polycarbonate crowns

Polycarbonate crowns (e.g. Directa, JS Dental Manufacturing Inc.) are tooth-coloured 'shells' which have a morphology to meet all anterior and bicuspid teeth (Figure 14.10). These products have been available for more than 35 years and in use are sublined with an acrylic such as Trim (PEMA temporary resin acrylic). First, a polycarbonate shell is selected that is slightly larger than the preparation dimension (Figure 14.11). A bur such as a large pink stone in a straight handpiece is then used to pare it back until it is of the correct preparation dimension and seats fully over the tooth preparation without bedding into the gingiva. A thin smear of petroleum jelly is applied to the tooth preparation and the acrylic resin (Trim) is spread into the fit surface of the crown. This is then seated over the preparation and positioned such that the aesthetic is satisfactory. When the acrylic has polymerized to a granular/dough stage, the shell is carefully removed and replaced, before finally removing to allow the acrylic to polymerize fully outside the mouth. The provisional restoration is then trimmed until the fit is acceptable (Figure 14.12). If the crown is overbuilt, blanching of the gingiva will occur and further trimming is indicated. Following impression taking, the provisional crown can be cemented with a temporary luting cement.

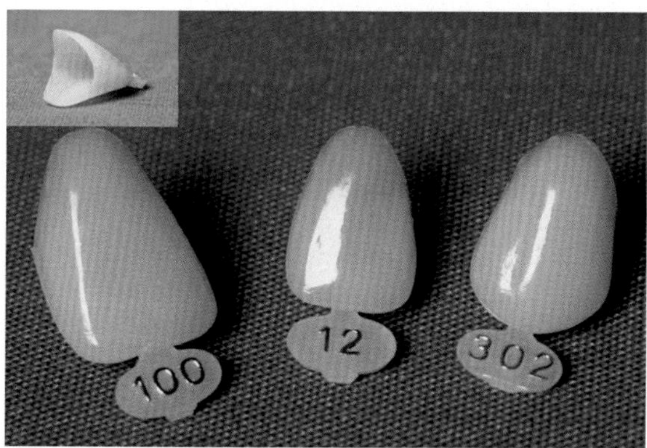

Figure 14.10 Polycarbonate Directa crowns.

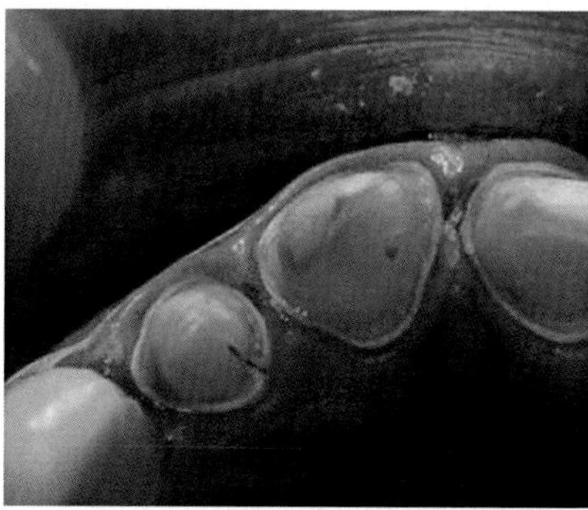

Figure 14.11 Adequate definitive restorations spawn from satisfactory tooth preparations and provisional restorations. These are the preparations for the provisional restorations as seen in Figure 14.12.

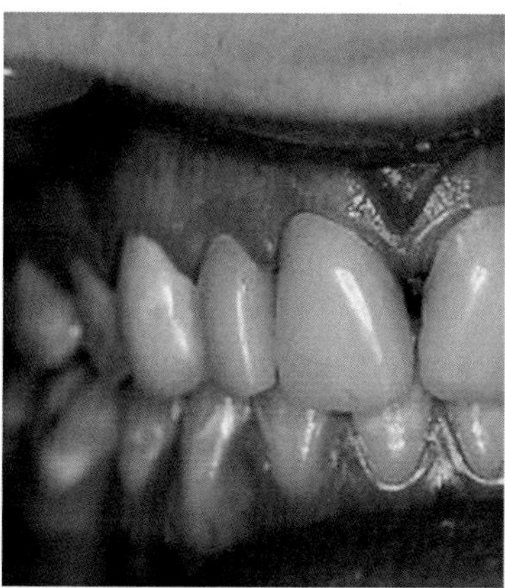

Figure 14.12 Adequate provisional restorations on the upper right central and lateral incisor made from polycarbonate Directa crowns. The buccal contour of the provisional restoration on the upper left central incisor is poor.

Other provisional restorations

In a similar way to the use of the polycarbonate crowns, clear plastic crown forms (Figure 14.13) can be selected and trimmed until they seat fully over the tooth preparation without traumatizing the gingiva. These are thin and can easily be trimmed with a scissors. Prior to filling with a bis-acryl composite resin, small holes can be made with a probe at the cusp/canine tips and incisal angles.

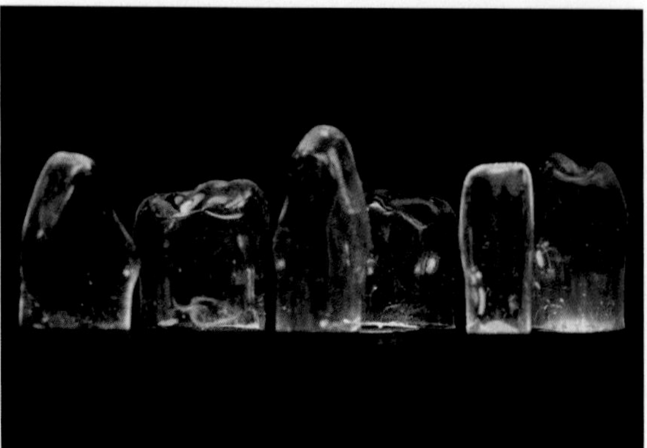

Figure 14.13 Clear plastic crown forms, suitable for use with bis-acryl composite resin.

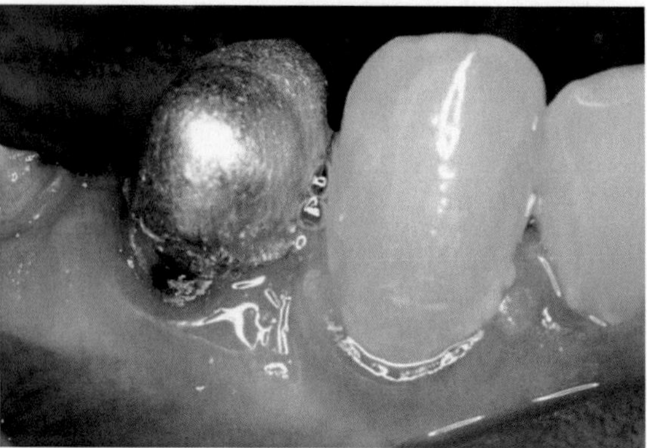

Figure 14.15 A poorly trimmed and contoured provisional aluminium crown. The margins are sharp and there is a ledge mesially.

This allows air to escape, reducing the risk of bubbles forming within the resin. Once the bis-acryl composite resin has set, the clear plastic crown form can be removed, the margins and occlusion can be checked and adjusted as necessary, and the crown cemented with a temporary cement.

Metal aluminium and stainless steel provisional crowns are also available for use on posterior teeth (Figure 14.14). Their margins are more difficult to adjust and ledges and sharp margins are more likely to cause soft tissue trauma (Figure 14.15). Some metal provisional crowns are provided with a crimping device that can be used to mould the margins of the crown to the tooth shape.

Occasionally, if replacing a crown, the original crown can be modified and used as a temporary. Consider the crown in Figure 14.16 which is being replaced because of distal caries. It has been partially sectioned, and following caries removal and refinement of the preparation, has been relined with a bis-acrylic composite resin and cemented temporarily.

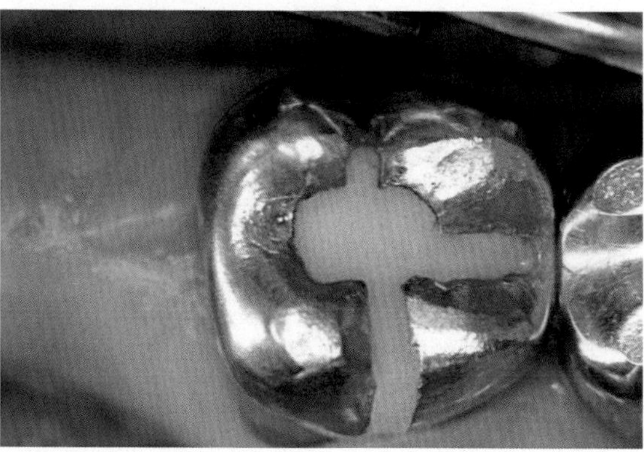

Figure 14.16 The partially sectioned crown on the molar tooth has been relined with a bis-acryl composite resin and cemented temporarily.

If the original crown is planned to be used as a provisional restoration, consideration should be given to its removal with a WAMkey (WAM). The WAMkey system is a set of three elevators, each with an oval end of increasing diameter. A hole is cut in the buccal aspect of the crown at the interface between the occlusal surface of the core and occlusal surface of the crown (Figure 14.17). The appropriate sized WAMkey is inserted at the interface and rotated, elevating the crown off the preparation with minimal risk of damaging the core and tooth preparation. Crown and bridge removers, such as pneumatic crown and bridge removers, that send a shock wave through the cement lute to shatter it, should be avoided as these can lead to decoronation of the tooth.

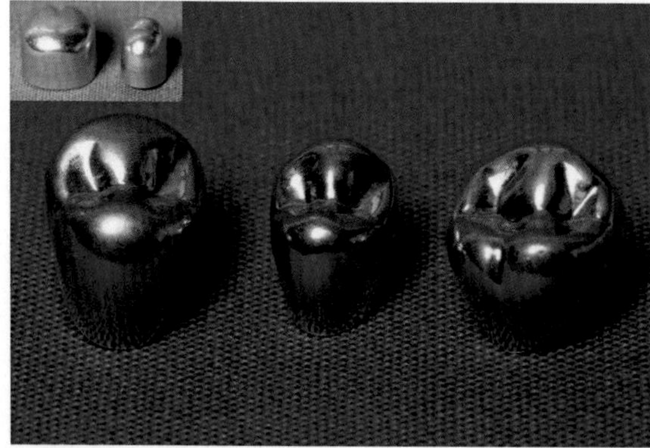

Figure 14.14 Metal provisional crowns.

More recently, preformed malleable composite crowns have been introduced (Protemp Crown Temporisation Material; Figure 14.18). These are soft and easily moulded to the tooth preparation in situ. Once the desired shape is achieved they can be partially light cured in the mouth. It is important to only partially light cure the crown in the mouth for about 2–3 seconds as complete cure can lead to difficulties in their removal from the tooth. The crown

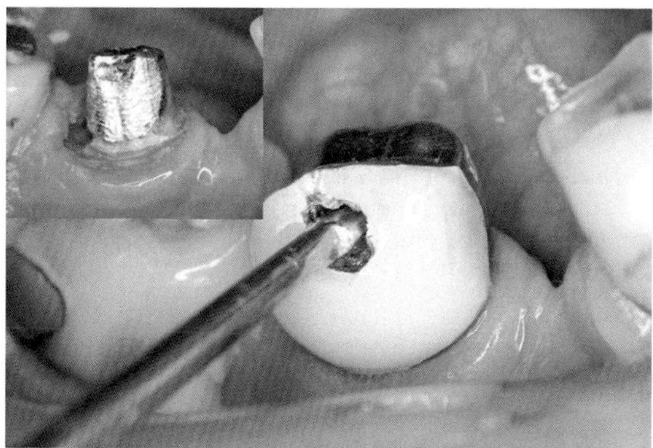

Figure 14.17 Use of a WAMkey to elevate off a metal–ceramic crown which has caries distally. The cast post and core beneath remain intact following caries removal and preparation refinement (Inset).

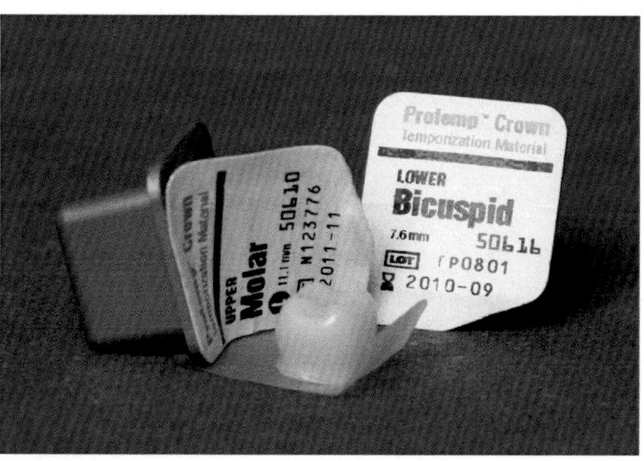

Figure 14.18 Protemp provisional crowns.

is removed and fully cured outside of the mouth. Final check of fit and any adjustment can be carried out prior to cementing with a temporary luting cement.

PROVISIONAL REPLACEMENT OF MISSING TEETH

Where full preparation, conventional bridges are concerned, provisional restorations can be made in a similar manner to custom-formed provisional crowns, using a diagnostic wax-up of the replacement tooth. Alternatively, a simple acrylic removable partial prosthesis can be used. This can be used if a minimum preparation bridge (resin retained) or implant retained restoration is planned; if adjacent teeth are to be prepared for a conventional bridge, the removable prosthesis can be used in conjunction with provisional crowns.

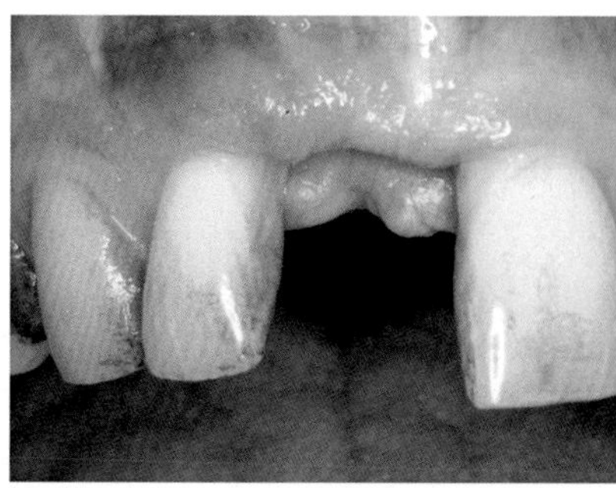

Figure 14.19 The upper right central incisor was restored with a post crown that catastrophically failed. This tooth was extracted and a bone-level implant placed 8 weeks later. Note staining due to the use of chlorhexidine following surgery.

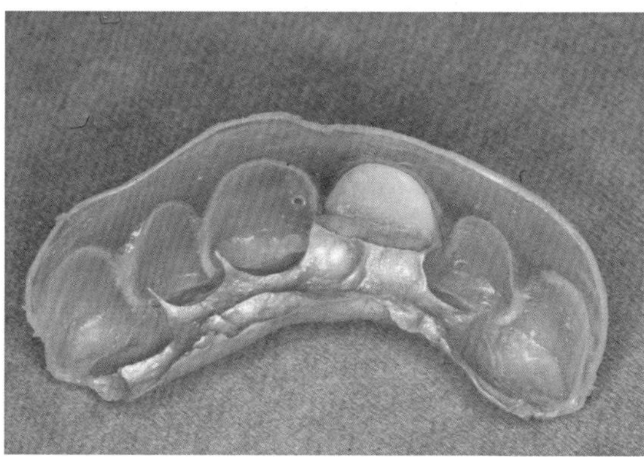

Figure 14.20 Ethylene vinyl acetate (EVA) copolymer splint with acrylic tooth replacing the upper right central incisor, secured in place with an adhesive.

Another method of provisionally replacing a missing tooth where no preparation of the adjacent teeth is planned (Figure 14.19) is to take an impression and place an acrylic prosthetic tooth in the edentulous space on the model. A plastic (ethylene vinyl acetate (EVA) copolymer) splint can then be made over this and the adjacent teeth (Figure 14.20). The acrylic tooth can then be secured to the splint using an adhesive, giving an acceptable appearance (Figure 14.21).

ADVICE DURING THE PROVISIONAL STAGE

A patient should be urged to disrupt regularly the plaque biofilm associated with provisional restorations, enlisting the full armamentarium of cleaning aids. One notable

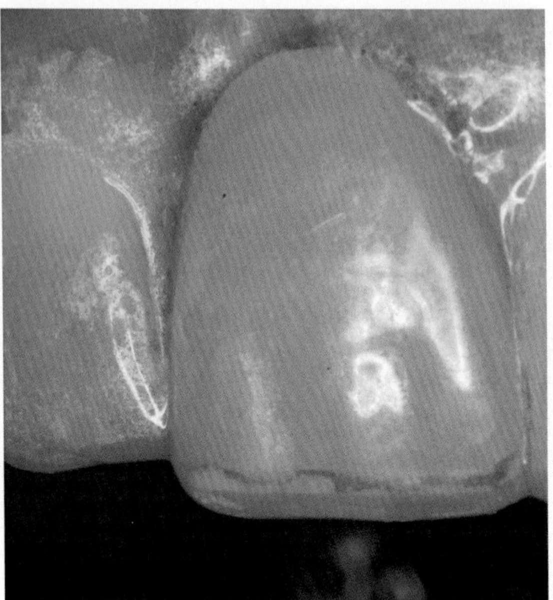

Figure 14.21 The acrylic tooth in clear splint has adequate aesthetics for a provisional tooth replacement (for patient seen in Figure 14.19). Oral hygiene has to be good.

caution is the use of dental floss which could pull out a provisional restoration if pulled back up through the contact point (it should be pulled out buccally). However, if the patient does not maintain adequate home care, gingival inflammation will result in an increased volume of gingival crevicular fluid or even gingival bleeding. At cementation this could lead to an inadequate cement lute. It is therefore good practice to advise patients to continue with routine dental home care.

SUMMARY

A carefully made provisional restoration should have all the characteristics of a definitive restoration. Unequivocally it is a surrogate marker for a dentist in determining the appropriateness of the tooth preparation and identifying errors. Custom-formed provisional restorations are also important when changes are planned to the appearance and occlusion. The demand for a quality provisional restoration is frequently overlooked in the focus to perfect tooth preparation and ensure an accurate impression; this is an error that should be avoided at all costs.

FURTHER READING

Wassell, R.W., St George, G., Ingledew, R.P., Steele, J.G., 2002. Crowns and other extra-coronal restorations: provisional restorations. Br. Dent. J. 192, 619–622, 625–630.

Chapter 15

Getting the appearance correct

Brian Stevenson

CHAPTER CONTENTS

INTRODUCTION

When making restorations that are visible in the smile line, and for some patients even when the restorations are not readily visible, appearance is critical. Creating a good appearance in a restoration depends upon matching the colour, shape and surface texture to adjacent teeth. Whilst selecting the correct shade requires an understanding of light and the science of colour, creating the shape and texture of teeth needs knowledge of tooth morphology, dimensions and proportion. This chapter addresses these issues so that the optimum appearance of aesthetic restorations can be achieved.

LIGHT

Visible light forms a small portion of the whole electromagnetic (EM) spectrum (Figure 15.1) and often takes the form of polychromatic light which is composed of electromagnetic radiation of more than one wavelength. The colour of an object that one observes is actually the reflection of the light that strikes it. For example, a red flower appears red because red light is reflected by the flower whilst the other colours of light are absorbed.

The unique appearance of teeth is due to the complex interactions between light and tooth tissue, and this makes shade selection difficult. The interactions that take place are as follows:

- *Reflection*. Light is reflected by mineralized tissue, mainly enamel rods and extratubular dentine. The amount of reflected light helps to determine the brightness of a tooth: the more light that is reflected, the brighter the tooth will appear.
- *Scatter*. Light entering the tooth tissue hits various tooth structures and is dispersed in all directions. Some light is returned towards the source and emerges from the tooth surface again in all directions. Scattering therefore reduces the intensity of the radiation being returned from the material. What

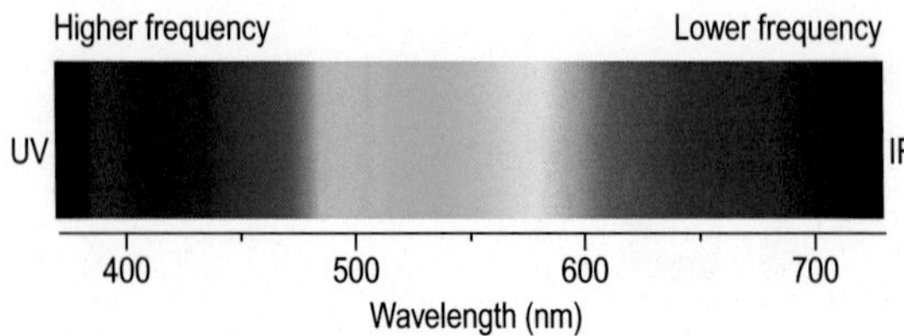

Figure 15.1 Electromagnetic spectrum.

causes the majority of scatter is different in each dental tissue. For example, in enamel a large amount of scatter is due to the enamel prisms, specifically the hydroxyapatite crystallites. However, most of the scatter in a tooth occurs in dentine and this is due to the dentinal tubules.

- *Absorption*. Light is absorbed by teeth and occurs to a greater extent in dentine than enamel. Energy that is absorbed does not emerge from the material and is converted to another form of energy. The amount of absorption is dependent on the light source and tooth.
- *Refraction*. The change in direction of a beam of electromagnetic radiation due to a change in the conveying medium is termed refraction. This occurs to a small extent in enamel (97% mineralized by weight) and to a greater extent in the less mineralized and tubular structure of dentine (approximately 70% mineralized by weight)
- *Transmission*. Light transmission occurs in both enamel and to a lesser extent in dentine. This is evident as neither material is opaque, unlike some materials used in dentistry (Figure 15.2). Transmitted light radiation passes through the incisal edge and approximal areas of a tooth following a number of the reactions described above. The number of these reactions is reduced at the incisal edge compared to the body of a tooth. This results in more light being transmitted at the incisal edge, occasionally giving the appearance of an almost transparent region. Enamel is almost translucent and if no dentine was present to block the transmission of light, teeth would appear glass-like.

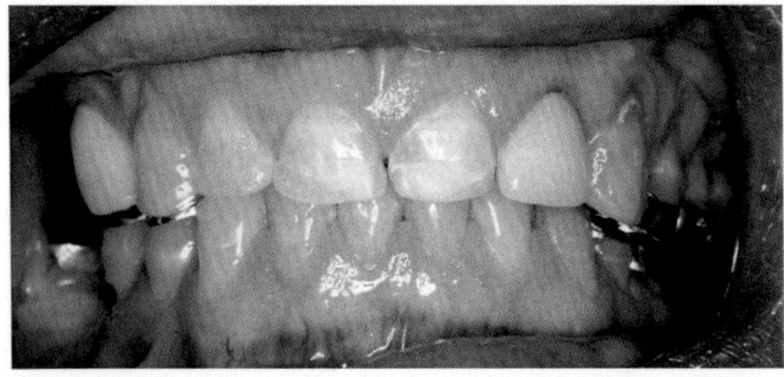

Figure 15.2 Opaqueness of the metal–ceramic crown on the upper left lateral incisor compared to the more translucent teeth and resin composite restorations.

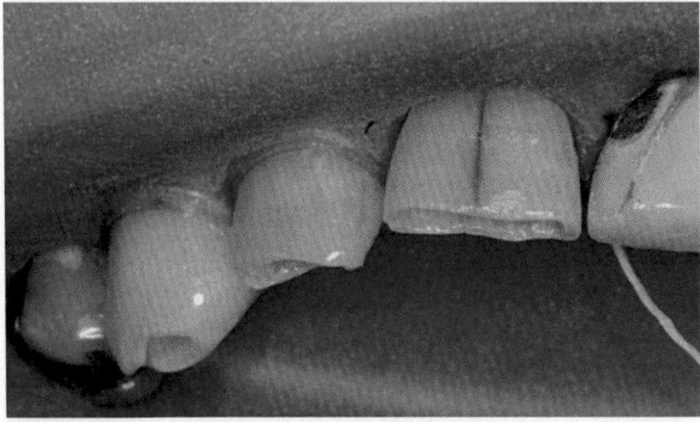

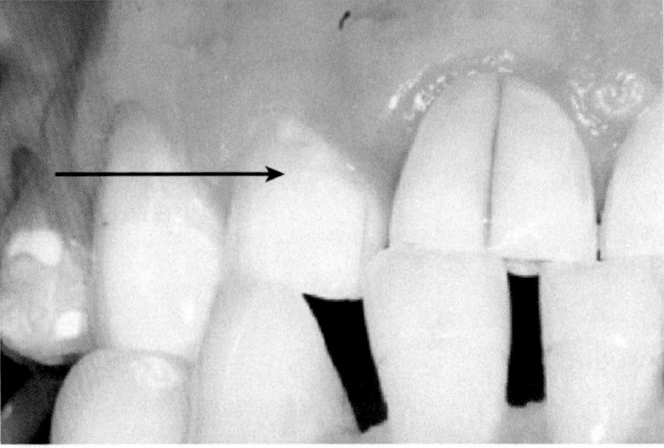

Figure 15.3 Image of teeth that have dehydrated under a rubber dam; the arrow shows where the rubber dam sat.

Dentine, however, provides the colour of a tooth that is evident in the body and cervical areas. When a tooth is dehydrated, it appears whiter and brighter due to dehydration of the collagen matrices. This can occur after impression making, rubber dam placement (Figure 15.3) and bleaching. It is therefore important to shade match at the beginning of an appointment rather than at the end when some temporary colour change might have occurred.

- *Translucency*. Translucency is defined as the ability to allow radiation to pass with little scatter. The degree of translucency varies with the wavelength of the light. Enamel is translucent due to the high level of mineralization and crystallite orientation. However, when enamel is hypomineralized as a result of developmental (fluorosis) or acquired (carious white spots – see Chapter 1 on caries) defects, greater scattering of light occurs and the enamel becomes opaque and less translucent.
- *Fluorescence*. Fluorescence is the property of a material to absorb light of a particular wavelength and then to emit light of a different wavelength and therefore colour. Teeth fluoresce bluish-white when exposed to ultraviolet radiation.
- *Metamerism*. Metamerism can have an effect on the appearance of a tooth or restoration. Metamers are

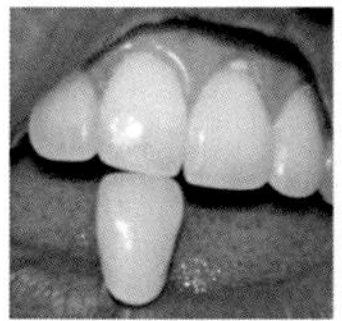
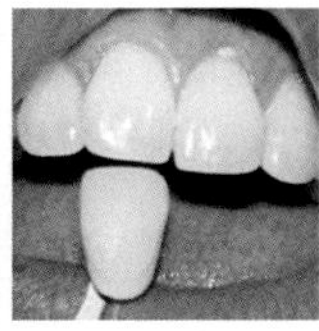
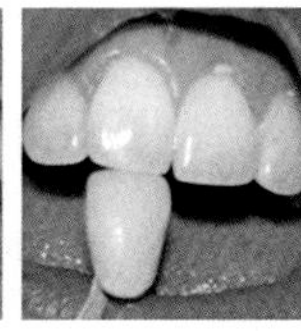
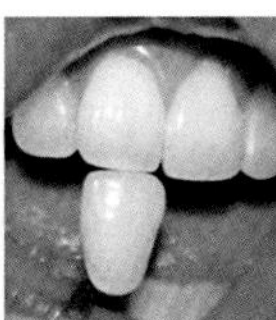
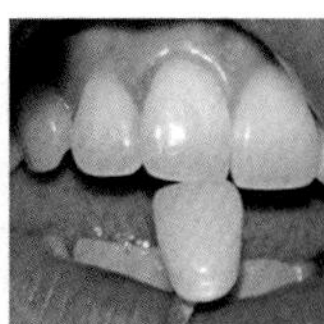

Figure 15.4 Metamerism: The same shade tab and tooth are matched under different light sources. It is observed that the shade match is better when viewed under the centre picture.

objects which match each other under one set of light conditions but mismatch under another as the light has different spectral properties (Figure 15.4).

- *Opalescence*. Opalescence is defined as having the property of opal stone. Natural teeth have the same properties as these stones: they appear yellowish-red in transmitted light but blue in reflected light.

HUMAN ANATOMY AND COLOUR VISION

The retina, on the internal posterior wall of the human eye, contains a complex network of nerve endings capable of detecting light. There are over 120 million light-sensitive receptors in the 0.2 mm thick retina. Two types of receptor cell are present: rods and cones. Rods far outnumber cones and are responsible for night vision which is monochromatic. Cones are responsible for medium to high level light vision in full colour and are found in the centre of the retina. Colour judgement is theoretically impaired if the operator views an object from the side of the eye. Three types of cone exist; each one has a different sensitivity to different wavelengths of light (blue, red and green).

Colour vision deficiency (colour blindness)

Colour blindness is usually a sex-linked inherited condition but is rarely due to an acquired defect of the retina; as a result, the majority of people who suffer from this condition are male. Approximately 8–10% of the male population suffers from a congenital colour vision defect (CVD) whilst the prevalence among females is much less (approximately 1%). Differences in prevalence of CVD have also been found between different racial groups. The affects of a CVD on shade selection is discussed below.

DESCRIPTION OF COLOUR

There are three main systems which can be used to describe and quantify colour, namely Munsell's colour order system, the 1976 C.I.E.L*a*b* uniform colour space system (C.I.E Commission Internationale d'Eclairage (International Commission on Illumination)) or the RGB (Red, Green, Blue) colour space system. The first system is the one most commonly used and quoted in clinical dentistry and is therefore the only system described in this text.

Munsell's colour order system

The Munsell colour system was devised by a painter, Albert Munsell, in 1905. The system's attributes are hue, chroma and value (Figure 15.5).

Hue

Hue is the quality by which we distinguish one colour from another – for example, red from yellow, or green from blue. There are 100 Munsell hues: 10 major hues with each placed 10 steps apart in a horizontal plane (z axis, Figure 15.5) around a central axis. Teeth are found in the yellow and yellow–red region but the exact range of hues varies with the method of assessment and is different for extracted teeth. Dentine provides the main source of hue in a tooth but this is modified by the enamel.

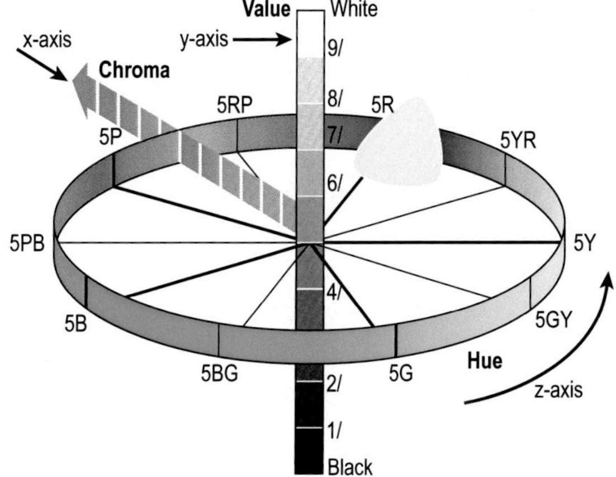

Figure 15.5 Framework of Munsell's colour order system.

Chroma

Chroma describes the intensity of the colour (hue) and distinguishes a strong colour from a weak one. The chroma scale starts at /0 and extends outwards; its maximum varies with each hue. The purest colours are found at the extremes of the colour cylinder (x axis, Figure 15.5). Reduced thickness or mineralization of dentine usually results in decreased chroma. The chroma of teeth is usually found within the range /1 to /5 but can range from /0 to /7.

Value

Value is the quality by which one distinguishes a light colour from a dark one and is therefore the brightness on a grey scale. The value symbol 0/ is used for absolute black and 10/ for absolute white (y axis, Figure 15.5). In a healthy young tooth there is less dentine thickness due to a reduced amount of secondary dentine and so the ratio of reflected to absorbed light radiation is increased compared to older teeth: as a tooth ages its value therefore decreases. Tooth value is usually found within the range 6/ to 8.5/ but can range upwards from 4/.

TOOTH SHADE SELECTION

'Selecting the shade' for a restoration belittles the complexity of the process of determining the shade and form for a restoration. Providing the technician with only the correct shade will not enable them to fabricate an aesthetic restoration, a substantial amount of additional information is required. Additionally, the clinician has to prepare teeth in such a way that the technician is able to recreate the desired shape and shade. (See chapter 10, 11 and 12). Methods of traditional and instrumental shade-matching will be described in this chapter, together with the supplemental information required for an aesthetic restoration.

Traditional shade matching

The basic shade for a restoration is usually selected using a shade guide. Most manufacturers provide a shade guide for use with their materials, whether they are for use with indirect or direct restorations. These allow transfer of information relating to tooth shade from the clinic to the laboratory. Ideally, shade selection would be completed by both the dentist and technician in conjunction with the patient. Unfortunately, this is often not practical as the laboratory is usually some distance from the dental clinic.

Value (brightness) is regarded as the most important and discernible aspect of colour when selecting a shade. Metal–ceramic crowns (MCC) have a higher value than natural teeth and are less translucent. The opaque ceramics that are required to mask the metal coping, which is obviously not translucent, give them their high value (see Chapter 10) and expose the restoration as fake compared to natural teeth (Figure 15.6). The increased value of crowns is usually due to insufficient tooth reduction (for adequate dentine and enamel ceramic) and laboratory shortcomings. A higher value also makes the tooth/restoration appear larger.

Shade guides for indirect restorations

The most commonly used shade guide for indirect restorations is based on the VITA classical shades. The VITA classical shade guide can be organized in two ways. First, the tabs can be grouped by similar hues (A–D), with these groups being divided via numerical values (1–4). Generally, the chroma (intensity of colour) increases and value (lightness) decreases as the numbers rise (Figure 15.7, above). Second, the shade tabs can be arranged by decreasing value (Figure 15.7, below).

The VITA System 3D-Master shade guide (Figure 15.8) arranges the shade tabs in a more logical fashion and is currently the only shade guide to meet the relevant American Dental Association (ADA) standard. The tabs are divided into five value groups (six if the three bleached shades are included). As value decreases, the tab group number increases. Within each value group, the chroma increases as one descends down the group. Moving from right to left alters the hue, making the tabs more red and yellow, respectively.

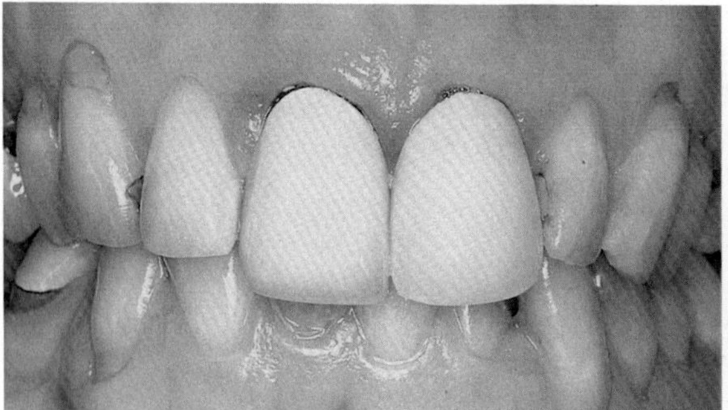
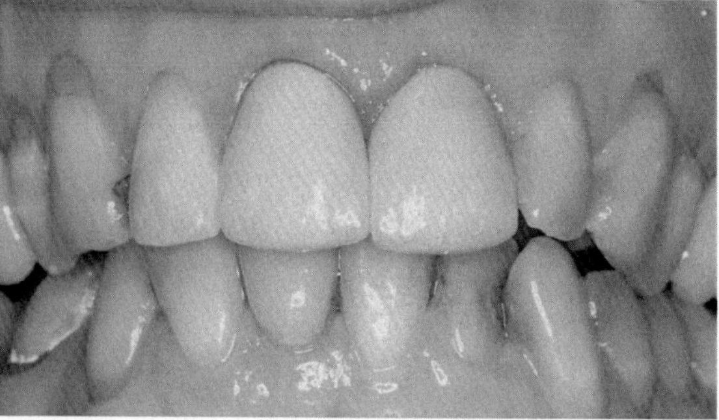

Figure 15.6 The effect of value on appearance. Metal–ceramic crowns on the central incisors (left) have too high a value and look bright. Replacement crowns (right) after correct tooth reduction and laboratory procedures give a more pleasing appearance.

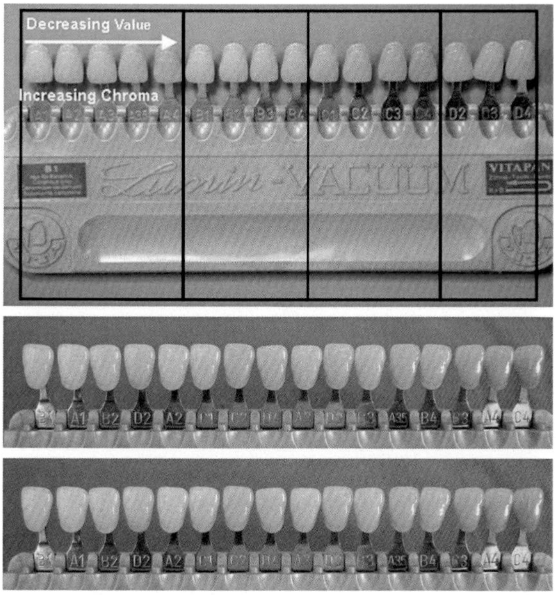

Figure 15.7 VITA classical shade guide arranged by hue (above) and value (middle and below).

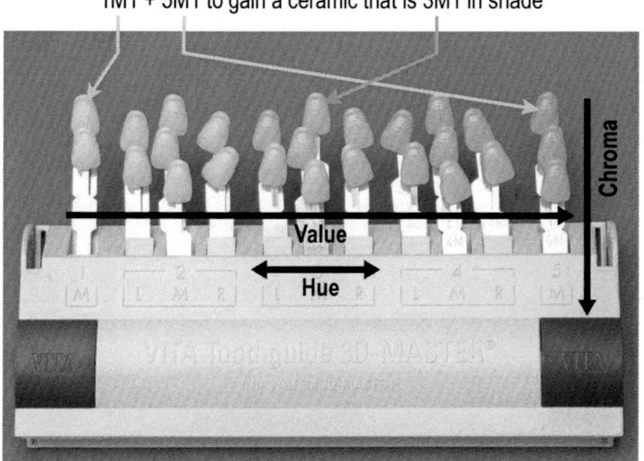

Figure 15.8 VITA 3D shade guide.

Unlike the VITA classical shade guide and most other shade guides, the manufacturer claims that each tab is equally spaced from the other, making intermediate shade selections possible. For example, 50% 1M1 plus 50% 5M1 will produce a 3M1 ceramic, or more relevant to the clinical setting, 75% 1M1 plus 25% 1M2 will produce a 1M1.25 ceramic. This allows a more objective selection of intermediate shades, making up to 96 different combinations possible. The fact that the tabs are equally spaced has been questioned, but despite this it has improved shade matching.

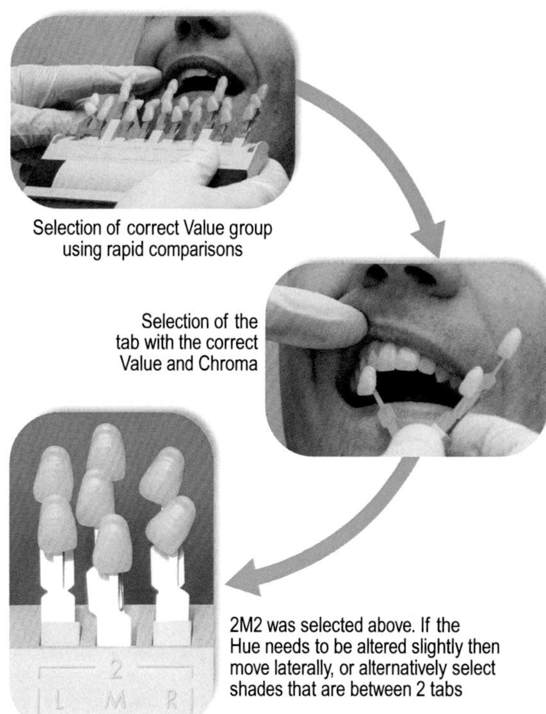

Figure 15.9 Shade selection using VITA 3D Master System.

The manufacturer's instructions should be used when selecting a shade with this shade guide (Figure 15.9). If the VITA System 3D-Master is used, it is important to ensure that the technician has the corresponding ceramic: if a 3D shade is selected, the restoration cannot be fabricated from VITA classical porcelains. Whilst a conversion table is available to convert VITA classical into 3D shades, this is only approximate.

Shade matching for teeth is notoriously difficult and is a result of a combination of problems:

- The unique properties of the teeth discussed previously
- Inconsistency in material manufacture
- Human observer errors.

There are many materials used to create aesthetic restorations; however, these do not always exhibit colour consistency. There are visible colour differences between batches and brands of ceramic and composite resin. Additionally, shade guides do not match each other, correspond to the colour of teeth or always match the materials they represent. Figure 15.10 shows three different A3 materials compared to a reference VITA classical shade tab and the VITA 3D shade tab that approximately represents A3. Custom shade guides manufactured from the batch of ceramic and composite resin to be used have been suggested, but these are not a practical alternative.

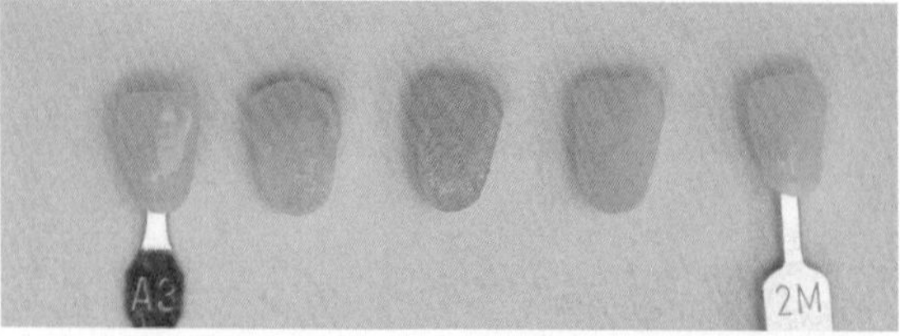

Figure 15.10 Two shade tabs and three materials all purporting to have an A3 shade. Obvious differences can be seen.

Humans are also unreliable when selecting shades: studies have shown that only between 20% and 73% of shade selections of the same material under the same conditions by the same observer were identical on different days. Different observers also vary in their shade selections of the same shade of material over time.

Figure 15.11 shows a flowchart that should facilitate a more repeatable shade-matching routine; the information in parentheses briefly justifies each stage.

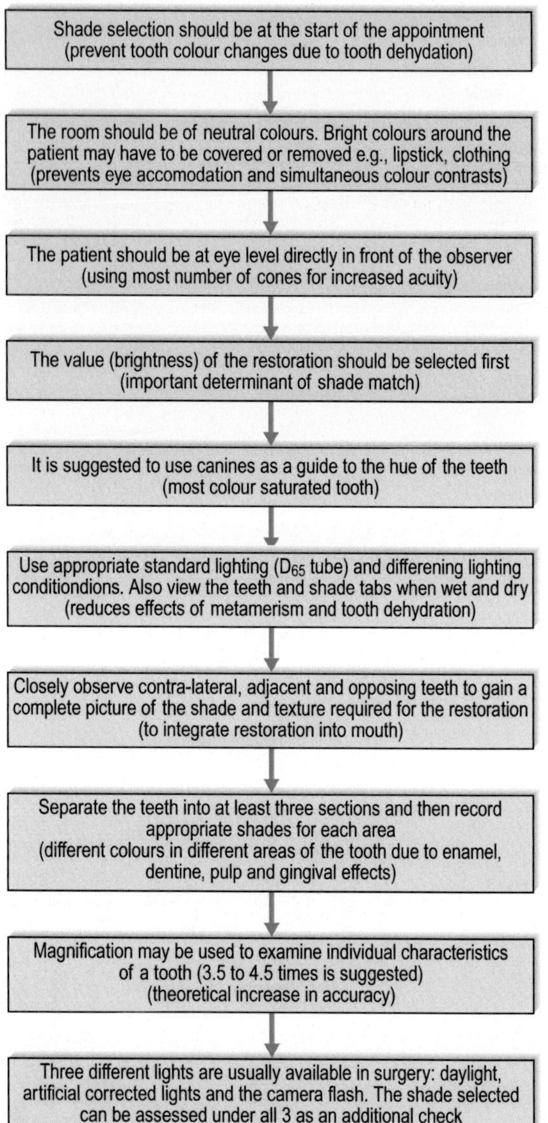

Figure 15.11 Traditional shade matching flow chart.

Effects of colour vision deficiencies

While colour vision deficiency has been shown to have an adverse effect on ability to match dental colours, it also appears to have an unequal effect on the descriptors of colour. When compared to colour-normal subjects, CVD subjects have difficulty in recording hue and chroma but not value. It is difficult to define the effect of CVD on the complete shade matching process but is worthy of consideration if problems are evident. In addition, a CVD may affect the ability of individuals to differentiate restoration margins in an impression depending on the colour of the materials. This is especially true if two materials of different viscosity and colour are used.

Instrumental shade matching

Shade-matching devices

Instrumental shade-matching systems make use of colorimeters, spectrophotometers or digital images to make measurements at one or a number of points on a tooth's surface (Figure 15.12). The devices that use a spectrophotometer or colorimeter require a precise technique, keeping the probe at right angles to the tooth surface whilst keeping a steady hand (Figure 15.13). It is recommended that three readings are made and the most common used as the shade to be transferred to the laboratory. The recorded shade is available to the dentist, patient and technician almost immediately and most devices are able to provide CIE data.

Little evidence is available about the use of these devices in clinical practice; however, they have the potential to improve inter- and intra-clinician repeatability with regard to their shade selections over time and to select shade matches that are more acceptable to patients and dentists. They can also be used by the technician to verify the shade of the restoration that has been fabricated.

Digital photography

Information relating to shade and the aesthetic details discussed below can be transferred in a more objective manner by digital images. The shade cannot be calculated from a

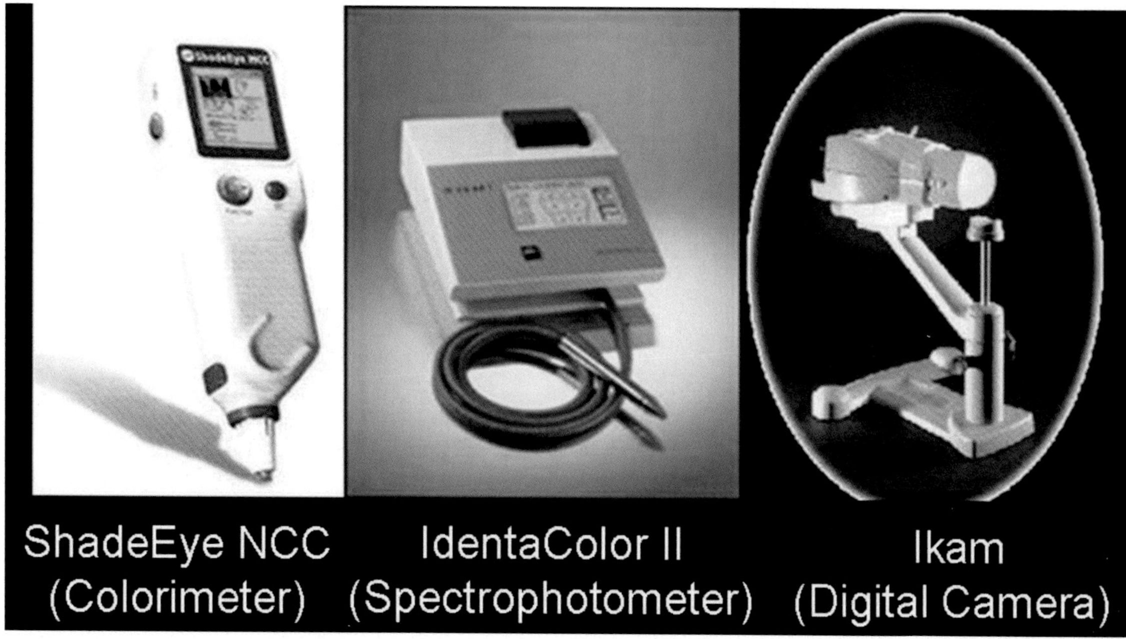

Figure 15.12 Instrumental shade-matching devices.

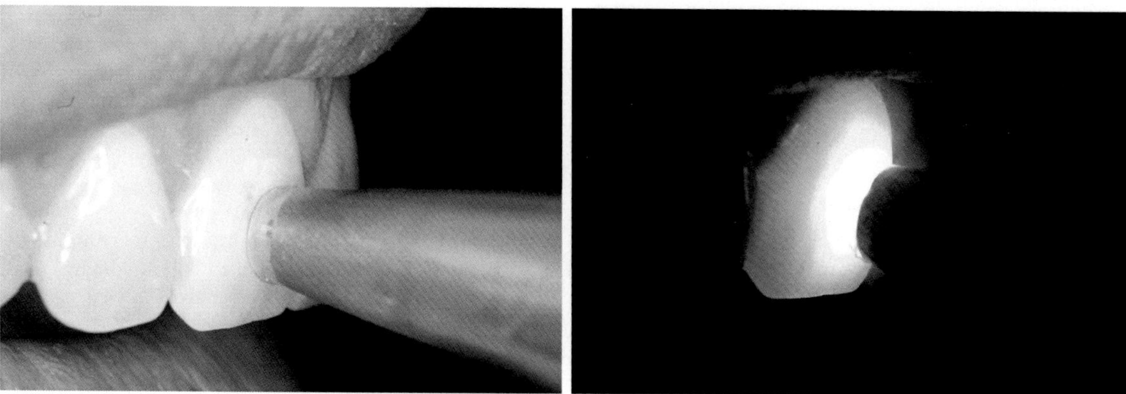

Figure 15.13 Probe of instrumental shade-matching device, being approximated to the tooth at right angles (left) and the device recording the shade (right).

digital image without a calibration tile and conversion software. If digital images are to be used, then a series of images are usually required (Figure 15.14). In Figure 15.14 the camera was held at right angles to the tooth to give an accurate representation of translucency, effects, etc.

The minimum requirements for making intraoral images are a single-lens reflex (SLR) camera with an appropriate macro lens and flash. Two main types of flash are used: ring and a dual-point light. The former produces images that have no shadows as the buccal corridors are illuminated, producing good all-round images. A dual-point light allows shadows to assess texture and subtle changes in tooth surface anatomy. Compact cameras may be used but the images are often less accurate and the macro (close-up) lens is not consistently accurate enough for intraoral images. In addition, the flash often gives teeth a washed-out appearance and prevents the reproduction of subtle tooth characteristics. If digital images are used, a secure memory card is also required to store images in a manner that conforms to data protection regulations.

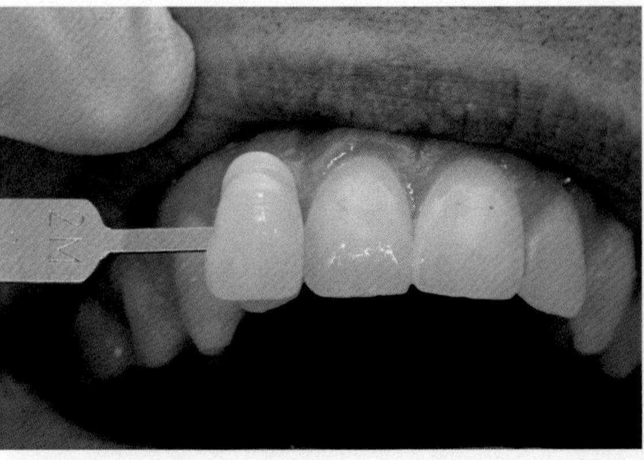
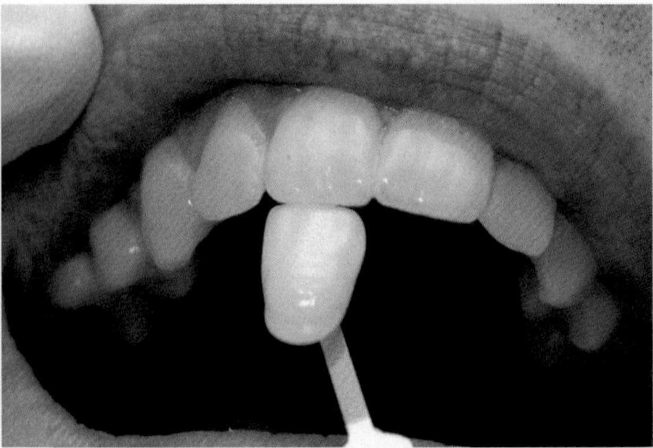

Figure 15.14 Digital photographs to aid the technician. It is important that several views are taken. Note the shade tabs are in the same horizontal and vertical plane as the reference tooth and the shade is visible to the technician on at least one of the photographs.

SUPPLEMENTAL AESTHETIC INFORMATION

Correctly matching the shade of a restoration to a tooth will not alone give an aesthetic result due to the complex structure of a tooth. Information relating to the subtleties of tooth form is also required. For example, vertical and horizontal tooth form need to be recorded, including specific characteristics such as transition lines, emergence profile, lustre, translucency, opalescence, dentine and enamel effects, stain lines, areas of hypomineralization, occlusal, cuspal/incisal and gingival colouration, root simulation, mammelons and lobe formation. In addition, conditions not related to tooth form have to be transferred to the laboratory and these should include tooth inclination (ideally progressive mesial angulation), gingival contours and levels, lip line and symmetry. Most of this type of information can be transferred via articulated study casts and diagnostic wax-ups during the diagnostic phase of treatment (see Chapter 5).

Aesthetic analysis

The aesthetic demands and expectations of individual patients vary considerably and are often different from those of the treating clinician. Personnel from dental specialities might be more discerning than laypersons; however, some patients can be quite critical. Individuals from different dental specialities may also have different perceptions of aesthetics, with orthodontists being more critical of minor deviations in symmetry than prosthodontists for example. It is therefore important that realistic results are discussed with patients as well as the potential shortcomings of certain treatment modalities.

The aesthetic demands of people range from low to individuals where their perception of appearance is altered by psychological conditions (body dysmorphophobia). The aesthetic demands of some of these patient groups can be impossible to achieve and part of the initial assessment should attempt to identify such patients.

Excellent aesthetic integration can be achieved by placing full coverage restorations on all teeth in the upper anterior sextant; however, adverse biological outcomes have to be discussed with the patient (loss of pulp vitality, possible gingival recession, extensive treatment, maintenance and replacement, etc.). It is much harder, but not impossible, to achieve consistent aesthetic results when individual teeth are treated and more conservative treatments are used.

Before embarking on treatments that are going to have a high impact on a patient's appearance, it is important to consider the facial, dento-facial and dento-gingival relationships to complete an aesthetic analysis as well as managing the patients' expectations.

Facial relationships

When viewed in the frontal plane, it has been stated that many face features are linked by orientation and size; however, rarely does one exhibit a perfectly symmetrical face.

Facial midline

Unfortunately, bilateral landmarks (eyes, ears, etc.) are often not exactly symmetrical: slight nasal deviations, small differences in the amount of eye opening and eye levels are found. This makes assessment of the facial midline difficult. Two reproducible points commonly used to identify a midline are nasion (midpoint between the two eyebrows) and the centre of the base of the philtrum. The direction of the midline can also be determined by these (Figure 15.15).

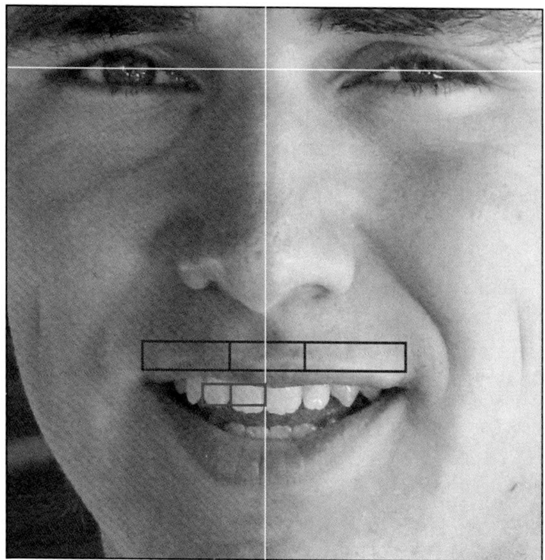

Figure 15.15 Horizontal and vertical lines showing the interpupillary horizontal line and facial midline. The boxes show aspects of dental golden proportion.

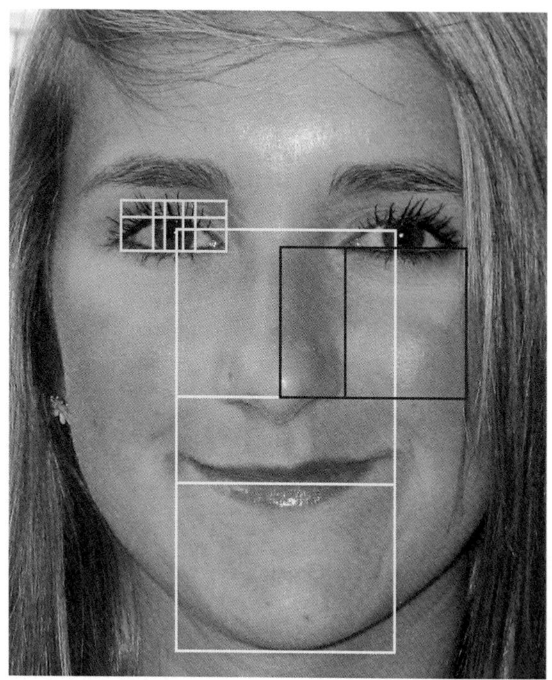

Figure 15.16 Facial golden proportions.

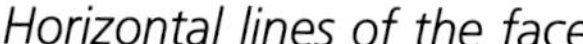

Horizontal lines of the face

It is often stated that the horizontal lines (interpupillary, commissural, nasal lines and occlusal plane) of the face should be parallel; however, this is often not the case. As the eyes are often at slightly different levels, it can be difficult to assess the relationship of the horizontal lines of the face using the interpupillary line as a guide. Therefore a better guide for the smile line is often to fabricate it at right angles to the facial midline (Figure 15.15).

Golden proportion

The ancient Greeks discovered a complex ratio they named the 'golden mean' or 'phi', equalling 1.618, which was considered the most aesthetically pleasing ratio. The human body is said to have many excellent examples of phi, or golden proportion: the combined length of one's hand and forearm divided by the length of one's forearm is said to produce phi. Several ratios in the head and neck are purported to exist and may indicate an aesthetically pleasing face (Figures 15.15 and 15.16). The relationship of facial structures in the sagittal plane must also be considered. Skeletal, and dental, Class II and III relationships often prevent facial features from conforming to the golden proportion and are therefore considered by some to be less aesthetic.

In reality, it appears few individuals conform to all of the ideal ratios; however, it is known that aspects such as marked asymmetry, substantial deviation of facial and dental midlines, changes in face height and lateral discrepancies such as retrognathia can cause patients to be concerned about their appearance.

Dento-facial relationships

Midline

As discussed, the dental and facial midlines should be coincident or at least parallel to each other (Figure 15.15). The dental midline (line between upper and lower central incisors) is often examined relative to the midpoint of the upper lip (the middle of the middle lobe of the upper lip), but this may not be coincident with the facial midline. The dental and facial midlines are not coincident in approximately a quarter of patients. A deviation of the dental midline from the facial midline of 2.2 ± 1.5 mm has been found to be acceptable by various dental and lay observers, with about half of observers being unable identify differences between the facial and dental midlines if the discrepancy is less than 2 mm.

Smile line

The relationship of the incisal edges of the maxillary anterior teeth and the lips can range from the parallel through to an inverted (reverse) relationship. When the upper central incisor and canine teeth rest on the lip curvature and the upper lateral incisors are above this line, the most pleasing outline is produced.

The smile line is assessed in several ways:

- The position of the upper lip to the maxillary gingival tissue (the most aesthetic smile is thought to exist when the full height of the maxillary teeth and the interproximal papillae are visible)
- The relationship of the curvature of the lower lip to the maxillary incisal tooth curvature
- The position of the maxillary incisal tooth curve relative to the lower lip.

These three factors can help determine the final contour and shape of restorations. It can be more difficult to treat patients with a high lip line as restoration contour, finish line placement and integration, gingival contour and colour are more critical. Assessing the lip line can be difficult as patients often produce a forced, unnatural smile. Asking a patient to say 'E' can help.

Vertical dimension

Vertical dimension relates to the proportions of the lower face height compared to the upper face height. Facial aesthetics may be affected by the dental occlusal vertical dimension (OVD); however, substantial changes in OVD are required to alter the facial height significantly. The lower face height would be expected to be reduced in cases of extreme wear; however, due to compensatory growth of the dento-alveolar complexes this is often not the case.

Dento-gingival relationships

The hard tissues

Teeth come in a large variety of shapes and orientations relative to other teeth in the same mouth and between individuals (Figure 15.17). In general, teeth should have progressive mesial inclination (Figure 15.18) to give a pleasing appearance. The position and length of the interdental contacts are paramount to a pleasing smile: the contact between maxillary central incisors is the most coronal and the contacts move apically as one moves more posteriorly. The 50-40-30 rule applies to the length of these contacts. This rule relates to the relationship of the interdental contact height between the maxillary central incisors, the central incisor and lateral incisor, and the lateral incisor and canine teeth relative to the height of the central incisor. Fifty per cent of the length of the central incisors should ideally be involved in the contact zone, 40% for the contact between the lateral incisor and central incisor, with 30% for the canine and lateral incisor teeth.

Incisal openings between teeth should increase in size starting at the midline and moving posteriorly. Tooth form helps contribute to this as maxillary lateral incisors often have a more rounded mesial edge than central incisors and the shape of the upper canine (cuspid) lends itself to a larger embrasure.

It is generally accepted that black triangles or spacing between teeth is less aesthetic than teeth with dental and gingival interdental closure (Figure 15.19). The cause of increased interdental spacing is usually periodontal disease or a tooth:arch size discrepancy. This spacing can be reduced by having long interdental contacts, but the excessive contacts can lead to a poor appearance ('tombstoning').

Teeth are individual and exhibit substantial variation in tooth form (Figure 15.17). Disorders of tooth formation (hypomineralization, hypomaturation, amelogenesis imperfecta, dentinogenesis imperfecta) can further affect the appearance (see Chapter 5) and lead to demands for extensive restorative work.

Tooth colour

When considering colour and creating the optimum appearance it is important to bear in mind that teeth within the same mouth vary – for example, the colour of canine teeth are often darker and more yellow than the incisors (Figure 15.20). In addition, the relative amount of value, hue and chroma varies across each individual tooth (Figure 15.20). There is obviously a considerable variability in the colour of teeth between individuals and within individuals; the range of colours of restorative materials is vast but still do not cover the range of tooth colours observed. It is worth re-iterating that teeth naturally darken with age.

Tooth size

The ideal width:length ratio of an upper central incisor is 0.75:0.8. Shorter and wider teeth have a smaller ratio. These ratios provide guidelines to achieve good dental aesthetics and if the ratio is repeated throughout the maxillary sextant then the appearance can be excellent. This ratio can be assessed using a golden proportion ruler/gauge (Figure 15.21). This proportion must be calculated when the patient is viewed directly from the front.

The size of teeth varies both between individuals and over one's lifetime. Many studies have measured tooth dimensions and the dimensions determined by Magne et al. (2003) are shown in Table 15.1. This table also demonstrates the changes that occur due to tooth wear, with the length of teeth obviously getting shorter as they wear. This alters the width:length ratio which may adversely affect appearance.

Bony factors

The alveolar bone may influence the appearance of a smile. For example, excess alveolar contours (buccal bony tori) and dehiscences/fenestrations leading to soft tissue defects may be present.

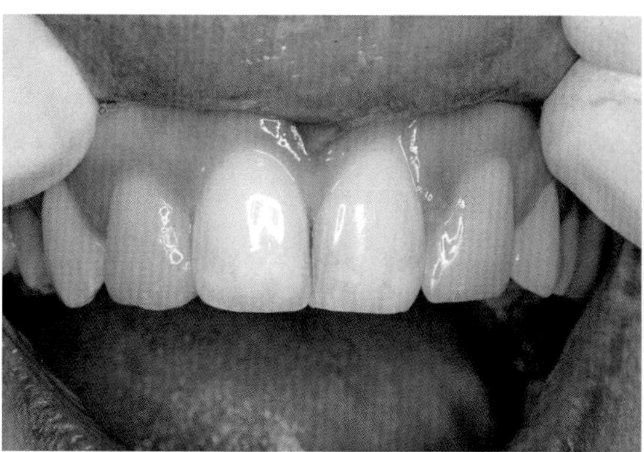
Congenitally absent lateral incisors with comouflaged canine teeth

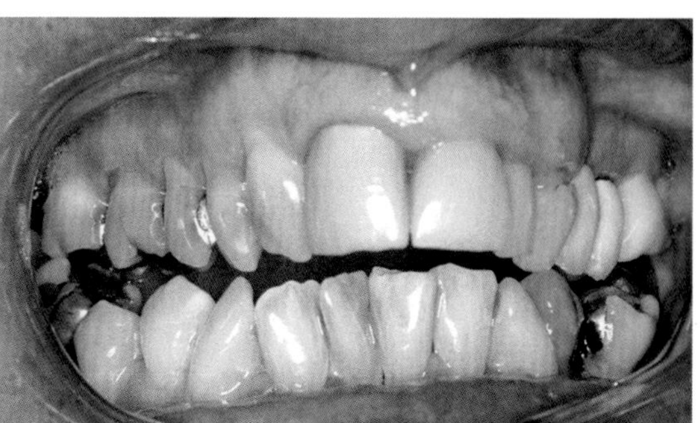
Absent upper right lateral incisor, retained deciduous canine, midline discrepancy and microdontic upper left lateral incisor providing a compromised aesthetic result

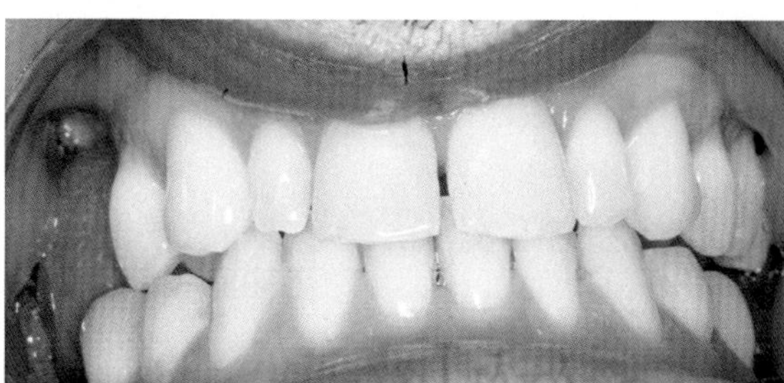
Microdontia of upper lateral incisors

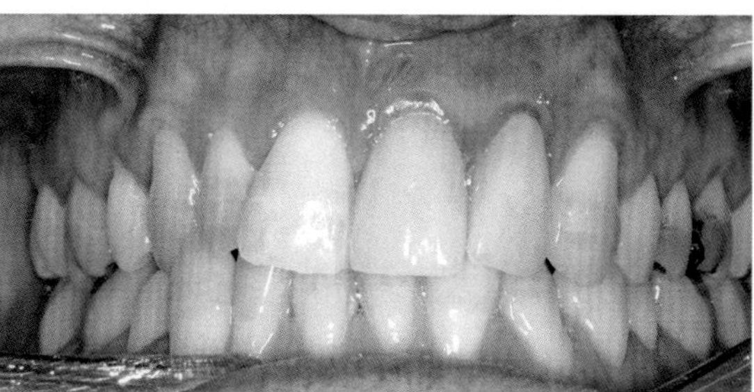
Distal inclination of upper right central incisor and excessive mesial inclination of upper left incisors giving a compromised aesthetic result

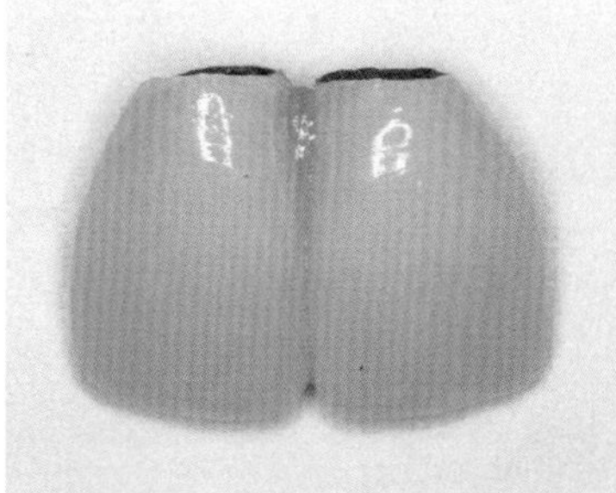
Restorative interdental closure: long contact points and pink ceramic

Figure 15.17 Variation in tooth form and appearance.

Soft tissues

Poor gingival health and a history of periodontal disease can lead to gingival aesthetic problems. Gingival health must be gained and established as a prerequisite to aesthetic success. Gingival health must be established prior to placing definitive restorations. The position of the free gingival margin, muco-gingival junction and the width of the attached gingiva have to be assessed and corrected if required.

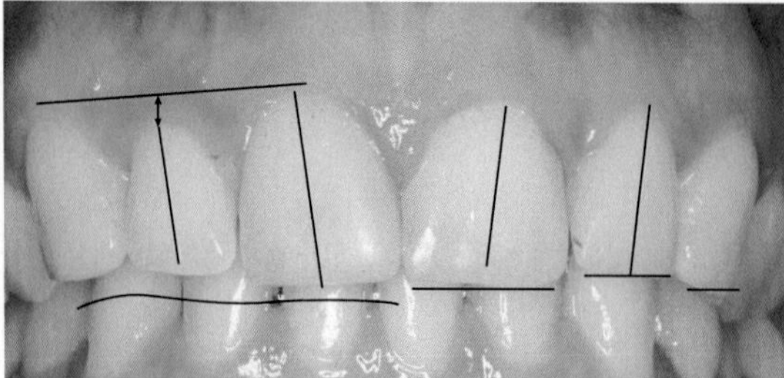

Figure 15.18 Pleasing appearance of the upper anterior sextant.

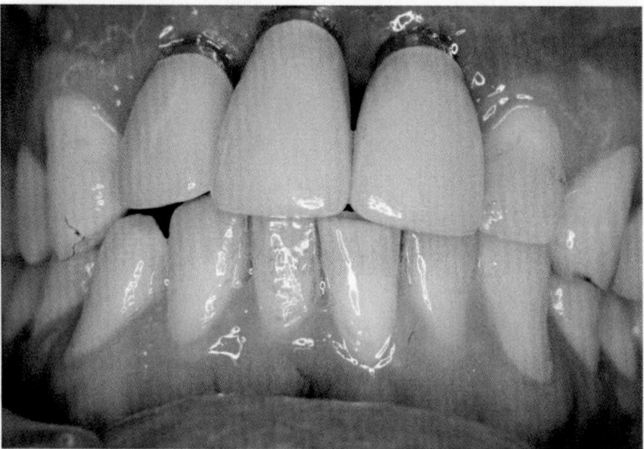

Figure 15.19 Poor contour of the central incisor implant retained crowns and loss of interdental papilla have led to unsightly black triangles between the restorations.

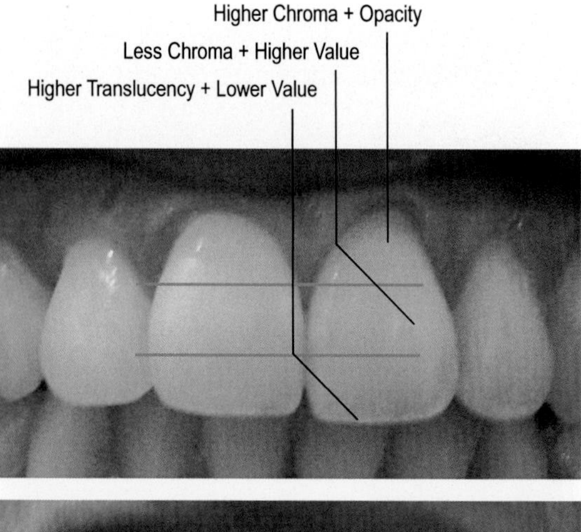

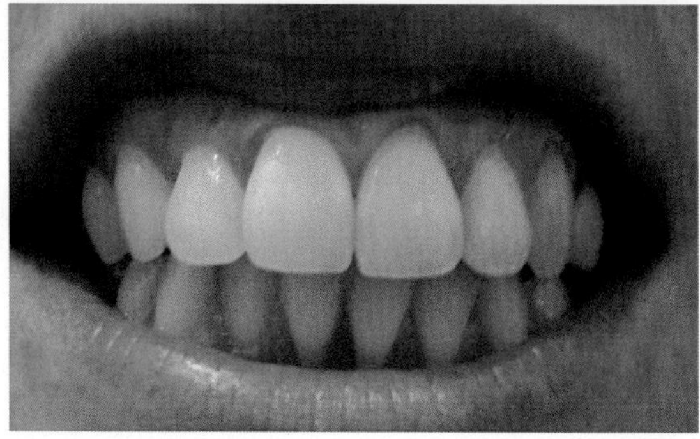

Figure 15.20 Tooth colour variation across a tooth (above) and between teeth (below).

Gingival contour

It is generally accepted that balance/symmetry and the correct proportions of the factors discussed are needed to create an aesthetic smile. In addition, the gingival contour is perhaps one of the most important factors in aesthetic dentistry. The example in Figure 15.22 shows that although the shade and size of restoration are acceptable, the gingival margins are not balanced. In addition to gingival health, complete gingival papillae, balanced gingival levels and correct gingival contours, colour and texture are required for a pleasing appearance (see Figure 15.18). It is generally accepted that the gingival margin should be more coronal around lateral incisors than central incisors or canines, and that the canine margin is the most apical of the maxillary anterior sextant. The gingival zenith should lie to the distal of each tooth's centre line (see Figure 15.18).

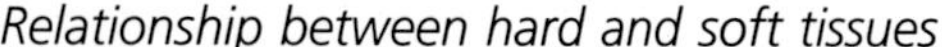

Relationship between hard and soft tissues

Periodontal characteristics have been studied in relation to crown shape. Two periodontal biotypes (thin and thick) have been identified which correlated to crown form (short-wide or long-narrow); patients with long-narrow teeth have been shown to be more prone to gingival recession than patients with short-wide teeth. This relationship has to be considered in patients with high aesthetic demands/high lip line as the risk of unsightly crown margins being exposed over time is increased.

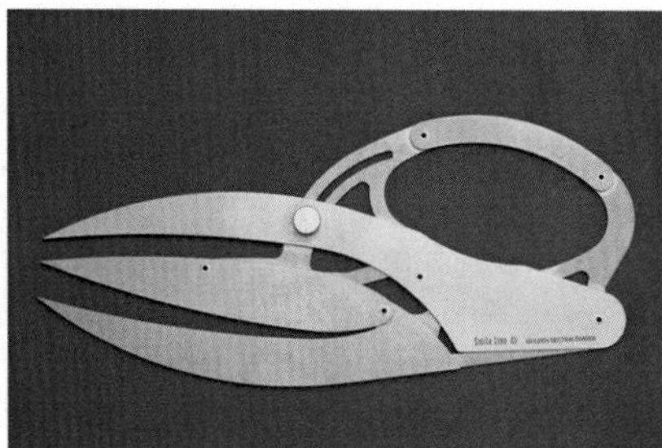

Figure 15.21 Golden proportion ruler.

Table 15.1 Tooth dimensions

	NO. OF TEETH MEASURED	WIDTH	LENGTH	W/L RATIO
Centrals, unworn (range)	18	**9.10** (0.62) (8.46–11.07)	**11.69** (0.70) (10.70–13.51)	**0.78** (0.03) (0.71–0.84)
Centrals, worn (range)	26	**9.24** (0.66) (8.21–10.34)	**10.67** (1.13) (8.56–13.42)	**0.87** (0.08) (0.74–1.10)
Laterals, unworn (range)	30	**7.07** (0.76) (5.51–8.22)	**9.75** (0.83) (8.19–11.51)	**0.73** (0.07) (0.57–0.83)
Laterals, worn (range)	11	**7.38** (0.52) (6.43–7.89)	**9.34** (0.80) (7.97–11.22)	**0.79** (0.06) (0.70–0.87)
Canines, unworn (range)	25	**7.90** (0.64) (6.80–9.02)	**10.83** (0.77) (9.71–12.94)	**0.73** (0.06) (0.60–0.82)
Canines, worn (range)	13	**8.06** (0.74) (6.60–8.72)	**9.90** (0.84) (8.83–11.77)	**0.81** (0.06) (0.72–0.91)
Premolars (range)	23	**7.84** (0.73) (6.61–8.84)	**9.33** (0.94) (7.66–10.45)	**0.84** (0.06) (0.65–0.95)

From Magne et al. (2003).

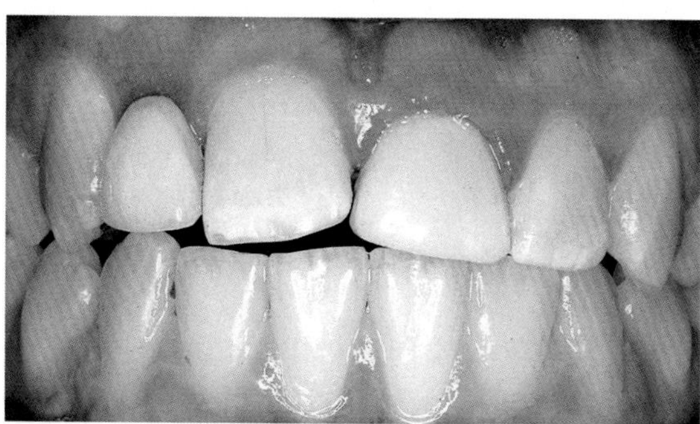

Figure 15.22 The aesthetic result for this patient is compromised by the unbalanced gingival margins, despite acceptable shade matches of the metal–ceramic crown on the upper left central incisor and the minimum preparation (resin retained) bridge replacing the upper right lateral incisor.

SUMMARY

Creating the best aesthetics in indirect restorations is a complex process and involves far more than simply colour matching. This chapter has looked in depth at shade matching as well as all associated features of tooth form and how this is framed within the supporting periodontal tissues, the smile line and facial features. Having an understanding of these will enable the dentist to achieve the highest aesthetics possible within a given situation, assess appearance critically and be able to inform patients about the limitations of possible treatment options.

FURTHER READING

Magne, P., Gallucci, G.O., Belser, U.C., 2003. Anatomic crown width/length ratios of unworn and worn maxillary teeth in white subjects. J. Prosthet. Dent. 89, 453–461.

Miller, A., Long, J., Cole, J., Staffanou, R., 1993. Shade selection and laboratory communication. Quintessence Int. 24, 305–309.

Wasson, W., Schuman, N., 1992. Color vision and dentistry. Quintessence Int. 23, 349–353.

Chapter 16

Complex multiple fixed and combined fixed and removable prosthodontics

David Bartlett, David Ricketts

CHAPTER CONTENTS

INDICATIONS

Complex multiple fixed and combined fixed and removable prosthodontics can be indicated to restore teeth damaged and depleted by the ravages of caries, tooth wear and inherited and acquired defects (outlined in Chapters 1–5).

COMBINED FIXED AND REMOVABLE PROSTHODONTICS

Many partial dentures are made using support from teeth restored with existing plastic restorations. Designing crowns and partial dentures at the same time helps to improve the retention, support and stability of the denture. The denture must be designed before crowns are made to ensure the rest seats, guide planes and undercuts are placed in the optimum position. A well-designed denture will need upper and lower study casts and ideally these should be mounted on an articulator. This can be an average value articulator which gives an indication of the intercuspal position and allows some degree of excursive movements, or for more complex cases involving multiple crowns, a semi-adjustable articulator should be used to more accurately allow assessment of functional movements of the mandible. The study casts should be surveyed to show the position of undercuts on the teeth or where undercuts are required in crowns. This process follows conventional prosthodontic procedures and is covered by the appropriate texts. Making crowns with guide planes, undercuts and rest seats increases their complexity and cost. Therefore, the design of tooth support, retention and stability for the partial denture needs to be carefully planned to be optimal and to ensure cost effectiveness.

Rest seats, guide planes and undercuts

Rest seats provide direct dental support for a partial denture. They need to be large enough to provide support and deep enough for the rest on the partial denture to fit into the cavity or rest seat in the crown (or tooth) without interfering with the occlusion. The size of the rest seats needs to be sufficient to provide support and normally about one-third of the proximal width of the tooth is sufficient. The shape of the cavity should avoid sharp internal line angles and follow the general shape as shown in Figure 16.1. There should also be sufficient occlusal clearance to allow a minor connection between the base of the partial denture and any rest seats and clasps around the same tooth (Figure 16.2).

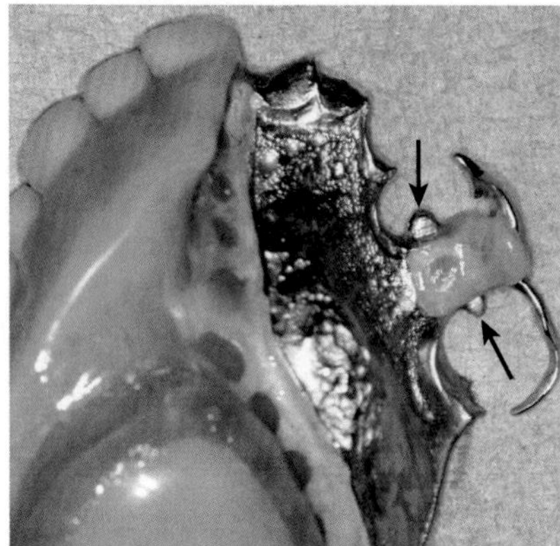

Figure 16.1 The fit surface of this partial removable cobalt chromium prosthesis shows the general outline of the rests (arrowed) having a rounded character in all dimensions. Note the obturator bottom left which seals a maxillary defect created following surgery to remove a tumour.

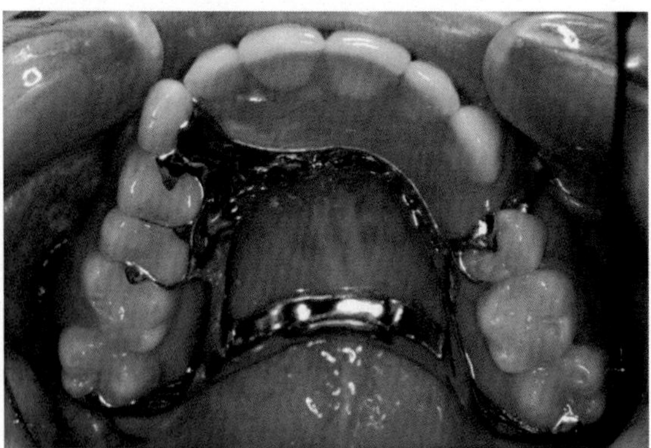

Figure 16.2 Sufficient occlusal clearance is required not only for the rest seat, but also the connector between the rest seat (and clasps if present) and base of denture.

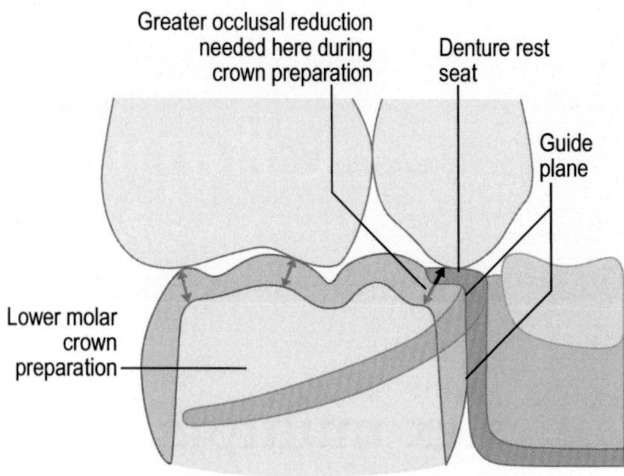

Figure 16.3 During crown preparation, the occlusal reduction in the region where a rest seat is planned has to be greater to allow for the thickness of the rest on the denture and the metal of the crown.

Knowing where the rest seat and connectors will ultimately be placed will therefore influence tooth preparation when a crown is planned. Occlusal reduction in the region of the rest seat and connector has to be greater than elsewhere on the occlusal surface as sufficient interocclusal space has to be provided for both the metal substructure to the crown and the thickness of the rest itself (Figure 16.3). Where crowns are concerned it is always important to place rest seats into metal as placement into ceramic will lead to shear fractures (Figure 16.4).

The retention of metal-based partial dentures relies heavily upon clasps. To create the necessary resistance to displacement of the clasps, an undercut, normally on the buccal surface of the crown (tooth), needs to be present. When designing crowns and partial dentures the depth of undercut required for cast cobalt chromium clasps is

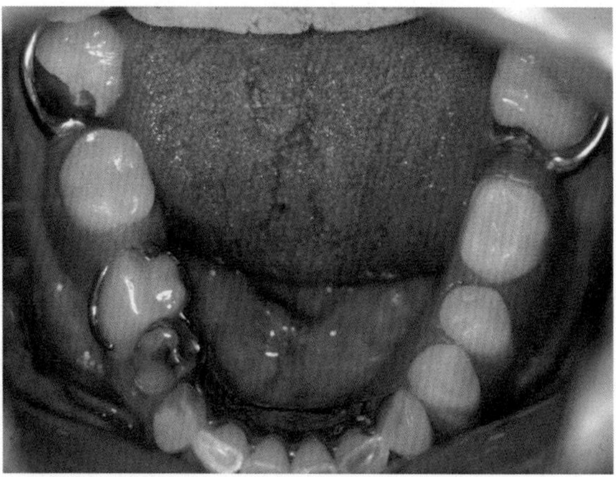

Figure 16.4 Inappropriate placement of rest seats onto ceramic in the metal–ceramic crowns on the lower molar teeth has led to ceramic fracture.

generally 0.25 mm; to a degree, however, this will depend on the length of the clasp arm (longer clasp arms can engage deeper undercuts). For wrought clasps a deeper undercut can be engaged (0.5 mm) as these have greater inherent flexibility. These undercuts have to be prescribed to the technician so that they can be incorporated into the crown contour.

Guide planes designed on the proximal surfaces of crowns increase the surface area in contact with the partial denture saddle area and increase the resistance to displacement and so retention. The guide planes, when present, need to be parallel to each other to maximize the retention. There is little value in having a single crown with a guide plane without reciprocating action from another crown or tooth.

This section emphasizes the importance of planning the denture design before any tooth preparation takes place. Figures 16.5 and 16.6 illustrate this point clearly.

Precision attachments

There are situations where precision attachments are still indicated when fixed and removable prosthodontics are considered together. The routine use of implants has, to some extent, reduced the need for precision attachments on teeth because the cost of the attachment and laboratory work can approach that of implant retained prostheses. Precision attachments linked to fixed laboratory-made prostheses can be used to retain and stabilize removable prostheses. There are a number of designs that can be considered, ranging from extracoronal stud or seeker (ball and socket) attachments to intracoronal movable joints similar to those used in conjunction with fixed–movable bridge designs (see Chapter 19). To illustrate how such precision attachments can be used, consider the following three clinical scenarios.

Patient 1

The patient seen in Figure 16.7 has missing lower posterior teeth with severe resorption of the edentulous ridge, making it difficult to tolerate a lower removable prosthesis due to the lack of retention and stability. To address this, the lower canine teeth have been prepared for metal–ceramic crowns which have distal cantilevered bars and stud attachments incorporated into the metal substructure (Figure 16.8). The lower removable cobalt chromium prosthesis has a corresponding female attachment (socket) embedded into the acrylic of the denture base (Figure 16.9). This 'ball and socket' arrangement provides sufficient retention and stability without the need for clasping anterior teeth (Figure 16.8).

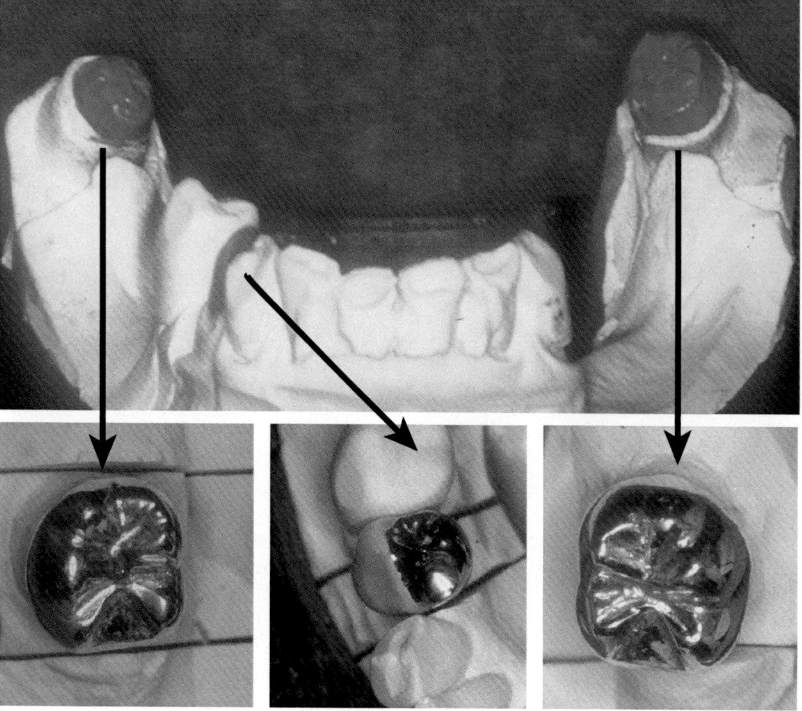

Figure 16.5 Having a denture design prior to preparation of the lower molar teeth and lower right premolar tooth for crowns has enabled appropriate prescription of rest seats, undercuts and guide planes in the indirect restorations.

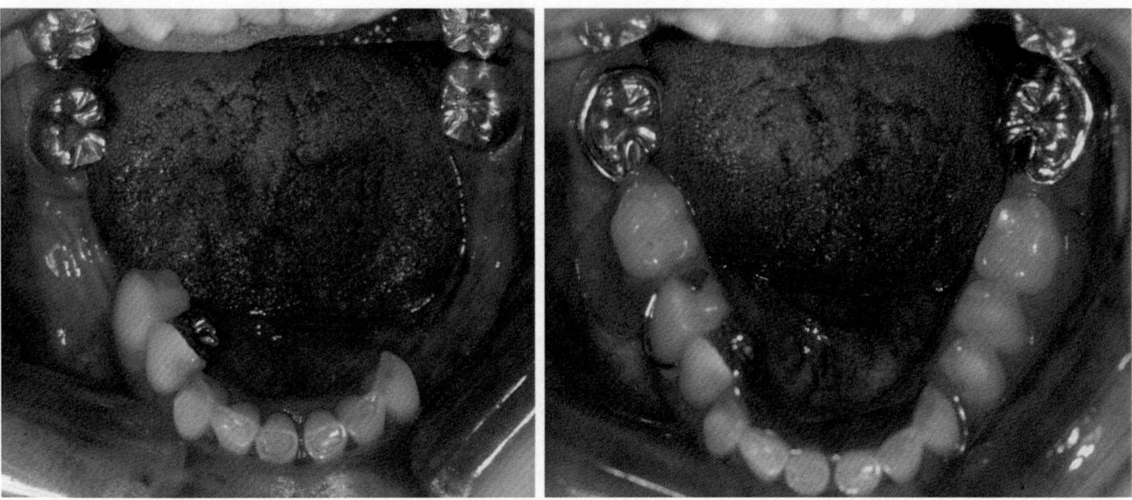

Figure 16.6 The crowns for the patient seen in Figure 16.5 cemented (left) and the new cobalt chromium denture (right).

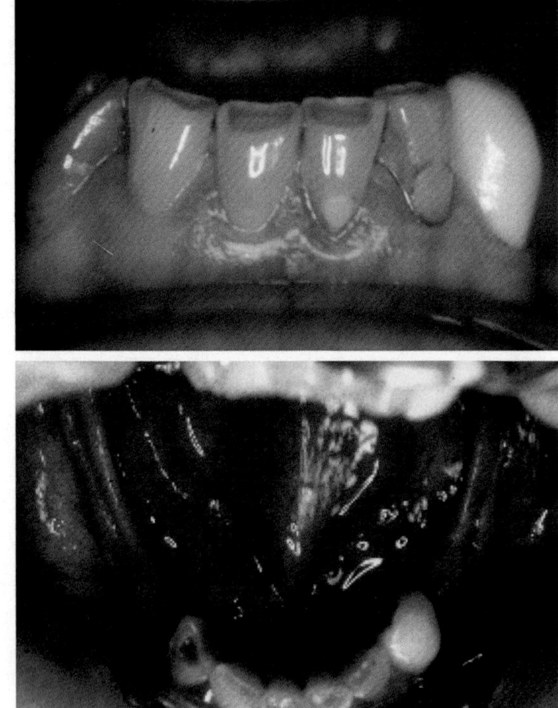

Figure 16.7 Patient with lower anterior teeth only. Due to the severe resorption of the lower edentulous ridge the patient is unable to tolerate their existing denture due to poor retention and stability.

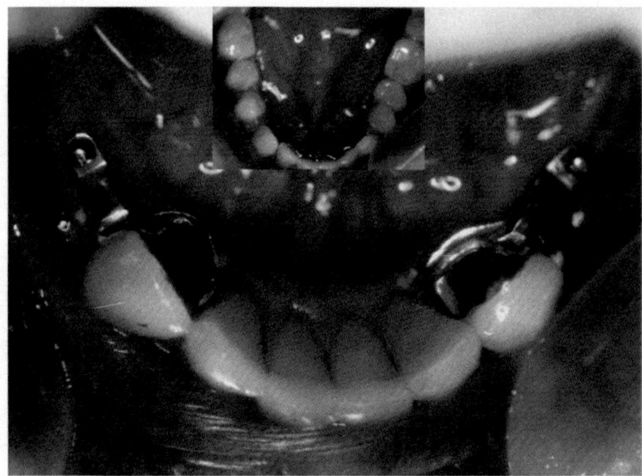

Figure 16.8 The patient seen in Figure 16.7 with crowns on the canine teeth that incorporate cingulum rest seats and distal extension bars with a stud attachment. The denture (inset) therefore avoids unsightly clasps in the anterior region.

Patient 2

Precision attachments can be used in conjunction with other conventional means of retention for removable prostheses. Consider the patient seen in Figure 16.10; gold crowns have been placed on the molar teeth incorporating rest seats, guide planes and undercuts to achieve support, stability and conventional retention; however, retention is not so easily achieved anteriorly without the presence of unsightly metal clasps. One way to overcome this is to use a precision attachment on the upper left

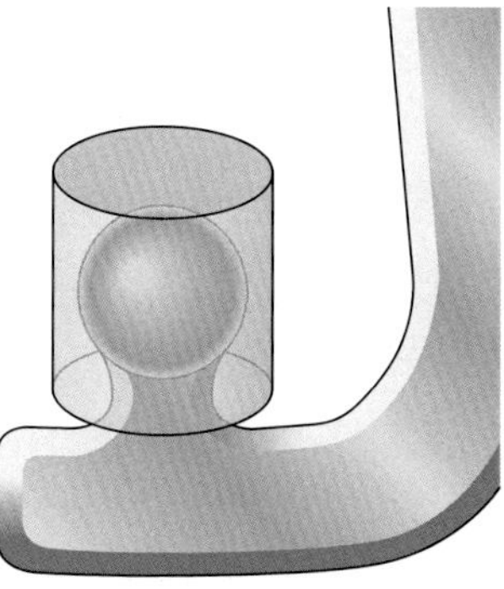

Figure 16.9 Diagrammatic representation of stud attachment on the distal cantilever arm. The metal housing for the socket joint is embedded into the denture base. The socket joint is provided by plastic colour-coded inserts of varying stiffness and hence retentiveness.

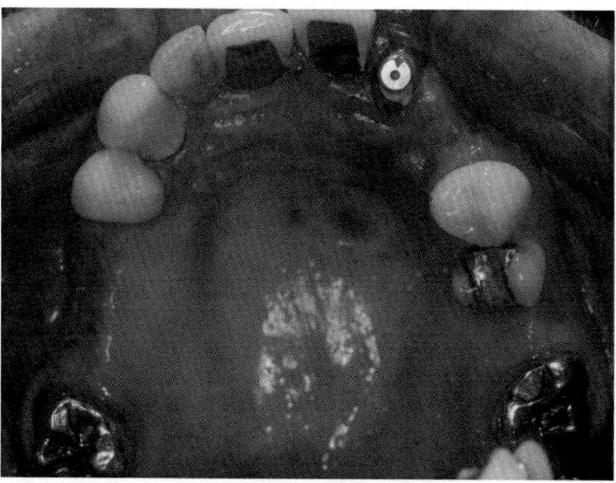

Figure 16.10 Patient for which an upper cobalt chromium prosthesis is planned. Gold crowns have been placed on the two molar teeth incorporating rest seats, guide planes and appropriate undercuts. Additional retention is gained anteriorly with a Rothermann-type precision attachment incorporated into a cast post and diaphragm on the left lateral incisor.

lateral incisor root. This tooth has been root treated and prepared for a cast post and diaphragm onto which is soldered the male component of a Rothermann type precision attachment; the female 'clip' attachment is embedded into the fit surface of the denture (Figure 16.11). The male component consists of a disc with a concavity around its periphery; the female clip seats into this concavity on insertion of the denture, giving good retention.

Patient 3

Figure 16.12 shows the die stone model of a patient who presented with multiple retained roots in the upper arch; the only teeth with natural crowns were the central incisors and the upper left second molar tooth. He was unable to wear a conventional denture due to a marked retch reflex. As for the previous patient the roots were root filled and prepared for cast post, diaphragm and Rothermann type attachments (Figure 16.13). The precision attachments provide excellent retention and allow a horseshoe cobalt chromium denture to be made with minimal palatal coverage.

With the advent of dental implants there is greater scope to retain, stabilize and support removable prostheses in edentulous patients. Studs, bars and magnets can be attached to implants with reciprocal components bedded into the denture base. Implant retained removable prostheses are outwith the scope of this text and the reader should refer to an appropriate source of information.

Shortened dental arch

The concept of the shortened dental arch is discussed in further detail in Chapter 17; however, of relevance to this section, it should be re-emphasized that not all missing teeth need to be replaced. If posterior teeth are extracted and the change in oral function is minor, there is little need for tooth replacement providing a stable occlusion is maintained. If the teeth are visible in the smile line, arguably there is a need to replace the teeth. The other important consideration when assessing the need to replace teeth is cost. From a health economic perspective anterior teeth and the first premolars provide adequate function for most of the population. Admittedly, this ignores the aesthetic and psychological components of replacing posterior teeth. Retention, stability and support for free-end saddles often results in poor compliance for these dentures, resulting in an unstable restoration compared to teeth.

MULTIPLE FIXED PROSTHESES

Most patients need crowns or bridges on only a few teeth. However, when patients need more extensive use of crowns and bridges, or a combination of fixed and removable prostheses that affect most of the occlusal table, careful planning is needed. For example, patients requiring extensive treatment are those suffering from severe tooth wear. When most or all of the teeth need restoration, a change to the intercuspal position can be planned, often at an increased occlusal vertical dimension due to short clinical crowns and the need to avoid further occlusal reduction. When this is done a *reorganized approach* to the occlusion is said to have been adopted and some refer to this as a 'full arch rehabilitation'. This is in contrast to when indirect restorations

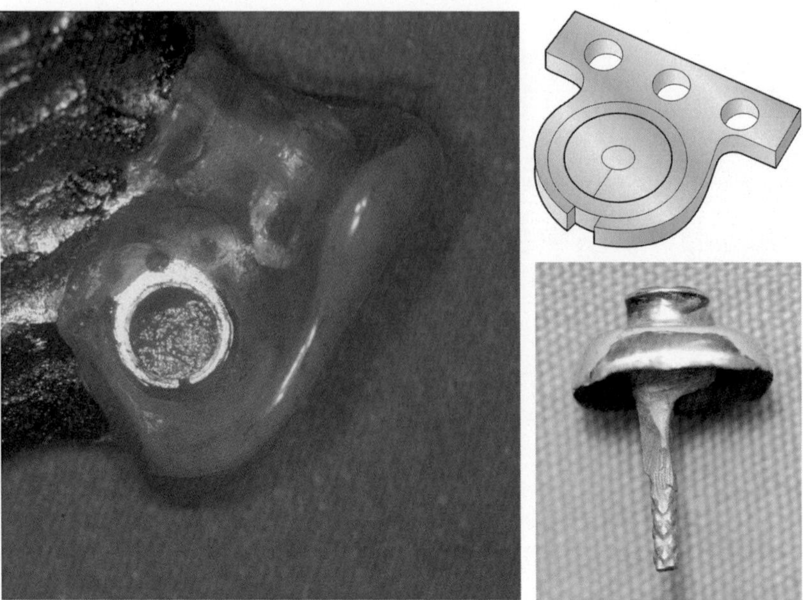

Figure 16.11 Female component of Rothermann-type attachment embedded in the denture base (left), the male component attached to the cast post and diaphragm (bottom right) and diagrammatic representation of how the female component clips into the recess on the sides of the male component (top right).

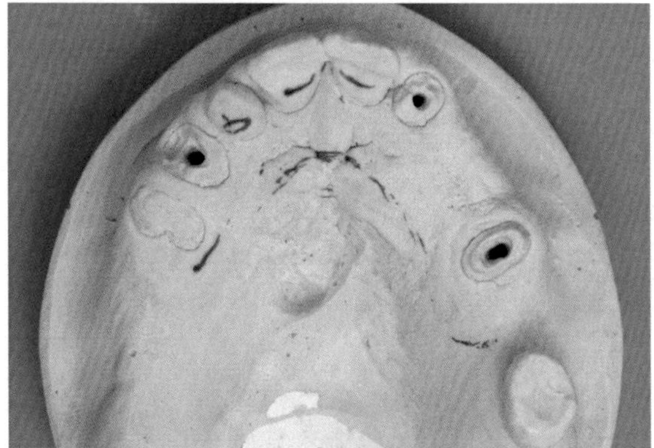

Figure 16.12 Model of patient whose retained roots have been root treated, and prepared for cast posts and diaphragms onto which precision attachments can be attached.

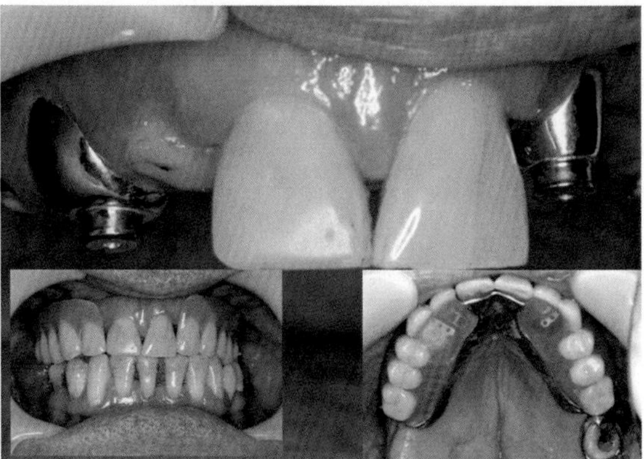

Figure 16.13 Patient whose working model is seen in Figure 16.12. The cast posts, diaphragms and precision attachments cemented (top) and horseshoe cobalt chromium partial denture fitted. The precision attachments provide adequate retention, support and stability to the upper partial prosthesis.

are provided to fit in harmony with the exiting intercuspal position, the so-called *conformative approach*. Restoring teeth adopting a conformative approach is sufficient for the majority of situations, as usually only smaller numbers of teeth are restored. The conformative approach is a simpler procedure whereas a full-mouth rehabilitation and reorganized approach will almost certainly need a semi-adjustable articulator and careful treatment planning and execution.

MANAGEMENT OF TOOTH WEAR

There is no justification to the concept that tooth wear inevitably leads to the total destruction of teeth. In some individuals the extent of the tooth wear may compromise the longevity of the tooth; however, in most patients, once prevention has been instituted, the process continues slowly and is part of the ageing process. For many patients monitoring of tooth wear is an effective and acceptable procedure, even though there is no attempt to restore the shape and appearance of the teeth. For the preventive management of tooth wear, see Chapter 4. The restoration of worn teeth is normally expensive and can require specialist levels of care, mainly because it rarely affects single teeth and more commonly involves quadrants or even whole dental arches.

Restorative management

The main indications for restorative management are to improve the appearance of teeth and to prevent intractable sensitivity (Figures 16.14 and 16.15). In some cases restorations are indicted to prevent wear compromising the survival of the tooth. Once the decision to restore teeth has been taken, the clinician needs to assess how much tooth height is present and whether or not there is sufficient vertical space for the restorations. The critical decision is whether there is sufficient proximal height of the teeth to allow conventional crown preparations, bearing in mind that additional occlusal reduction may be needed to make space for a crown (Figure 16.14).

Surgical crown lengthening

Crown preparations on already shortened teeth due to tooth wear may result in an unacceptable retention. If insufficient tooth height remains, crown lengthening will be needed to reposition the gingival margin in a more apical direction. In this procedure a muco-gingival flap is raised, crestal alveolar bone is removed and thinned slightly, and the flap replaced in a more apical position. Surgical access makes the procedure easier to provide on the buccal surfaces of upper anterior teeth and more difficult lingually and palatally. The palatal mucosa is also more firmly attached to the underlying bone, increasing the difficulty in reflecting the tissue to gain access to the alveolar bone. Normally, crown lengthening of upper anterior teeth is possible because of their relatively long roots but lower incisors have shorter roots and are more challenging (Figures 16.16 and 16.17).

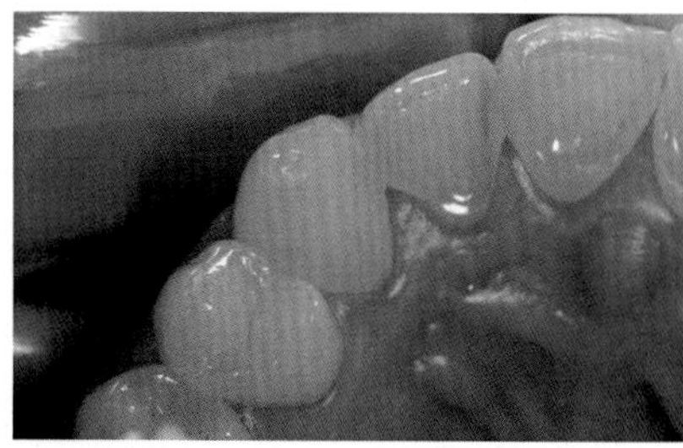

Figure 16.15 Intractable sensitivity in relation to tooth wear is rare but can justify restorations, particularly if the pulp might be compromised if delayed any further.

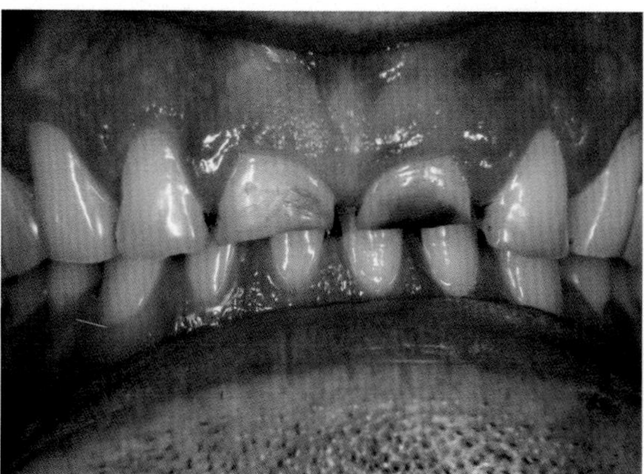

Figure 16.14 Extensively worn upper central incisors leading to a poor appearance. The mesial and distal height of both teeth is insufficient for conventionally prepared crowns. During crown preparation approximately 1–2 mm of occlusal and incisal reduction will be required to create space for the metal and porcelain if a metal–ceramic crown is chosen. In this case further reduction of the tooth would produce unretentive preparations.

Crown lengthening is not without its disadvantages. Whilst a longer clinical crown is achieved, interocclusal clearance is not, and further occlusal or incisal reduction is required, often necessitating elective root canal treatment (Figure 16.17). Once crestal alveolar bone is removed, bone support is lost and an adverse crown:root ratio may be produced. Additionally, as the longitudinal shape of roots, particularly of anterior teeth, is tapered, the more apically the gingival margin is placed, the larger the interdental

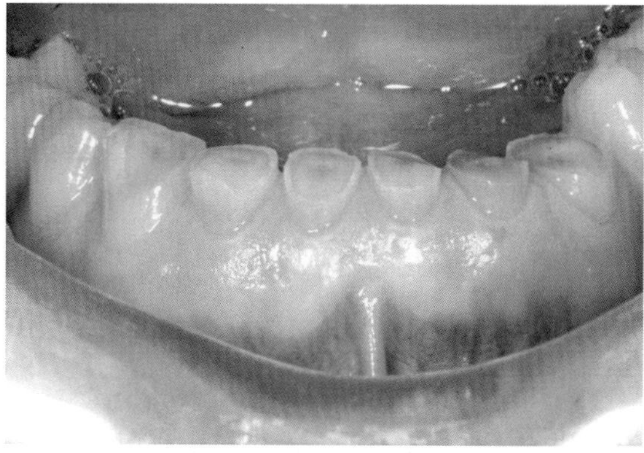

Figure 16.16 These teeth are too short for conventional restorations and need crown lengthening.

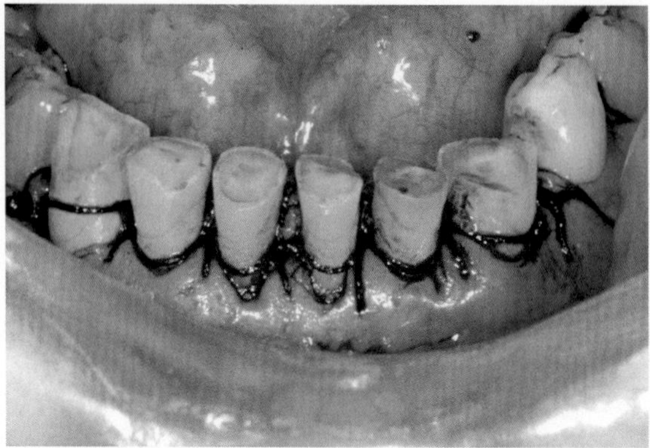

Figure 16.17 The results after crown lengthening for the patient seen in Figure 16.16. To place crowns on these teeth will require incisal reduction, which is likely to necessitate elective root canal treatment as the reactionary (tertiary) dentine is already visible.

space becomes (Figure 16.18) and crowns are either produced with poor emergence profiles to overcome this or large interdental black triangles have to be accepted. Finally, surgical crown lengthening is an uncomfortable procedure that some patients may find unacceptable.

Overdentures

If the clinical crown height and root length are too short for crown lengthening, then either the teeth can be preserved as overdenture abutments (Figure 16.19) or extracted and replaced by dentures or implants.

Creating occlusal clearance

In patients with tooth wear that requires operative intervention, how they are managed will, to a large extent, depend on whether the tooth wear is localized or generalized and how heavily restored the remaining dentition is.

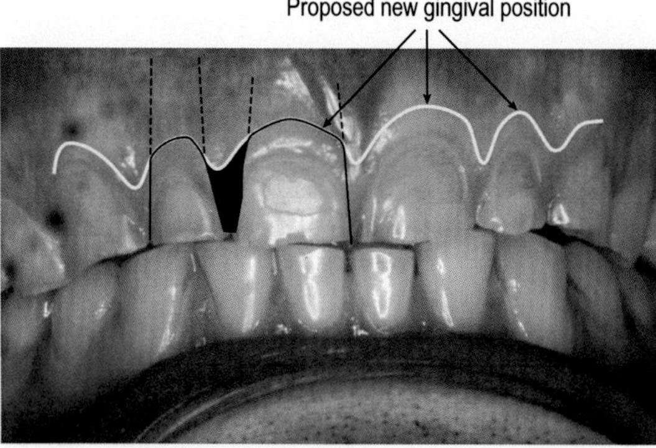

Figure 16.18 Crown lengthening in the upper anterior region can lead to unsightly interdental black triangles due to the tapered roots (outlined in broken lines).

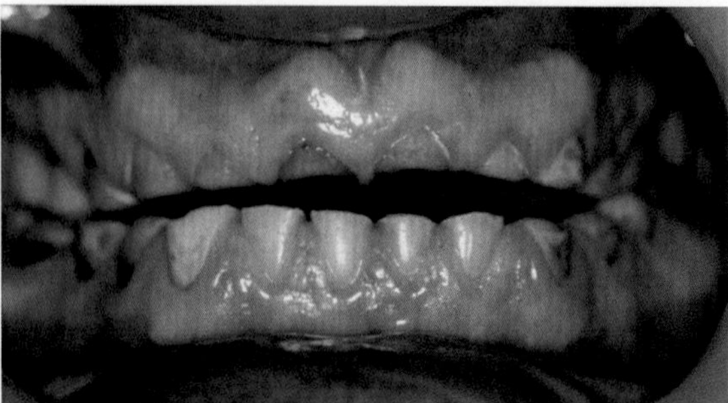

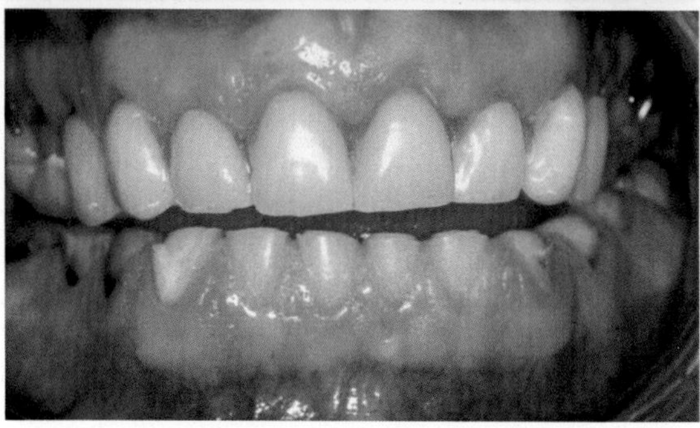

Figure 16.19 Severely worn teeth (top) where crown lengthening was not considered and restored with an overdenture (bottom).

Localized tooth wear

Localized tooth wear is often seen confined to the upper and/or lower anterior teeth. Despite the amount of wear the teeth are commonly in occlusal contact in intercuspal position; this is due to dento-alveolar compensation (Figure 16.20). If the worn teeth are in occlusal contact there is insufficient space to place restorations; however, occlusal (incisal) reduction to achieve interocclusal space would foreshorten the teeth even more and to a level that crowning would be impossible. Interocclusal space can be created either with conventional orthodontic intrusion/extrusion using fixed appliances or with a bite plane – the Dahl concept.

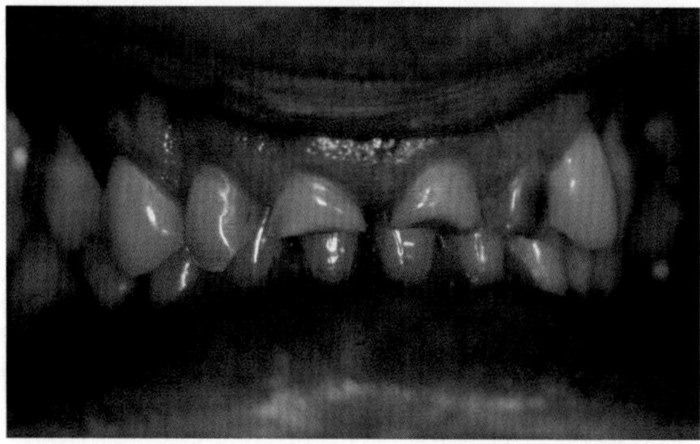

Figure 16.20 Patient with severe tooth wear of the upper anterior teeth; however, there is no interocclusal space in intercuspal position due to dento-alveolar compensation.

The Dahl concept utilizes intrusive forces and the eruptive potential of teeth to create differential movement between groups of teeth, so creating sufficient occlusal vertical space necessary for a crown without any significant occlusal reduction. The Dahl concept has received considerable attention and been shown to be a reliable and effective management for short clinical crowns. In preserving occlusal/incisal tooth tissue the added benefit can be preservation of pulpal health which would otherwise be compromised if additional tooth reduction was necessary.

Early Dahl appliances were made using partial dentures or metal occlusal splints which were placed between the worn teeth (Figures 16.21 and 16.22). The anterior plane encourages the intrusion of the opposing teeth and as the splint prevents contact of the remaining teeth it allows their overeruption. Research by the Dahl group showed that the initial tooth movement was mainly intrusion of the teeth opposing the splint, followed by overeruption of the teeth propped apart. Commonly at the end of treatment overeruption exceeded intrusion which resulted in a small increased vertical dimension. Usually sufficient interocclusal space is created in 3–4 months (Figure 16.23).

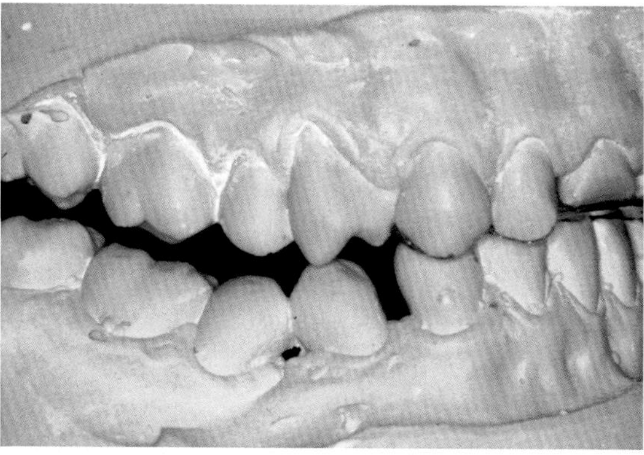

Figure 16.21 Construction of a fixed metal Dahl appliance for the anterior teeth of the patient seen in Figure 16.20. Note the degree of separation of the posterior teeth.

In the experience of clinicians using this technique, precipitation of symptoms of mandibular dysfunction does not occur. However, the presence of symptoms before treatment normally contraindicates the use of the Dahl principle. A common clinical finding with patients suffering from severe tooth wear is good periodontal health; however, poor oral hygiene or increased periodontal probing depths over 3 mm also contraindicate the use of this technique.

Whilst early work on Dahl appliances concentrated on removable or fixed bite planes, most clinicians today use composite build-ups shaped to the ideal contours of the teeth to create the space (Figures 16.24 and 16.25).

The Dahl movement is only applicable when the tooth wear is localized to a few teeth. The differential movement of the teeth produces the space necessary to crown the worn teeth and removes the need to remove additional tooth tissue to provide occlusal clearance. If the tooth wear is generalized the movement is ineffective and a full-mouth rehabilitation is indicated.

Stages in the treatment of localized tooth wear

Articulated study casts mounted on a semi-adjustable articulator using a retruded contact position interocclusal record will provide the clinician with an opportunity to plan the patient's care. The probable reason why Dahl movements are successful is that patients with tooth wear resulting in short clinical crowns and no interocclusal space have a proven dento-alveolar adaptive capacity. Therefore, they are more likely to respond favourably and without symptoms if the height of the teeth is restored to their original dimensions. Articulated study

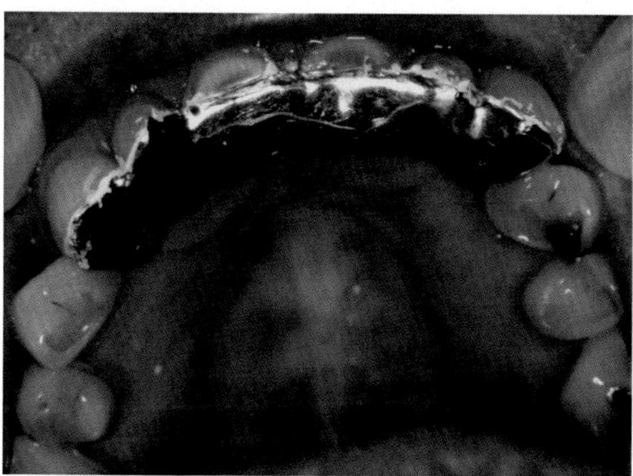

Figure 16.22 Patient seen in Figure 16.20 with the fixed metal Dahl appliance cemented to the upper anterior teeth.

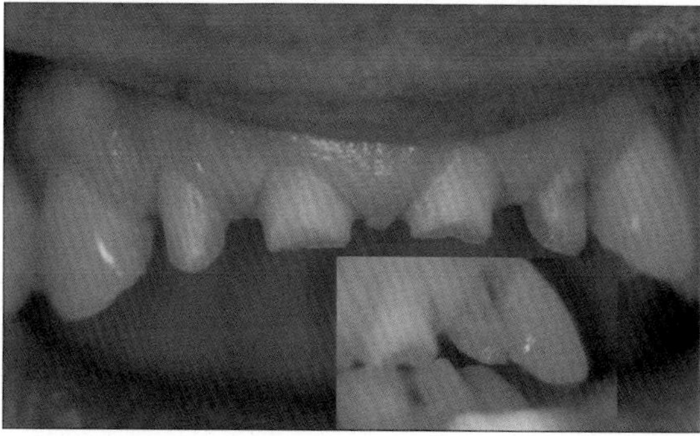

Figure 16.23 Patient seen in Figure 16.20. Preparation of the upper incisors for crowns has been possible without incisal or palatal reduction as the Dahl appliance has created sufficient differential tooth movement and interocclusal space (inset). The canines were restored with palatal gold veneers (see Chapter 12).

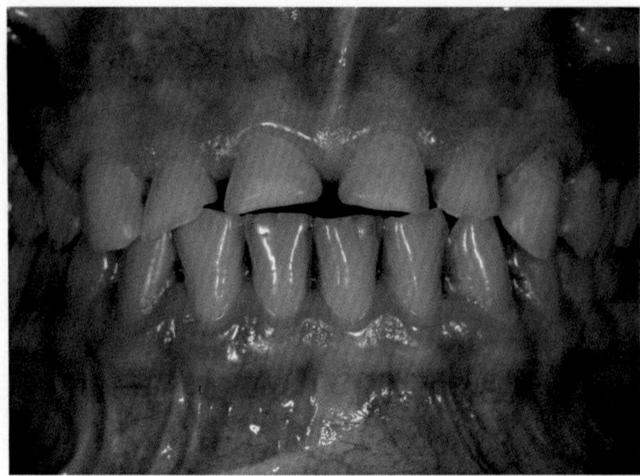

Figure 16.24 Patient with tooth wear and dento-alveolar compensation. Most Dahl movements are now created by restoring the teeth to their ideal shape and appearance by using composites.

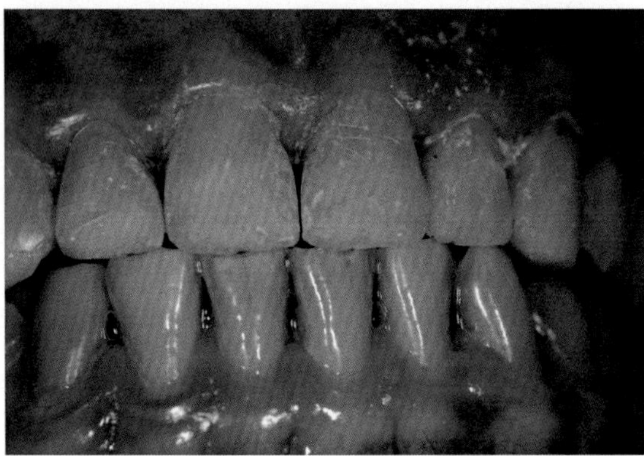

Figure 16.25 The composite Dahl appliance for the patient seen in Figure 16.24. Note the posterior teeth are separated to allow overeruption.

casts allow the technician and clinician to plan the tooth shape in wax and determine how much interocclusal clearance is required. This diagnostic process is driven by the ideal shape and height of teeth (see Chapter 15). Previous photographs and other visual aids may provide some idea of the original tooth dimension; however, if not, then the shape of the tooth needs to be formed using basic principles. There will obviously be individual variations but the diagnostic wax-ups should be made to conform to the shape and size of the patient's teeth.

The next phase of treatment will depend on the clinician's personal preference. Although some practitioners still use a fixed Dahl appliance, most prefer to restore the teeth with composite prior to crowns (Figures 16.24 and 16.25). The advantage of using composite, particularly in the anterior part of the mouth, is that the build-ups act as the Dahl appliance and also act as a provisional restoration. If the diagnostic wax-up has not fully predicted the ideal shape and size of the teeth, an intraoral adjustment of the restorations creates the optimum appearance. Once built up, the composites need to have an even occlusal contact with the opposing teeth (Figure 16.26). The adjustment is critical to the survival of the restorations. If, after the composite additions, only a few teeth have occlusal contacts, there is an increased risk of fracture of the restoration as they become overloaded and are more likely to cause discomfort to the patient than is otherwise necessary. There is reasonable evidence to suggest that composites used to restore worn anterior teeth will survive between 3 and 5 years (Gow & Hemmings, 2002; Hemmings et al., 2000; Redman et al., 2003). During that time a certain amount of adjustment with composite additions may be necessary to preserve the restorations.

At some point the composites will need replacing and this is often managed using crowns. In some patients the transition to crowns occurs more quickly, particularly if repeated fractures of the composite occur. Once the decision to restore the teeth with crowns is made, either the original diagnostic wax-up can be reused or a new one can be created, or indeed the existing composites can be used to plan the shape of the indirect restorations. A custom-formed incisal guidance table as described in Chapter 14 can be used to ensure the anterior guidance is reproduced if necessary.

A fundamental indicator to the success of restoration of worn teeth is the amount of tooth structure remaining. The Dahl movement only creates interocclusal space but if the height of the natural teeth is too short there will be insufficient retention of crowns. Following crown preparation any residual composite remaining on the tooth cannot be considered reliable retention for crowns in the long term (Figure 16.27). Although composite additions give the illusion of the ideal shape and height of a crown

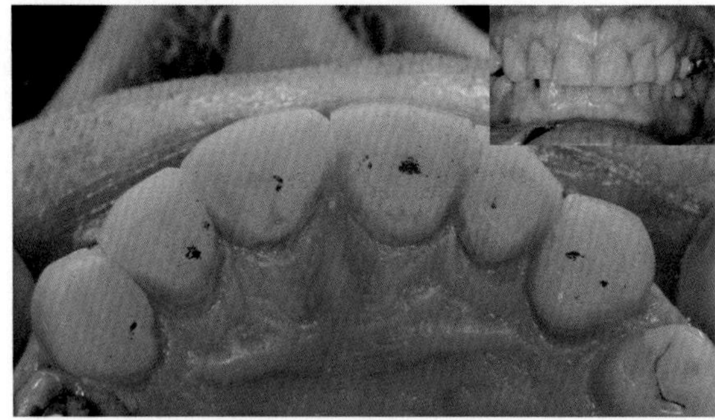

Figure 16.26 Composites to build up worn teeth. The composites were initially used as a Dahl appliance and even occlusal contact on all the Dahl teeth is essential. Inset: posterior tooth contact achieved.

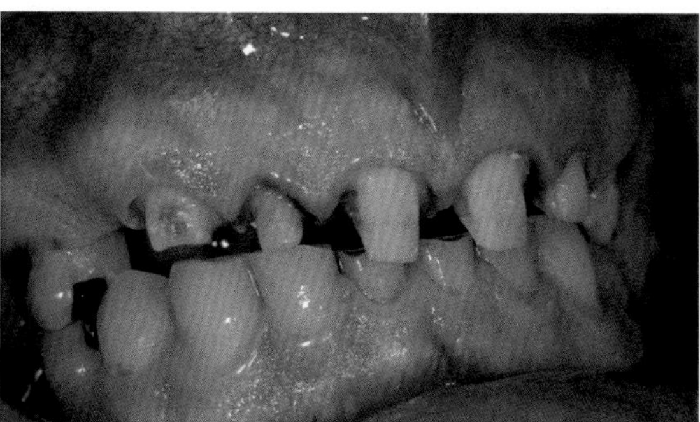

Figure 16.27 The tips of the two central incisors have composite additions. The bond between composite and tooth cannot be relied upon over the long term.

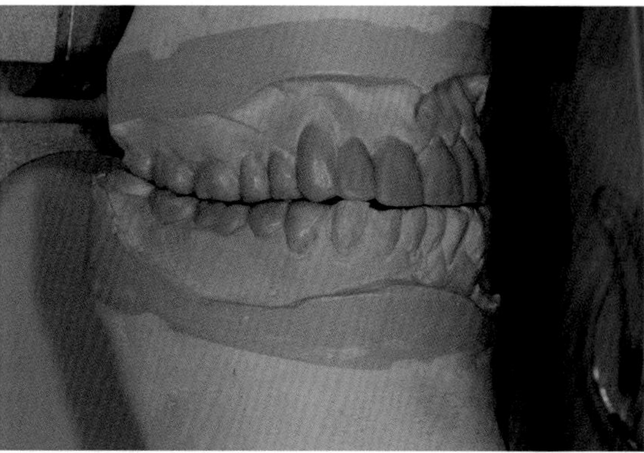

Figure 16.28 A diagnostic wax-up of a patient requiring multiple crowns. The shape and the height of the teeth are created not only from the basic shape of the standing teeth but also using the width and height ratio.

preparation, their bond to tooth is insufficient over the lifetime of the crown.

There is a mounting evidence base to support the use of Dahl movements to restore worn teeth. The technique is not universally accepted and there is scepticism, particularly in North America. However, many other parts of the world have adopted the technique. The work by Gough and Setchell (1999) suggests that the time needed for the adaption and occlusal changes ranges from 3 to 9 months. The time increases when the incisal relationship is a Class II Division II and is less successful with Class III and Class II Division I relationships. If insufficient teeth meet in the intercuspal position, a Dahl movement is unlikely to be successful and more radical intervention is necessary.

Generalized tooth wear

Where the tooth wear is generalized and affects most teeth the differential movement using a Dahl restoration is inappropriate. In these more severe cases the distribution of tooth wear is rarely restricted to one arch or one quadrant. Often there is a mixed outcome, with some severely worn teeth in one arch opposed by less worn teeth in the other. The restoration of the mouth should be aimed to increase the height of the worn teeth but to leave, where possible, the less severely worn without restorations.

The procedure for restoring a dentition with an increased number of restorations follows a similar procedure to the work-up needed for the Dahl appliance. Upper and lower study casts mounted on a semi-adjustable articulator using a retruded contact position interocclusal record provide the opportunity to plan the treatment. The diagnostic wax-up (Figure 16.28) allows the height and shape of the teeth to be predicted and to determine the increased occlusal vertical dimension that is required. Provisional restorations can then be made based on the wax-up, either in composite directly built up in the mouth or from provisional crowns. The provisional crowns can be made from a vacuum-formed splint made on a duplicate model of the wax-up. These provisional restorations can then be used to assess the appearance, occlusion and function over a period of time. An individual assessment of the available tooth structure of each tooth is required and an estimate made of the effect of tooth preparation for a crown. If that assessment predicts there will be insufficient tooth remaining to provide adequate retention, crown lengthening could be considered. Once the provisional restorations are fitted, further occlusal adjustment is needed to ensure the shape conforms to the patient's expectations and that there is even occlusal contact. Provided the patient and dentist are happy, the definitive crowns can be made based on the shape and contour of the provisional restorations.

When a full arch rehabilitation is considered and a reorganized approach is adopted to manage the occlusion, restorations should be made using a terminal hinge axis position at a set occlusal vertical dimension. The terminal hinge axis is used as it is the most reproducible jaw relationship and it facilitates alteration of the occlusal vertical dimension (see Chapter 6). The most demanding part of making crowns for a full arch rehabilitation is the need to ensure even occlusal contact and smooth guidance.

In a full mouth rehabilitation at an increased occlusal vertical dimension the procedure can either be planned according to groups of teeth or teeth in one arch can be prepared and restored all at once. The latter is demanding and extremely time consuming for the dentist, and arduous for the patient. A quadrant or sextant approach overcomes this problem and can be carried out in two ways:

- Teeth can be prepared in groups at different appointments with two lots of provisional restorations being made, the first set at the original vertical dimension and conforming to the existing occlusion and the second at the reorganized occlusion at an increased vertical dimension. The first set will be used until all preparations are carried out and at this stage the second set will be used to assess the increased occlusal vertical dimension and occlusion according to the diagnostic wax-up. A single impression can then be taken of all the prepared teeth and all restorations made on one model. This has the benefit that all the characteristics and shade of tooth-coloured restorations will match. All of the restorations will then be fitted at the subsequent appointment, ensuring even occlusal contacts throughout to prevent any overeruption of teeth. This process is dependent upon accurately articulated study casts. Once all the interocclusal contacts are removed, the demands on the technician making the crowns and the dentist fitting them increase significantly.

- Teeth can be prepared in groups, an impression taken and then the provisional or definitive restorations made in groups. If the definitive restorations are cemented, the occlusal clearance created for the remaining arch has to be maintained. This can be with composite build-ups on the remaining teeth which have to be placed at the same appointment the crowns are cemented or more simply by using an occlusal splint which is adjusted accordingly. Consider the patient in Figure 16.29: the teeth in the upper arch are worn and the posterior

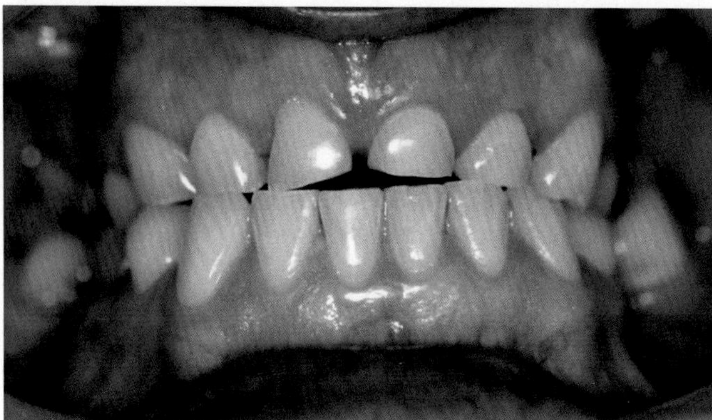
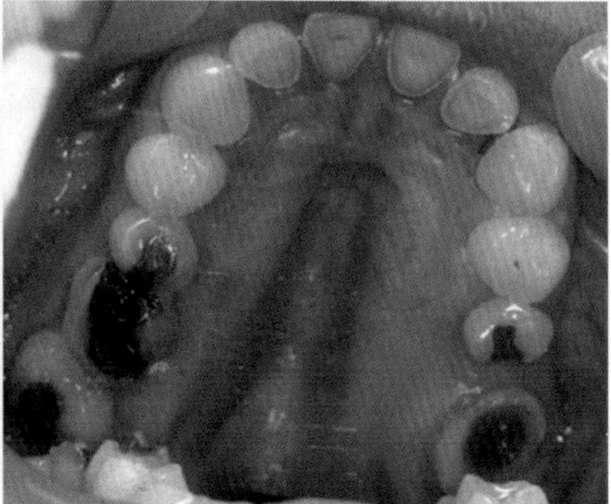

Figure 16.29 Patient with marked tooth wear and heavily restored posterior teeth for whom a full upper arch rehabilitation is planned.

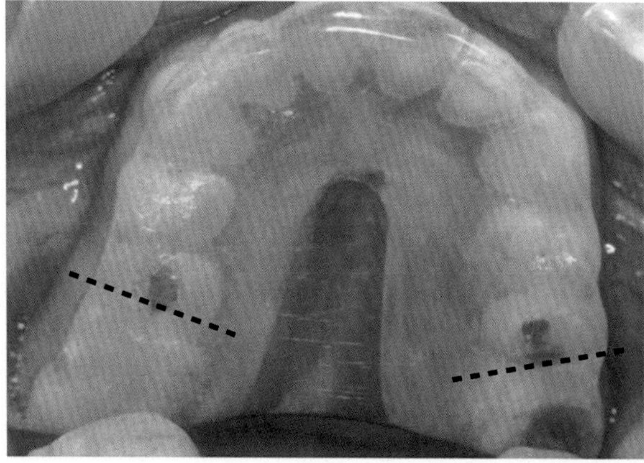
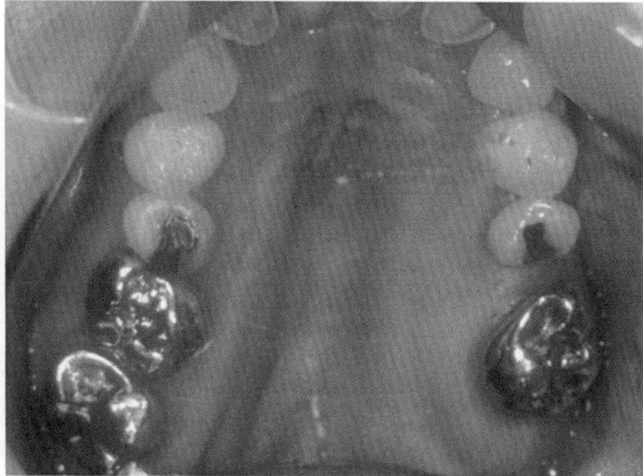

Figure 16.30 Patient seen in Figure 16.29 with Michigan splint at the desired increased occlusal vertical dimension (left). Once the gold crowns and onlays are cemented on the molar teeth (right), the splint can be cut back to the dashed lines. Wear of the splint over the premolar, canine and incisor teeth will maintain the occlusal clearance created. Even occlusal contact on crowns and splint must be ensured.

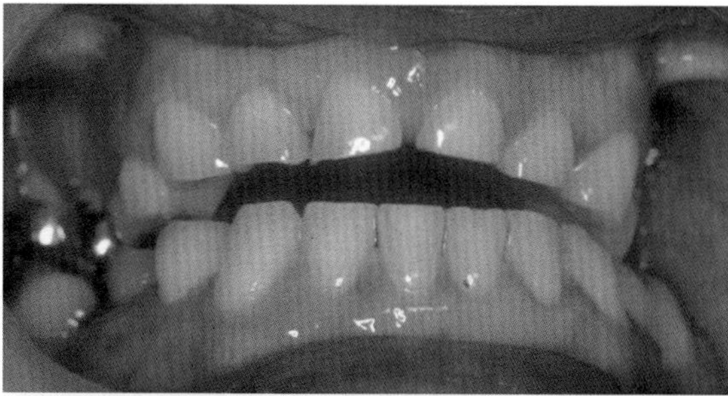

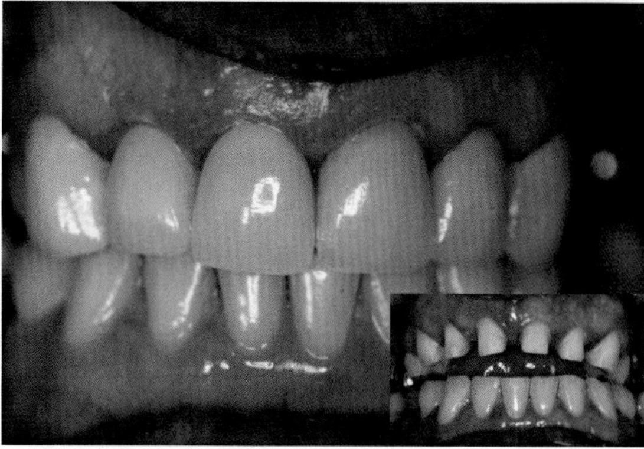

Figure 16.31 Patient seen in Figures 16.29 and 16.30. The Michigan splint retained anteriorly has maintained the occlusal clearance created by the posterior gold restorations, allowing sufficient space for dentine-bonded crowns.

teeth are heavily restored. An upper full arch rehabilitation is planned. A Michigan splint is made to assess the increased occlusal vertical dimension planned (Figure 16.30). The molar teeth are prepared for onlays and crowns at the increased vertical dimension. The crowns are made and tried in to ensure bilateral occlusal contact and cemented. The splint is then cut away from over the new gold crowns so that it sits over the premolar and anterior teeth only, maintaining the occlusal clearance achieved over these teeth (Figure 16.31). These teeth can then be prepared at a subsequent appointment for composite onlays (premolar teeth) and dentine-bonded crowns (anterior teeth) (Figure 16.31).

SUMMARY

The restoration of dentitions with multiple fixed or a combination of fixed and removable prostheses is complex and requires careful decision making and planning. It also comes with a cost in both monetary terms and maintenance of oral health in the long term. Such complex dentistry should not be considered lightly and should only be undertaken with the full informed consent of the patient.

FURTHER READING

Gough, M.B., Setchell, D., 1999. A retrospective study of 50 treatments using an appliance to produce localised occlusal space by relative axial tooth movement. Br. Dent. J. 187, 134–139.

Gow, A.M., Hemmings, K.W., 2002. The treatment of localised anterior tooth wear with indirect Artglass restorations at an increased occlusal vertical dimension. Results after two years. Eur. J. Prosthodont. Restor. Dent. 10, 101–105.

Hemmings, K.W., Darbar, U.R., Vaughan, S., 2000. Tooth wear treated with direct composite restorations at an increased vertical dimension: results at 30 months. J. Prosthet. Dent. 83, 287–293.

Redman, C.D., Hemmings, K.W., Good, J.A., 2003. The survival and clinical performance of resin-based composite restorations used to treat localised anterior tooth wear. Br. Dent. J. 194, 566–572.

Ricketts, D.N., Smith, B.G., 1993a. Minor axial tooth movement in preparation for fixed prostheses. Eur. J. Prosthodont. Restor. Dent. 1, 145–149.

Ricketts, D.N., Smith, B.G., 1993b. Clinical techniques for producing and monitoring minor axial tooth movement. Eur. J. Prosthodont. Restor. Dent. 2, 5–9.

Chapter | 17 |

When and how to replace missing teeth

David Ricketts

CHAPTER CONTENTS

DO WE NEED TO REPLACE MISSING TEETH?

The loss of any tooth does not automatically mean the need for a prosthetic replacement. Patients should be aware that tooth replacement has a biological and financial cost with a long-term commitment to maintenance. Complications can arise with any restorative intervention and a sound justification for tooth replacement is required. Patients should always be informed of the alternatives, irrespective of cost, for tooth replacement and they should be informed of the potential advantages and disadvantages to each. It is only then that informed consent can be given by the patient.

WHEN TO REPLACE MISSING TEETH?

Appearance

Tooth loss can have a devastating effect on a patient's appearance, self-confidence and motivation. The loss of an upper central incisor is an obvious indication for prosthodontic replacement (Figure 17.1), but the technical challenges of designing the restoration must be taken together with the impact of the 'smile line'. This assessment should be undertaken when the patient is talking and smiling in a relaxed environment and not from under forced conditions! For some patients the replacement of an upper premolar tooth may be unnecessary, but for those with a wide and high smile line tooth replacement may be justified. Whatever the clinical situation, it is advisable that tooth replacement based on appearance should be led by the patient and not the dentist.

Occlusal stability

When a tooth is missing the occlusion can change, with overeruption, tilting or drifting of opposing or adjacent

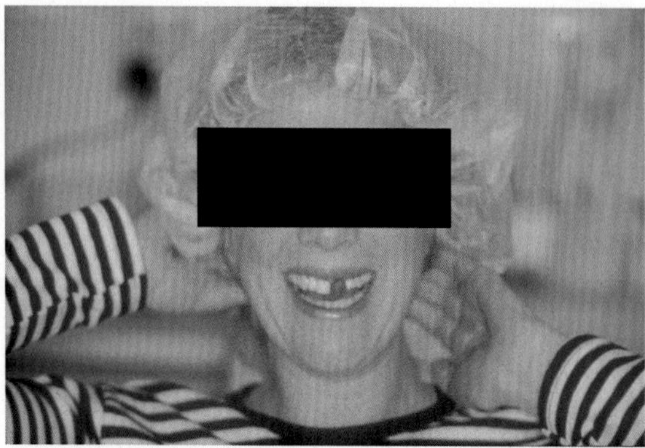

Figure 17.1 A patient with a missing upper left central incisor tooth which poses a major aesthetic problem. The patient also has a high and wide smile line involving both first and second premolar teeth.

teeth, causing a condition commonly referred to as an unstable occlusion. Consider the 25-year-old patient in Figure 17.2. The loss of the upper first and second premolar and lower first and second molar teeth has led to an unstable occlusion. The failure to replace these missing teeth led to overeruption of the lower second premolar and upper first and second molar teeth into the opposing edentulous spaces. This now complicates prosthodontic replacement as there is inadequate space between the teeth and opposing edentulous ridge.

The overeruption of teeth into edentulous spaces does not always occur and is impossible to predict. Therefore, if restoration of occlusal stability is the only clinical indication for tooth replacement following an extraction, it is advisable to monitor tooth movement over time. This tooth movement or dento-alveolar compensation can occur quickly in some patients and the tooth movement seen in the patient in Figure 17.2 occurred after 6 months. To avoid such a clinical situation, review appointments should be advised and a suggested timing would be after 3 months in the first instance. Baseline study models taken soon after the extraction may also be useful in confirming any tooth movement.

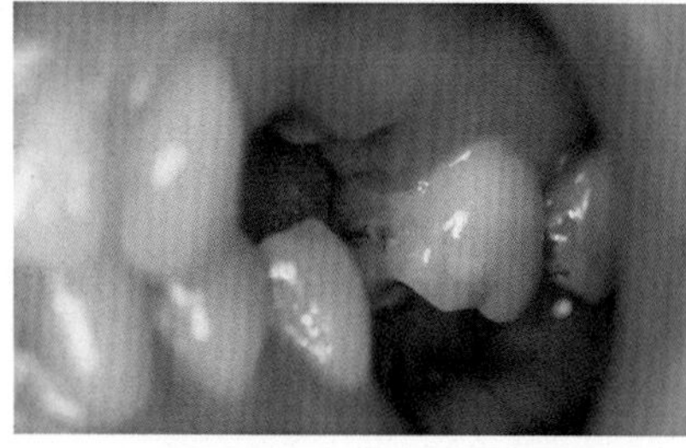

Figure 17.2 A patient with an unstable occlusion and overeruption of the lower premolar and upper molar teeth. Note the alveolar tissues have accompanied the tooth movement, hence the term dento-alveolar compensation.

Function

Mastication

Patients frequently complain of difficulty in eating and trauma to the edentulous ridges following tooth loss. The latter problem can only be addressed with a prosthodontic replacement but the former is subjective and individual to each patient. There is little evidence to confirm that loss of molar teeth is accompanied by a significant loss of masticatory function. To the contrary, there is a large body of evidence to support the concept of the shortened dental arch (SDA) (Kanno & Carlsson, 2006). The posterior teeth are mainly involved in mastication and the SDA was proposed as a treatment option if molar teeth had been extracted. The minimum number of occluding pairs of teeth was the four premolar teeth or two pairs of occluding molar teeth. Today, the SDA is generally accepted as a premolar to premolar occlusion, following the loss of the molar teeth.

Opponents to the concept of the SDA have cited loss of masticatory function, mandibular displacement and problems such as temporomandibular dysfunction (TMD). There is some evidence to suggest that these complications are more likely in younger patients and those with unilateral tooth loss. In addition, some patients have reported difficulty in chewing harder foods though they tend to modify their diet accordingly. The other important factor in assessing the role of the SDA is the challenges associated with the prosthodontic replacement of molar teeth. For many patients replacing molar teeth with implants is prohibitively costly and the alternative of removable prostheses, particularly in the mandible with free-end saddles, means denture-based solutions are often not successful. The strength of evidence strongly supports the concept of adopting the SDA when the molar teeth have been extracted.

Does the SDA lead to increased wear of remaining teeth?

It would seem logical that if patients have missing molar teeth and a lack of 'posterior support', there would be increased tooth wear of the remaining teeth as these take the entire functional load. This is a frequent comment and perhaps misconception of many dentists. In those patients with tooth wear the rate generally increases over a lifetime but those without evidence of wear are unlikely to develop wear following the loss of the teeth.

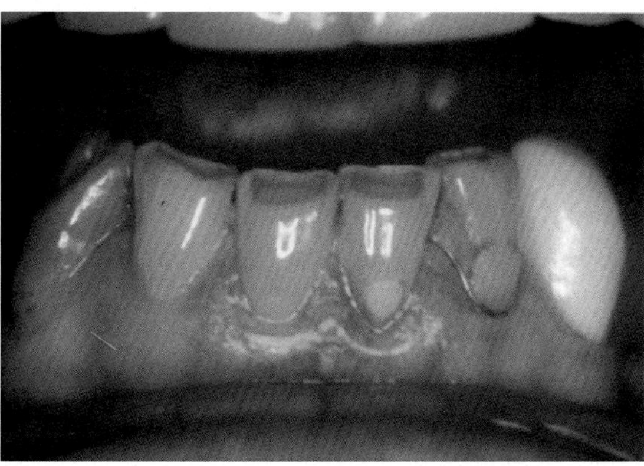
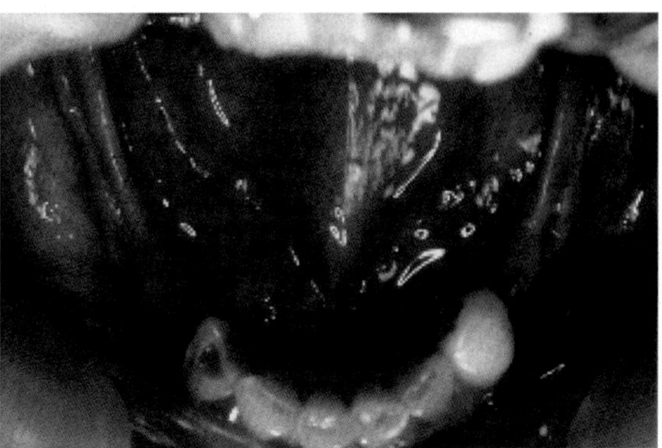

Figure 17.3 A patient with missing posterior teeth. The remaining anterior teeth are worn, mainly as a result of erosion (cupping out of the incisal edges is seen) and not lack of 'posterior support'.

The patient in Figure 17.3 has lost all their posterior teeth and due to the severity of posterior alveolar ridge resorption is unable to wear a successful removable prosthesis. The lower anterior teeth are worn, with cupping of the incisal edges resulting from erosion, though attrition might be a contributing factor to the tooth wear. Whether the tooth wear would have reached the same severity if the posterior teeth were present is unknown.

In general terms, provided the severity of the wear does not result in short clinical crowns, the prosthesis can be made with conventional techniques. However, if short clinical crowns are present the complexity of care increases significantly.

Speech

Missing maxillary incisor teeth often lead to difficulties with speech, especially those with lip to tooth and tongue to tooth sounds. However, for most this is a temporary condition which slowly improves as adaption occurs. However, for a small minority the difficulties continue and contribute to challenges in their social interaction. Whilst missing anterior teeth have the greatest potential impact on speech, the over-riding reason to replace the teeth will be, for most patients, the impact on appearance. Patients with congenital or acquired dental and skeletal defects (e.g. cleft lip and palate) and oncology patients require special consideration as it is not only the loss of teeth that impacts upon speech.

Psychological/quality of life

It can be seen from the preceding sections that the loss of teeth can have an impact on a patient's quality of life, particularly those teeth within the smile line, leading to impact on their appearance, lack of confidence and social withdrawal, and in some instances loss of function. The loss of a tooth or teeth is an emotional event for many patients, seen as a sign of old age and takes time to adapt to. The decision on tooth replacement should be driven by the patient and not the dentist. Patients should be informed of the disadvantages associated with the tooth's prosthodontic replacement and so are fully able to give informed consent.

HOW TO REPLACE MISSING TEETH?

The question of 'How to replace missing teeth?' can only be answered on an individual patient basis, taking into consideration the patient's expectations and each clinical situation and presentation.

Removable prostheses

Removable prostheses have a number of advantages over fixed prostheses and can be used in situations that are unsuitable for a fixed alternative. In general, the provision of removable prostheses is less invasive and therefore conservative of tooth tissue and is often quicker and cheaper to provide, especially acrylic-based prostheses. Whilst a removable prosthesis potentially might be seen as an opportunity for patients to thoroughly clean their appliance and teeth, studies have shown that removable prostheses lead to deterioration in oral hygiene, not only in the arch in which the appliance is placed but also in the opposing arch. The distribution of plaque accumulation also changes as the potential plaque stagnation areas within the mouth are altered by the appliance (Figure 17.4). As this will predispose the patient to periodontal problems and caries, careful attention therefore needs to be given to prevention of dental disease.

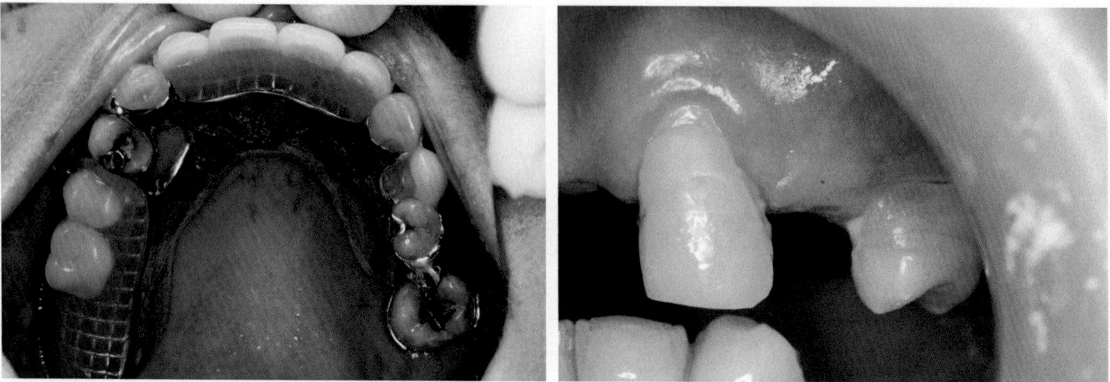

Figure 17.4 The wearing of this upper removable partial cobalt chromium prosthesis may have contributed to this patient's poor oral hygiene and change in the distribution of plaque accumulation on the proximal tooth surfaces.

Multiple edentulous spaces, long spans and free-end saddles

Removable prostheses are more likely to be considered where there are multiple edentulous spaces, for example as seen in Figure 17.5. It could be argued that each individual edentulous span could be restored with a fixed prosthesis (bridge) if care was taken with the occlusion. However, this would require extensive operative intervention and dismantling of existing crown work, with concomitant risks to the abutment teeth. A removable prosthesis allows all edentulous spaces to be restored with a cobalt chromium denture that can be removed for ease of maintenance.

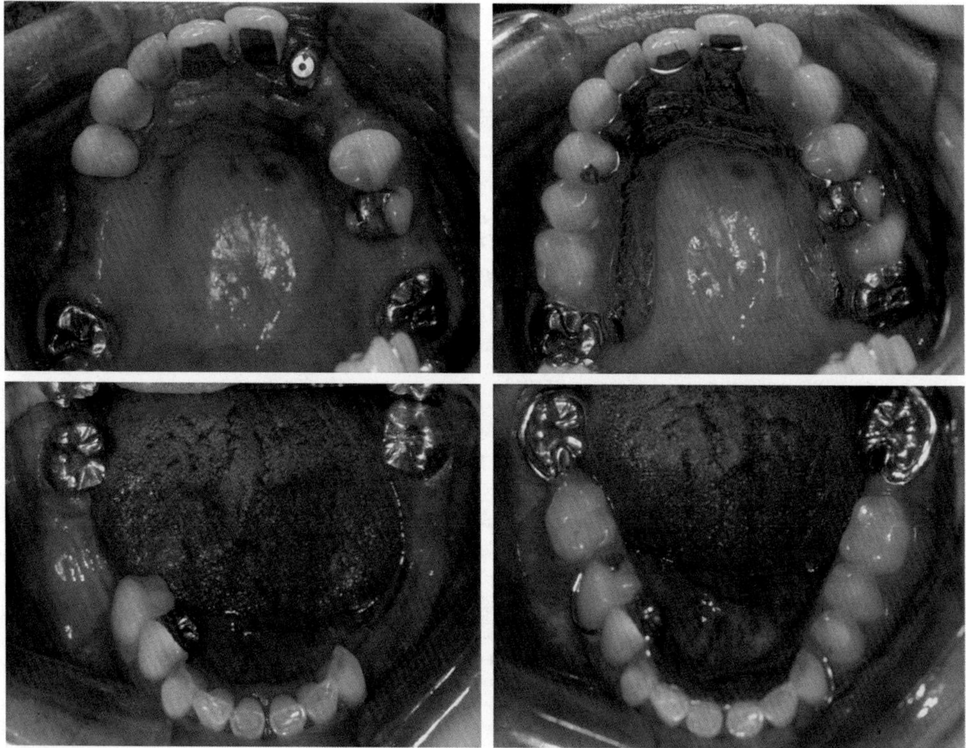

Figure 17.5 Multiple edentulous spaces and long edentulous spans make this patient unsuitable for fixed bridges. Removable cobalt chromium prostheses are a preferred option.

Where long edentulous spans are concerned, conventional fixed bridges may be contraindicated due to the excessive loads applied to the abutment teeth (see Chapter 19) and increased demands on retention for the retainers. The length of the span also increases the difficulty of achieving parallel preparations on the abutment teeth, increasing the risk of creating undercuts. This would pose a problem if fixed–fixed bridge designs were planned. Consider the edentulous spans in the upper right and lower left quadrants for the patient in Figure 17.5. In this situation removable prostheses are preferred where support for the occlusal load and retention can be obtained not only from the adjacent teeth, but also other teeth in the same arch and mucosa.

A unique situation occurs when there is a single or bilateral free-end saddle (Figure 17.6). In these circumstances the only fixed prostheses possible to replace all or the majority of teeth would be implant retained restorations (Figure 17.7). Surgical placement of implant fixtures can be complicated by the presence of anatomical features such as the inferior dento-alveolar neurovascular bundle in the lower arch and the maxillary sinus in the upper arch. Distal cantilever conventional or minimal preparation (resin retained) bridges are limited in most situations to a single premolar unit replacement (Figure 17.8). As such, the restoration of choice is most commonly a removable partial prosthesis.

Ridge resorption

Following an extraction, alveolar ridge resorption takes place. Therefore, if a fixed prosthesis is planned, it is important that the definitive restoration is delayed until most of the resorption has occurred. Whilst ridge resorption following tooth loss continues over a lifetime, most resorption occurs during the first 3 months. The rate of resorption slows but continues over many years; however, the rate and extent of resorption over time will depend on numerous factors, such as:

- The anatomy of the residual ridges, including the quantity and quality of bone (e.g. bone density)

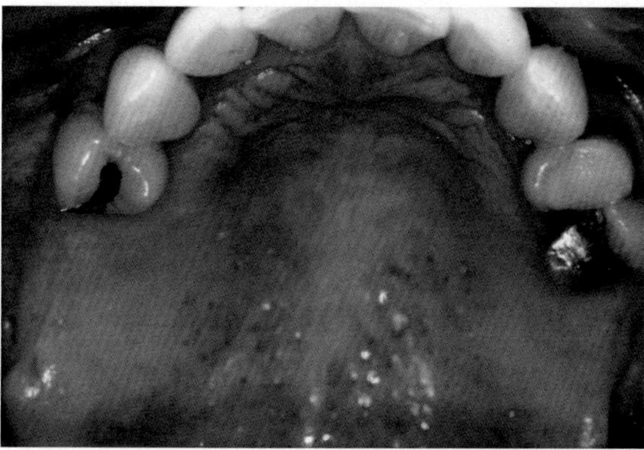

Figure 17.6 Bilateral free end saddles. Treatment options include a removable prosthesis, implant retained restorations or distal cantilever bridges off the premolar teeth. The last option would only allow replacement of a single premolar unit and could be minimum preparation (resin retained) in design on the patient's right and conventional on the left.
(Courtesy of Dr Brendan Scott)

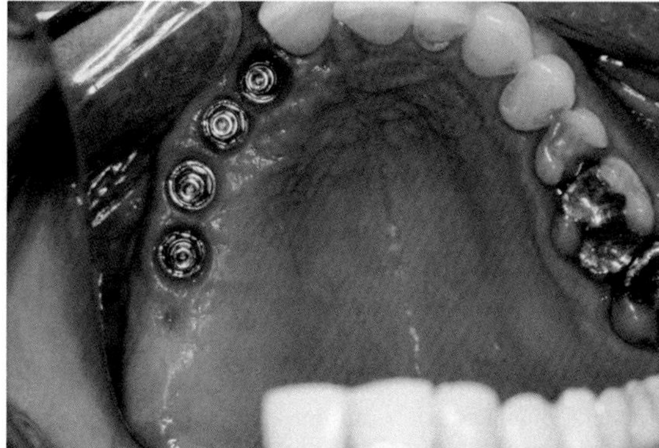

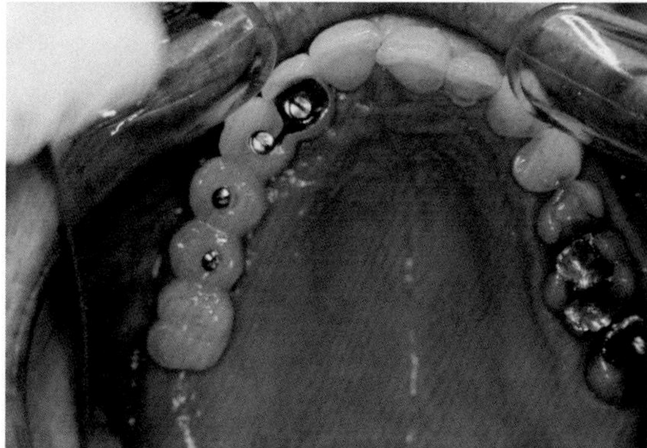

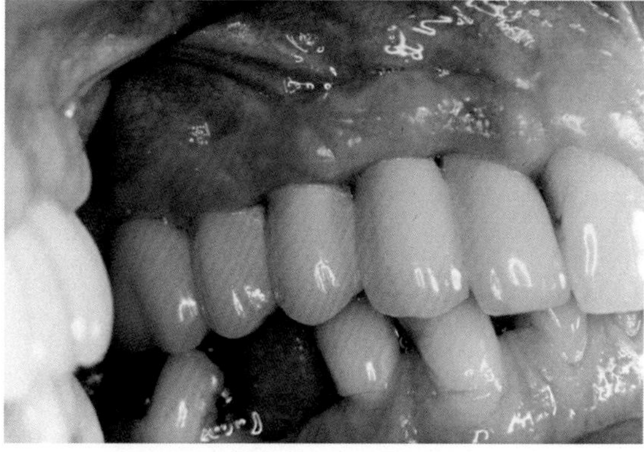

Figure 17.7 Loss of teeth in the upper right quadrant has led to an extensive unilateral free-end saddle. The only fixed prosthesis possible is an implant retained bridge. Care in treatment planning and implant placement is required to avoid the maxillary sinus.

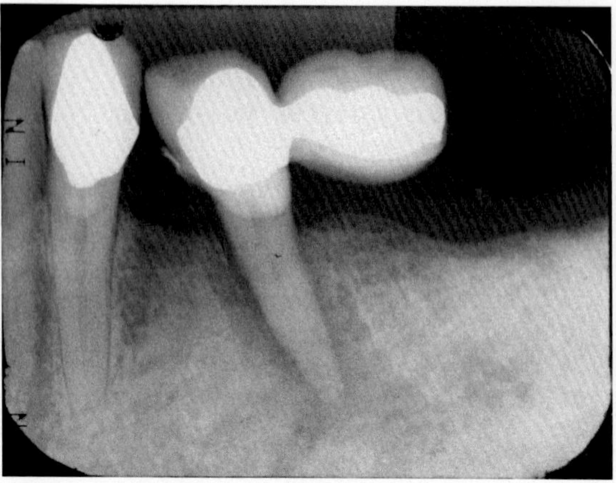
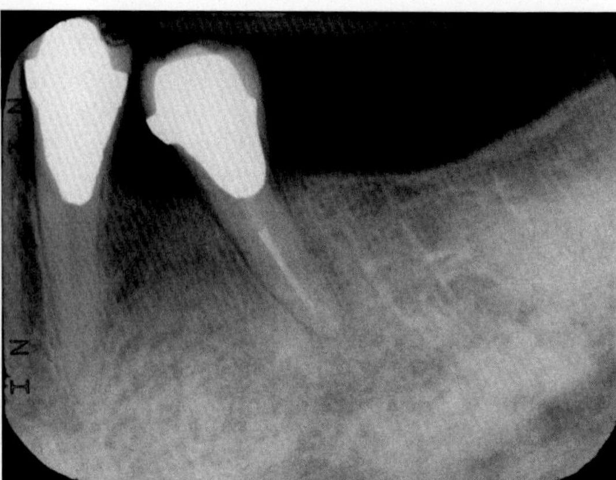

Figure 17.8 A molar pontic has been cantilevered off this premolar tooth. Excessive occlusal forces together with loss of vitality of this tooth have led to increase mobility and bone loss (left). Root canal treatment and removal of the pontic has resolved these problems (right).

- Advanced periodontal disease resulting in severe alveolar bone resorption
- Metabolic factors: for example, the imbalance in sex hormones can result in an imbalance in bone resorption and bone formation, leading to osteoporosis and more rapid alveolar resorption
- Functional forces: it is not uncommon when heavy loads are applied to an edentulous ridge to see a marked increase in resorption leading to atrophy. Such a situation can be seen when a mucosal-borne removable prosthesis is opposed by a natural dentition. The excessive forces generated by the natural teeth to the opposing edentulous ridge via the prosthesis are sufficient to cause marked ridge resorption (Figure 17.9).

Where bridges are planned

It is generally accepted that the rate of ridge resorption following an extraction will have slowed sufficiently after 6 months to allow placement of a fixed prosthesis (bridge). Placement of a fixed prosthesis before this runs the risk of continued ridge resorption beneath the bridge pontic and formation of an unsightly gap.

Where implants are planned

The timing of implant fixture placement is influenced by the health of the bone surrounding the planned site. Sufficient time is needed for resolution of any infection or tissue damage, and soft tissue and bony healing prior to implant placement. Where there is no infection and stability of the implant can be achieved, an immediate implant placement into the extraction socket is possible. There is little evidence on the long-term outcomes of immediately placed implants compared to delayed implant placement following extraction. Careful case selection is required with immediate implant placement and compared to delayed conventional implant placement there would appear to be a higher risk of

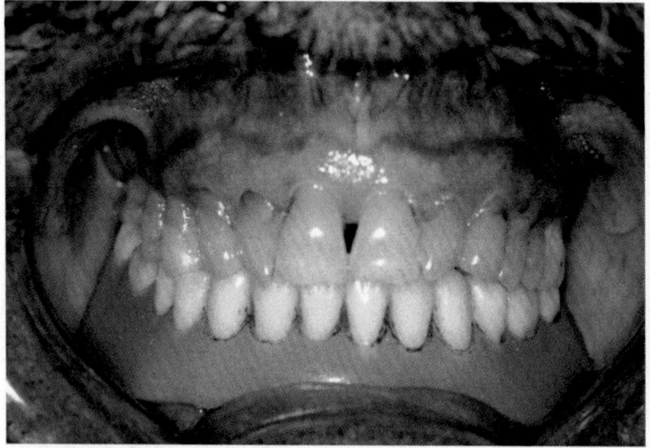
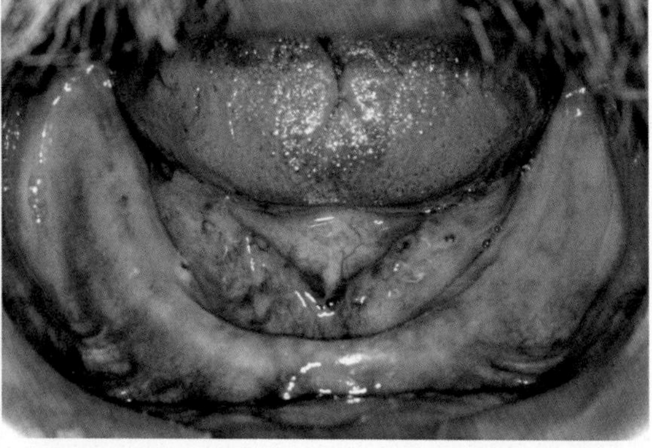

Figure 17.9 A natural dentition in the upper arch opposing a complete removable prosthesis can lead to marked alveolar ridge resorption in the lower arch over time.
(Courtesy of Dr Brendan Scott)

failure (Schropp & Isidor, 2008). Immediate loading of implants has also been suggested but this takes a great deal of planning and again the risk of failure is likely to be higher.

Whether implant placement is immediate or delayed a provisional restoration is needed in the majority of cases; if a removable prosthesis is used as a provisional tooth replacement, excessive loading of the implant site immediately after placement should be avoided. This is particularly true if a single-stage surgical procedure is carried out and the transmucosal abutment is visible.

Immediate prostheses

The extraction of anterior teeth and the immediate replacement with a removable prosthesis eliminates some of the aesthetic problems associated with tooth loss. This clinical technique is relatively straightforward for single tooth replacement but becomes more challenging as the number of teeth extracted increases. An impression is taken of both dental arches prior to the tooth extraction, the technician then removes the tooth that is to be extracted and associated undercuts from the resultant working model, and an acrylic prosthesis is processed. Once the tooth has been extracted the denture is fitted immediately into the edentulous space, avoiding an unsightly gap for any time (Figure 17.10).

Severe alveolar bone loss

Occasionally there can be marked bone loss following tooth removal. This may be due to a number of reasons such as the adverse factors previously mentioned, significant preoperative periradicular pathology, following surgical extraction and bone removal (Figure 17.11) or where teeth have been lost through trauma with associated loss of alveolar bone. Other patients may have a deficit of bone if teeth are congenitally missing, if there is a developmental defect such as a cleft palate or if surgery has been required for removal of pathology (Figure 17.12). In these patients not only can the teeth be replaced with a removable prosthesis, but the lost bone and soft tissue can also be replaced with an acrylic flange or obturator.

Single missing teeth with spacing

Some patients have a spaced dentition simply due to a dento-skeletal discrepancy (Figure 17.13). Anterior tooth replacement in such patients poses a particular problem. To place a tooth of equal width to the contralateral counterpart, in the middle of a larger space, can only be achieved with a removable prosthesis (see Figure 17.10 with immediate denture) or an implant (Figure 17.14). Historically, spring cantilever bridges were used but these are now obsolete (Figure 17.15).

Transitional prostheses

Where teeth are lost and there are other teeth of a poor prognosis within the dentition, fixed prostheses are usually contraindicated and a removable acrylic prosthesis can be used as a transitional prosthesis. This can be designed so that it is easy to add any further teeth lost in the future.

Fixed prostheses

For most patients a fixed solution to replace missing teeth is preferred. This might be due to the fact there is no palatal or lingual connector or that they are smaller and do not cover extensive areas of alveolar ridge. Some patients may simply not be able to tolerate a removable prosthesis

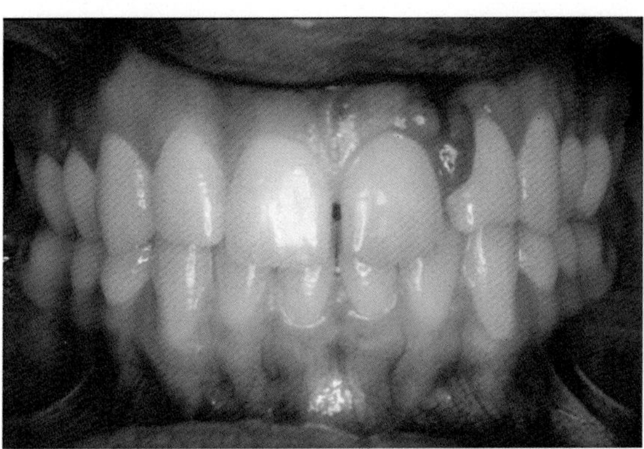

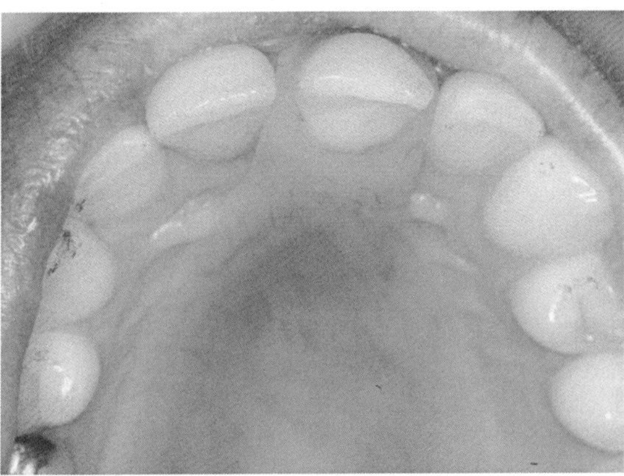

Figure 17.10 The upper left central incisor has suffered a root fracture and requires extraction. An immediate removable acrylic prosthesis has been made and fitted immediately after the tooth was extracted, avoiding the patient having an unsightly space for any period of time.

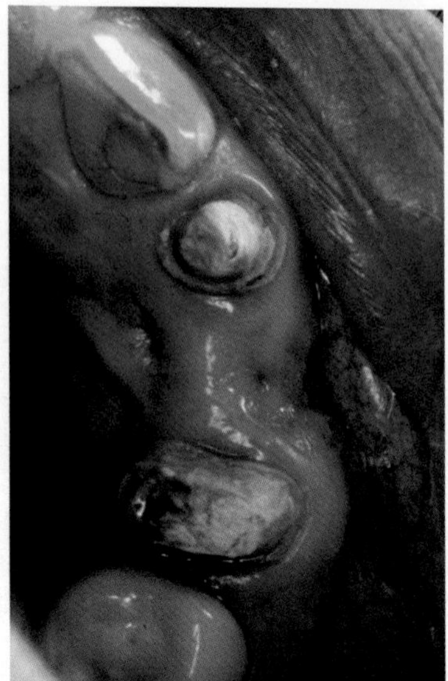

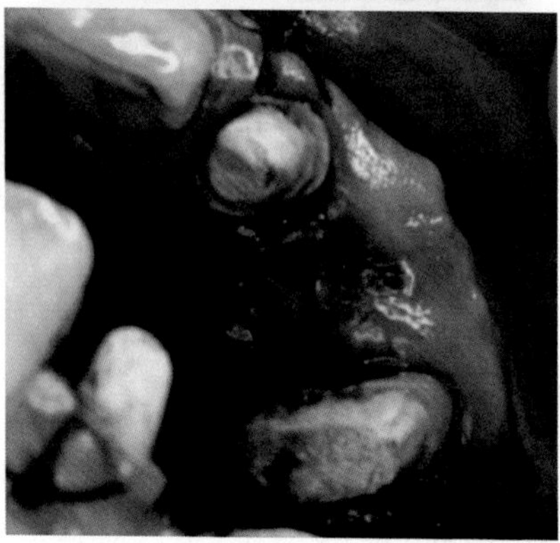

Figure 17.11 This patient has had an upper left canine surgically removed leaving a marked alveolar defect (top). To avoid an unsightly relationship between the bridge pontic planned and the edentulous ridge, an alveolar bone graft has been performed (bottom).

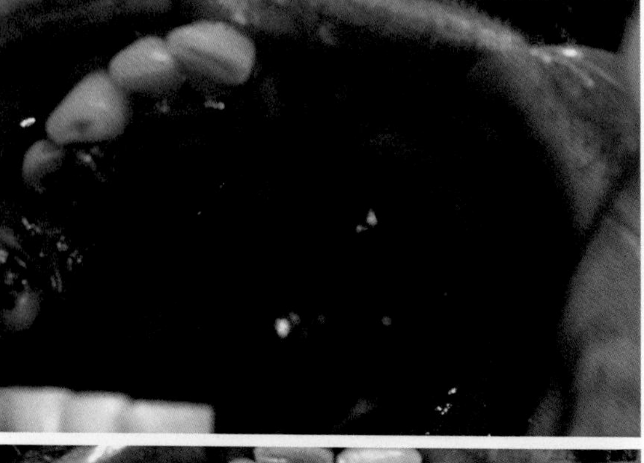

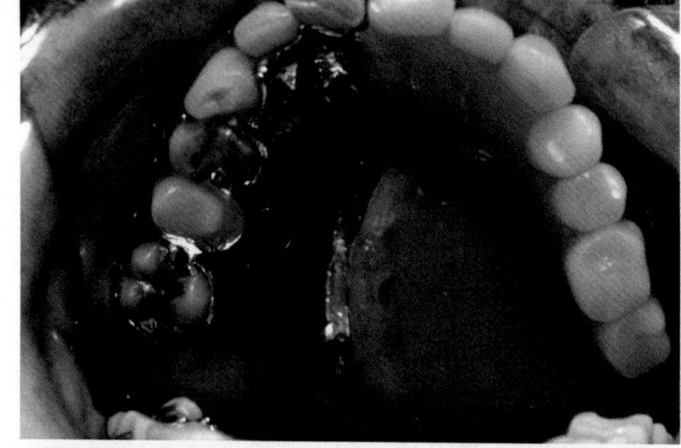

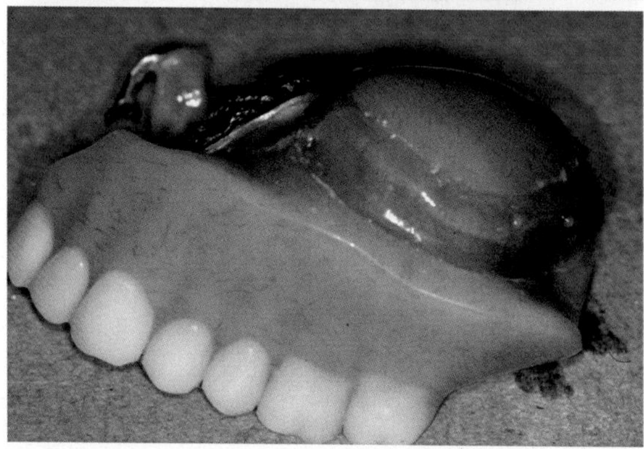

Figure 17.12 This patient has had surgery to remove a tumour leaving a large defect in the maxilla. The removable prosthesis not only replaces the missing teeth, but it also replaces the lost tissues and seals the oro-nasal communication.

due to a retch reflex for example. A fixed restoration gives patients added security and psychologically becomes an integral part of the dentition but generally increases cost. There are two types of fixed restoration that can be considered: bridges and implants.

Bridges

There are two main types of bridges available to the dentist: conventional bridges and minimal preparation (resin retained) bridges. Irrespective of the type of bridge, both of which will be described in detail in the subsequent two chapters, the terminology used to describe the components is common to both.

Conventionally prepared bridges

Conventional bridges are usually indicated when the abutment teeth are extensively restored, requiring preparation of the teeth for conventional retainers, normally full coverage crowns. Full coverage retainers protect the remaining coronal tooth tissue of the abutment teeth and the core material from occlusal loading, and provide optimum retention for the bridge.

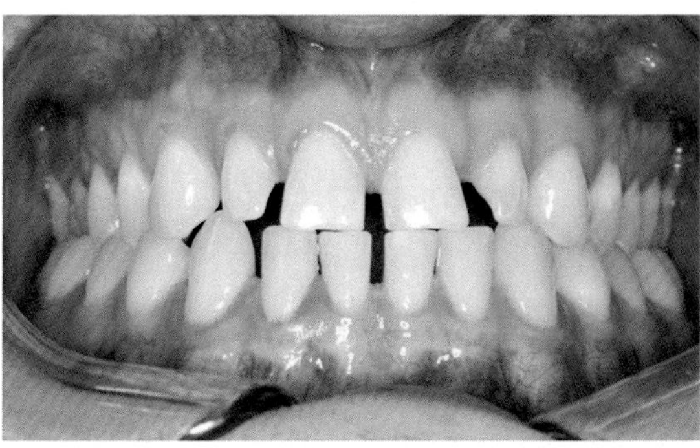

Figure 17.13 Patient with dento-skeletal discrepancy leading to spacing. Loss of an anterior tooth will require a removable prosthesis or implant retained restoration to produce the same appearance.

Minimal preparation (resin retained) bridges

Minimally prepared (resin retained) bridges are indicated when the abutment teeth are unrestored or minimally restored. Rather than preparing virgin teeth for full coverage retainers, the abutment teeth are minimally prepared and the primary retention for the bridge is achieved from adhesive cements (see Chapter 18). It could be argued that with improved dental health and fewer heavily restored teeth, minimally prepared (resin retained) bridges are, or may become, the more 'conventional' of the bridge designs. However, with the rapidly growing market in implants, these too may become the restoration of choice for the minimally restored dentition in the future.

Implant retained restorations

Both conventional and minimally prepared (resin retained) bridges use adjacent teeth to gain support and retention for the prosthetic tooth or pontic. As such, caries

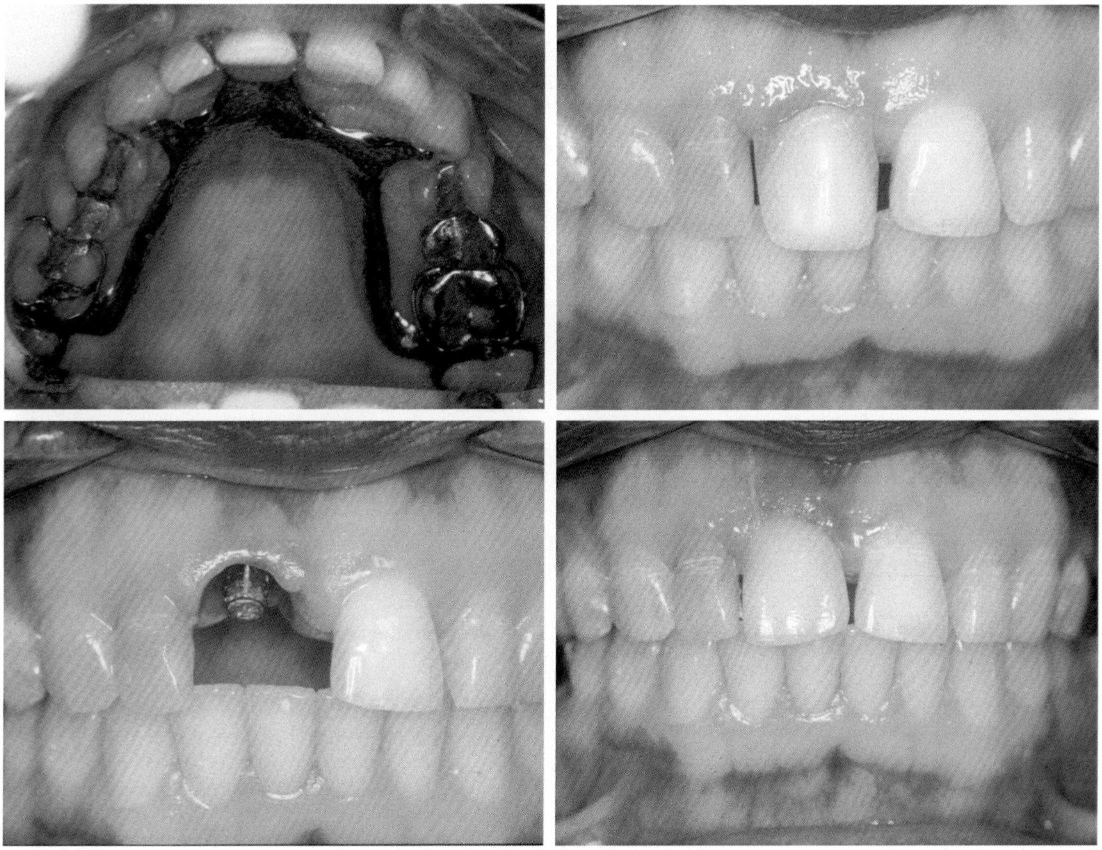

Figure 17.14 A missing central incisor tooth initially replaced by a cobalt chromium removable prosthesis and latterly by a single tooth implant. Both treatment options preserve the midline diastema.

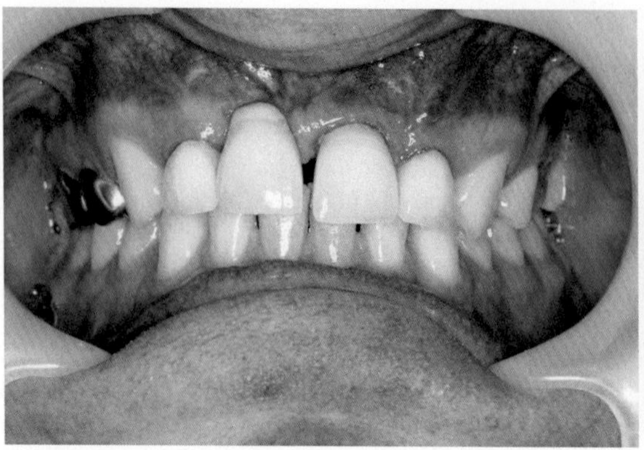

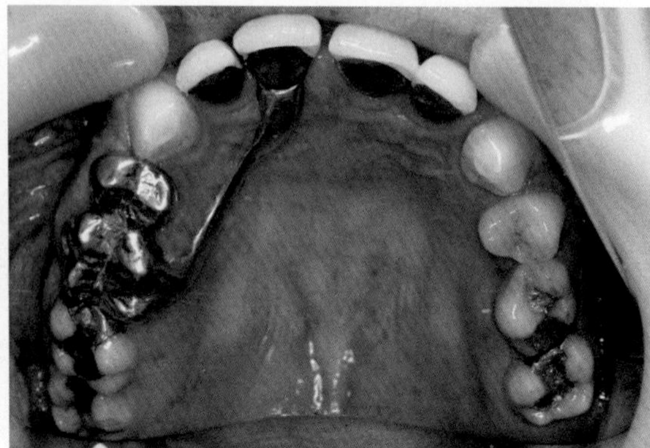

Figure 17.15 This patient had a midline diastema which has been preserved by placement of a spring cantilever bridge. A single tooth implant would be the preferred treatment option today.

can occur at the margins of the restoration and periodontal problems can arise in susceptible patients (Figure 17.16). In most situations this risk can be reduced by effective preventive management given preoperatively and postoperatively and throughout any reviews and maintenance. In some situations the adjacent teeth are unsuitable for bridge abutments by virtue of the tooth size (crown and/or root) and periodontal support compared to the length of the edentulous span. Such situations can be treated with implant retained crowns, bridges or dentures (Figure 17.17).

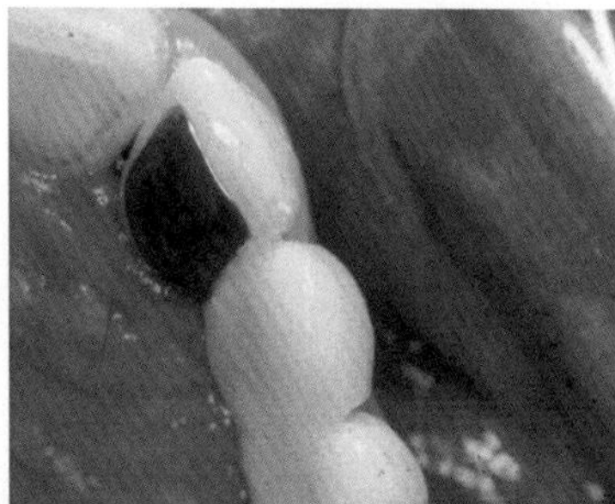

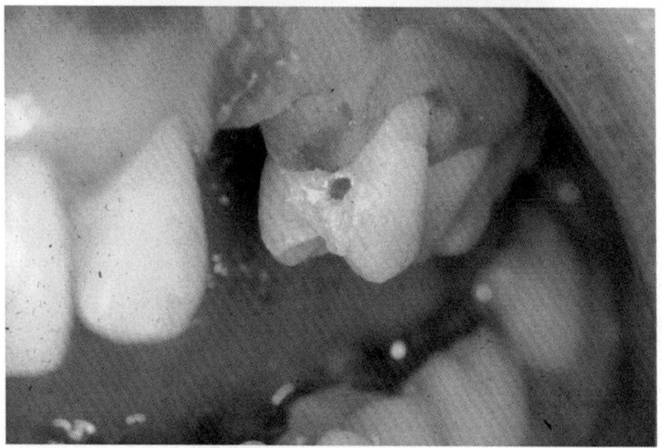

Figure 17.16 The resin retained bridge on the upper left premolar tooth has failed due to secondary caries.

Orthodontic treatment and replacing teeth

Whenever a patient is provided with a restoration of any kind, and in particular costly indirect restorations, it is important to emphasize that they will require maintenance and possible repair or replacement throughout life. For some this prospect is not acceptable and the spaces can be closed orthodontically. A typical example is the management of congenitally missing upper lateral incisor teeth. A decision has to be made as to whether to close the space orthodontically or to open up sufficient space to place prosthetic lateral incisor teeth. The former avoids prosthetic replacement but the appearance may be compromised by darker coloured, pointed and bulbous canine teeth adjacent to the central incisor teeth. Whilst the shape of the canine teeth can be altered to some degree by addition of composite resin and judicious tooth adjustment, gingival contour, canine eminence and lack of canine guidance cannot be overcome (Figure 17.18).

A superior appearance can be obtained by creating space for a prosthetic tooth (Figure 17.19); however, this may involve extraction of a sound tooth more posterior to the canine tooth, providing space for distal tooth movement. It also relies on a co-operative patient who is prepared to undergo a more protracted course of orthodontic treatment and accept a prosthetic replacement and its maintenance throughout life.

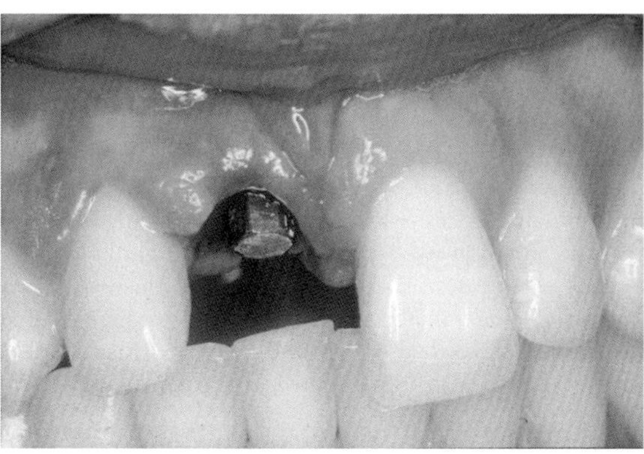
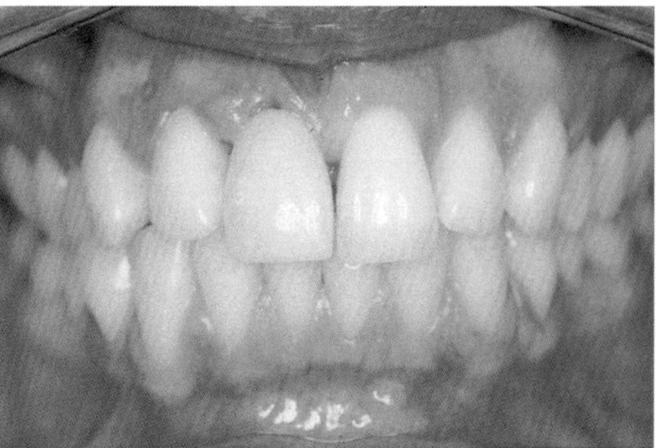

Figure 17.17 Replacement of upper right central incisor with an implant retained crown in a patient with an unrestored dentition and no periodontal disease.

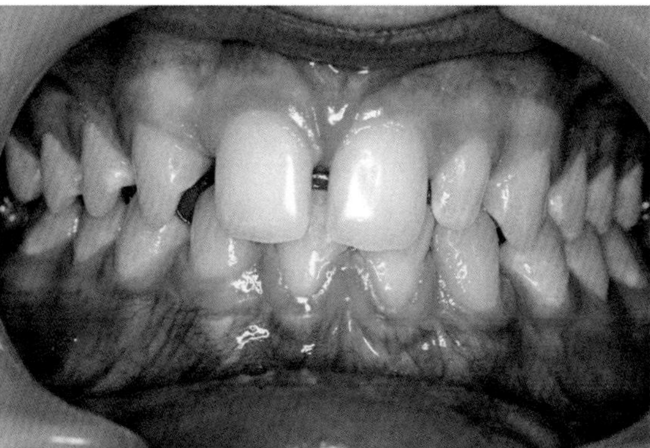
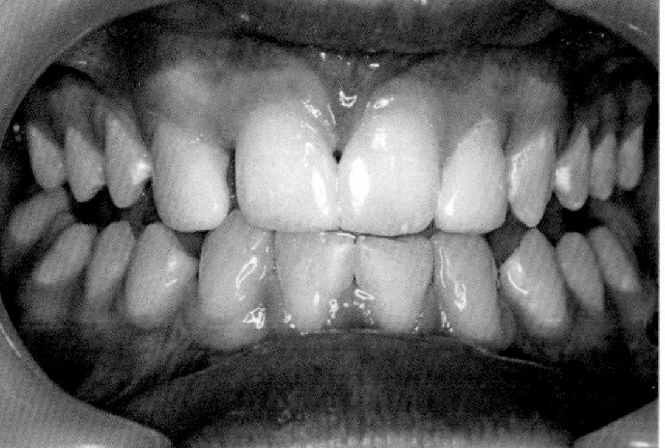

Figure 17.18 The upper right lateral incisor is congenitally missing, the upper left is diminutive in size and there is a midline diastema. As the patient did not want orthodontic treatment the upper anterior teeth have been restored with composite. The result is a reasonable compromise.

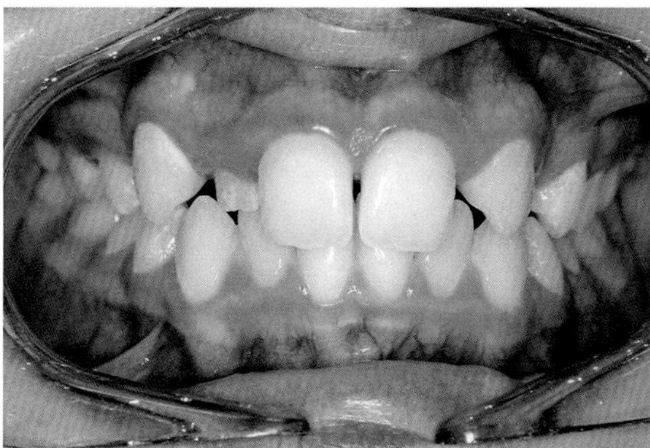
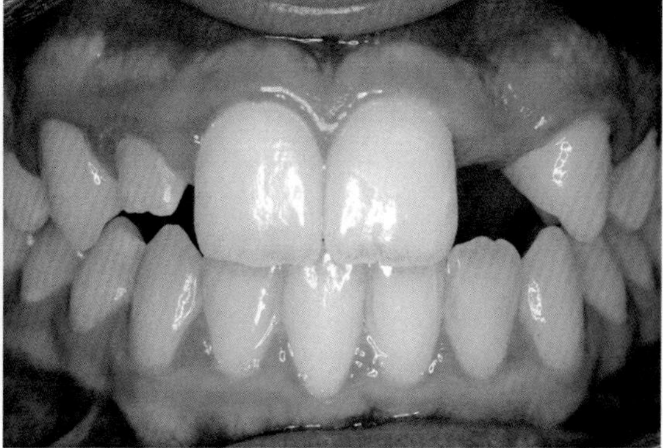

Figure 17.19 Patient with congenitally missing upper left lateral incisor and diminutive right lateral incisor tooth. Orthodontic treatment has produced sufficient space for a resin retained bridge on the left and a composite build-up on the right.

(Continued)

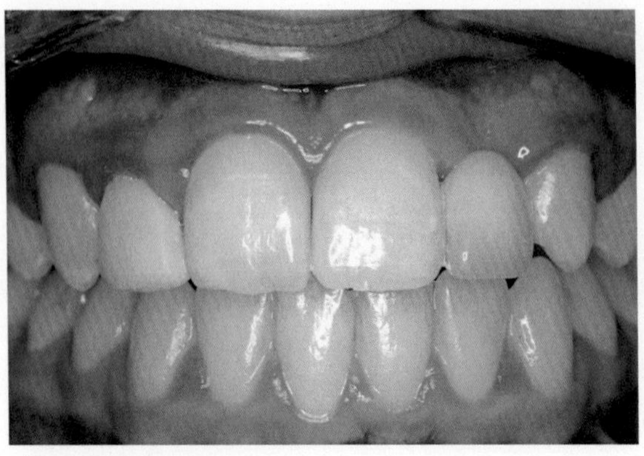

Figure 17.19—cont'd

SUMMARY

When a patient loses or has a missing tooth or teeth, their replacement needs to be considered carefully in light of the advantages and disadvantages of doing so. Once a decision to replace missing teeth has been made, each clinical situation needs to be evaluated carefully with the aid of appropriate special investigations such as radiographs and articulated study models. The ways of how to replace the teeth should then be discussed, paying particular attention to the prognosis of each.

FURTHER READING

Fiske, J., Davis, D.M., Leung, K.C., McMillan, A.S., Scott, B.J., 2001. The emotional effects of tooth loss in partially dentate people attending prosthodontic clinics in dental schools in England, Scotland and Hong Kong: a preliminary investigation. Int. Dent. J. 51, 457–462.

Jahangiri, L., Devlin, H., Ting, K., Nishimura, I., 1998. Current perspectives in residual ridge remodeling and its clinical implications: a review. Prosthet. Dent. 80, 224–237.

Kanno, T., Carlsson, G.E., 2006. A review of the shortened dental arch concept focusing on the work by the Käyser/Nijmegen group. J. Oral Rehabil. 33, 850–862.

Schropp, L., Isidor, F., 2008. Timing of implant placement relative to tooth extraction. J. Oral Rehabil. 35 (Suppl. 1), 33–43.

Chapter 18

Minimal preparation (resin retained) bridges

David Ricketts

CHAPTER CONTENTS

WHAT ARE MINIMAL PREPARATION (RESIN RETAINED) BRIDGES AND WHEN ARE THEY USED?

Minimal preparation bridges have also been referred to in the literature as resin retained bridges, adhesive bridges and resin-bonded bridges. In this text the term minimal preparation (resin retained) bridge will be used. These are bridges that require minimal preparation of tooth tissue and rely on adhesive cements for their primary retention, unlike conventional bridges that require significant tooth reduction to make retentively shaped preparations which provide the primary retention and then rely on a cement lute for secondary retention.

Minimal preparation (resin retained) bridges are therefore used when the potential abutment teeth are unrestored or minimally restored and there is a need to reduce unnecessary tooth preparation. Consider the 22-year-old patient in Figure 18.1: preparation of the vital upper right central incisor tooth for a metal–ceramic retainer has been destructive of tooth tissue as this tooth only had a small fractured incisal edge. A cantilevered minimal preparation (resin retained) bridge using the central incisor as an abutment tooth would have been much more conservative. However, in this patient both lateral incisors are missing. Conventional bridge retainer preparation of the non-vital upper left central incisor tooth has been necessary not only to retain a pontic but also to disguise the appearance of the discoloured tooth. Furthermore, this patient had orthodontic treatment to close a midline diastema and since this treatment tends to be unstable, the conventional retainers were linked to also act as an orthodontic retainer.

HISTORY OF RESIN-BONDED BRIDGES

It is useful to understand the history of the development of minimal preparation (resin-bonded) bridges as some principles and applications can be useful in contemporary practice.

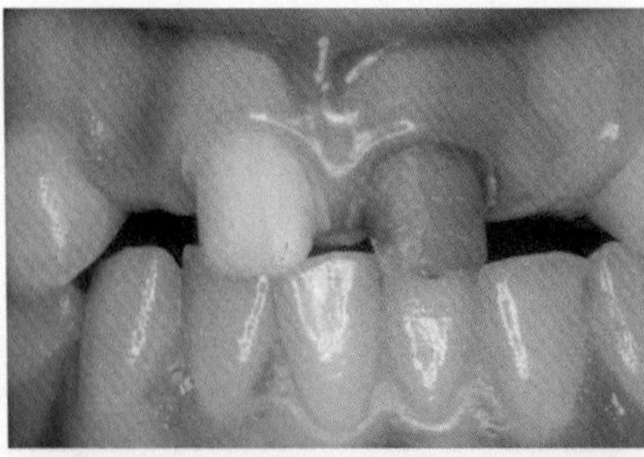

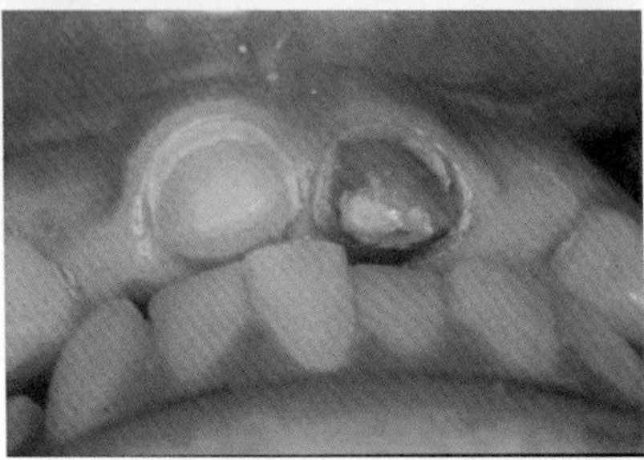

Figure 18.1 This is the patient seen in Figure 19.2, Chapter 19. Preparation of the upper right central incisor for a metal–ceramic retainer has not been conservative of tooth tissue.

Macromechanical retention

Natural tooth pontic

This technique can be used for a tooth that needs to be extracted. Once extracted, the root is resected and then the crown is cemented to the adjacent tooth/teeth using composite resin cement. At the resected root end the root canal should be opened and restored with either a glass ionomer or composite resin to prevent food and plaque stagnating within the tooth. To bond the extracted tooth the corresponding approximal surfaces are acid etched, bond applied and then composite used to cement the crown in place. Figure 18.2 illustrates diagrammatically how this procedure is carried out and Figure 18.3 shows an example where this has been done. In the author's opinion this technique has been remarkably successful for the patient in Figure 18.3 as this 'temporary' measure had been carried out many years previously.

If a patient presents with a missing tooth, which is either lost or not reusable, a replacement tooth can be made from composite resin using a crown former or simply an appropriately sized acrylic denture tooth can be used. Additional retention can be obtained, if required, by embedding a contoured orthodontic wire, wire mesh or fibre-reinforced ribbon in composite to the lingual surface of the extracted tooth and the tooth or teeth to which it is being bonded.

Laboratory-made bridges using macromechanical retention

Rochette bridges

A Rochette bridge consists of a pontic connected to a metal wing retainer which covers the lingual surface of the abutment tooth. Within the wing, countersunk holes are cut which allow retentive composite plugs or rivets to form when the bridge is cemented in situ (Figure 18.4). When Rochette bridges were originally described, they were designed to act as permanent fixed prosthodontic restorations (Figure 18.5). However, to achieve composite plugs of adequate strength they had to be of a significant

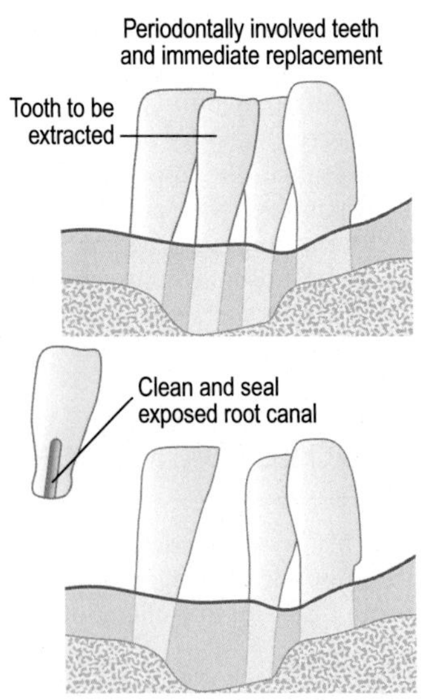

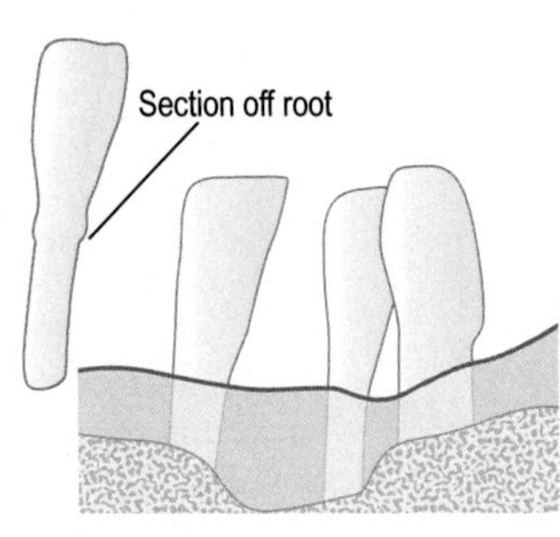

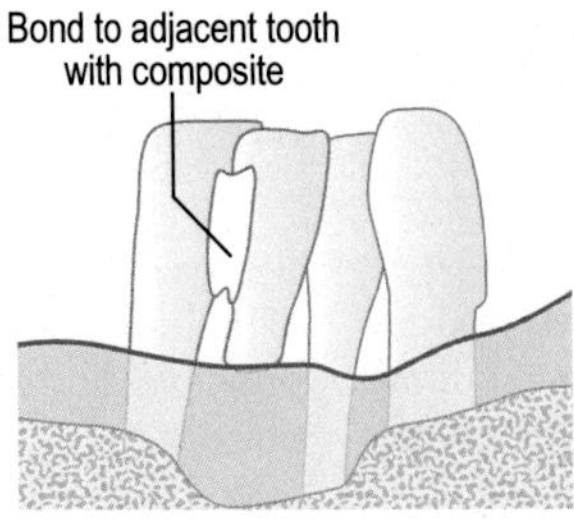

Figure 18.2 Diagrammatic representation of the patient seen in Figure 18.3. The teeth are periodontally involved and the lower right central incisor requires extraction. Following extraction the root is resected (top right), the root canal is cleaned from the resected end and the canal restored with composite resin or glass ionomer (bottom left). The tooth is then bonded to the adjacent tooth with composite resin cement (bottom right).

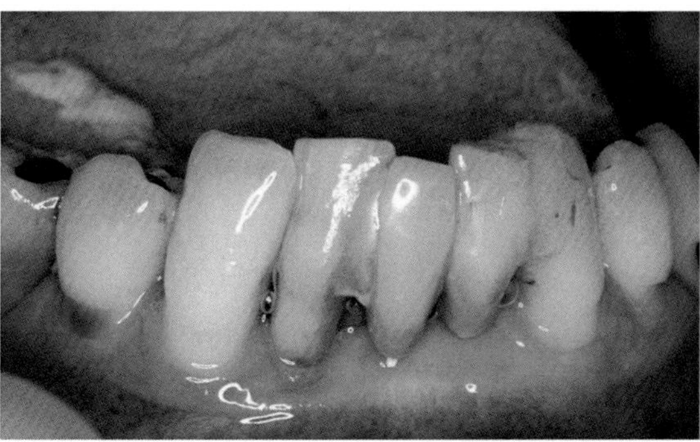

Figure 18.3 Lower central incisor resin retained natural tooth pontics cantilevered off the lateral incisors.

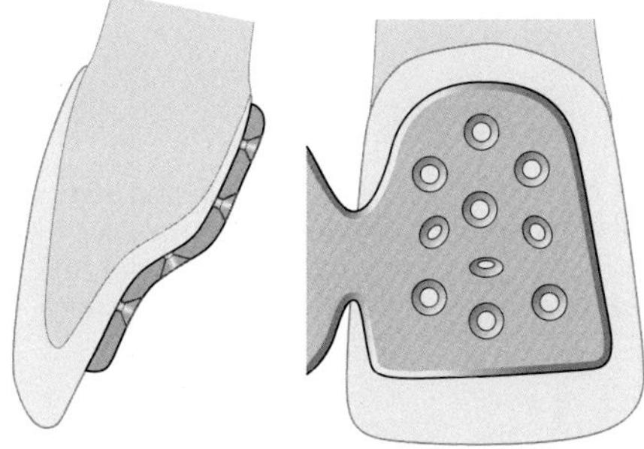

Figure 18.4 Diagrammatic representation of a Rochette bridge. The cross-section shows the countersunk holes and retentive composite 'rivets'.

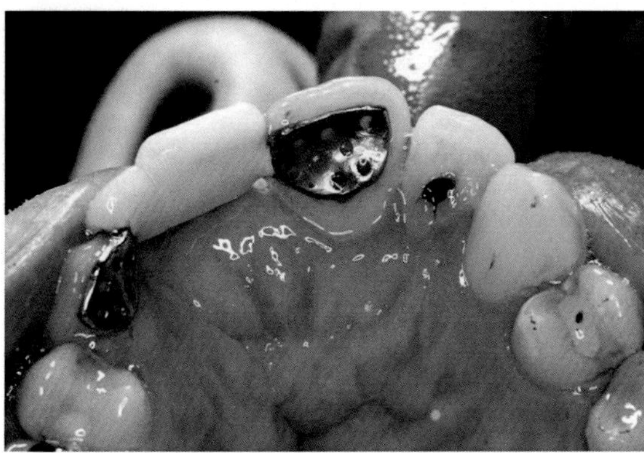

Figure 18.5 An example of a fixed–fixed Rochette bridge. This bridge had been in situ for over 20 years.

diameter and depth, the latter necessitating a thick wing which caused problems in relation to the occlusion, especially when placed in the upper anterior region. In addition, occlusal stresses were concentrated on a limited number of composite plugs, predisposing to them to fracture and, as such, retention rates were often poor in the long term.

Today, Rochette bridges can still be considered as an immediate provisional tooth replacement when ease of removal is a benefit. For example, if a patient was unable or unwilling to wear a removable prosthesis and an upper central incisor required extraction, its immediate replacement with a cantilever Rochette bridge, using the contralateral central incisor as an abutment, could be considered. The tooth could be extracted, rubber dam applied and the Rochette bridge cemented without any blood contamination from the socket.

Provided the bridge is cemented in place with a *non-adhesive*, dual or chemically cured composite resin luting cement, such as Nexus luting cement (Kerr/SDS), removal is achieved by simply removing the composite from the holes within the wing. It is important to note that if the permanent tooth replacement is to be a minimal preparation (resin-bonded) bridge using the same abutment tooth, the superficial enamel will be impregnated with resin and this will also have to be removed, otherwise the subsequent bond for the permanent bridge will be compromised. Therefore, this technique is preferred when either a different tooth is to be used as an abutment for the definitive bridge or if the final replacement is an implant which is not reliant on a tooth for support and retention.

Micromechanical retention and solid wing retainers

Rochette bridges suffered from a number of problems, namely potential degradation of the exposed composite (wear) and areas of stress concentration within the countersunk holes and composite rivets. In an attempt to retain a solid wing with reduced thickness and provide an improved retention for minimal preparation (resin retained) bridges Thompson and Livaditis in 1982 described a method of electrolytically etching the fit surface of non-precious alloys. The acid, its concentration and etching time were different for different alloys. In each case, however, an etch pattern was produced that allowed micromechanical retention of the bridge when a chemically cured non-adhesive resin was used for cementation. This bridge became known as the 'Maryland bridge'. The Maryland bridge technique required acid baths in the laboratory, and was a technique-sensitive procedure. Attempts were made to use chairside acid etch gels for the metal frame; however, the introduction of adhesive resin cements in the late 1980s superseded their further development.

Adhesive resin luting cements

Unlike resin luting cements, adhesive resin luting cements have the ability to bond to metal in addition to etched

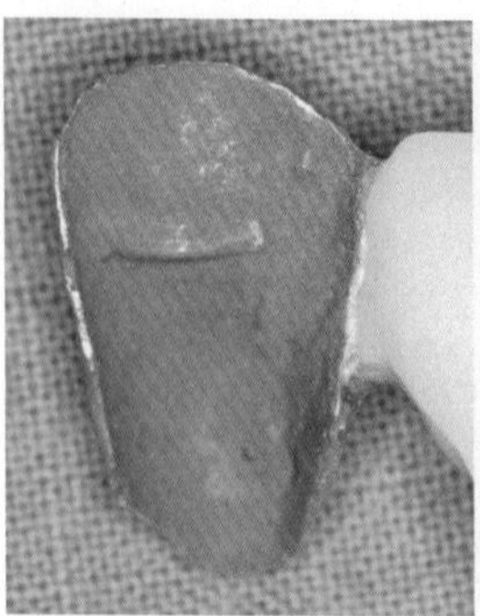
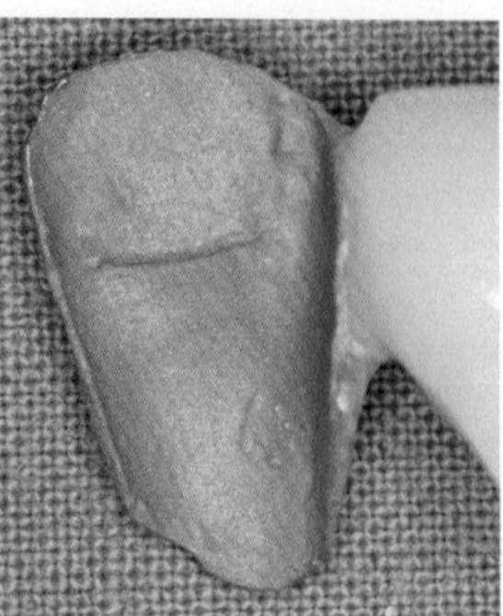

Figure 18.6 Resin retained bridge. Fit surface of wing before (left) and after sandblasting (right).

tooth tissue. Such cements include those that contain 4-META (4-methacryloxyethyl trimellitate anhydride) or phosphate groups (e.g. Panavia) which allow a chemical bond to form with metal. Superior bonding of these cements occurs with surface-abraded non-precious metal alloys such as cobalt chromium or nickel chromium. Whilst the latter allows a more rigid casting to be formed, there are problems associated with allergies (to nickel) for laboratory workers, dentists and patients. Precious metal alloys have therefore been used despite earlier reports of inferior bond strengths to precious metals.

To improve the bond strength of adhesive resin luting cements to precious metal alloys, various surface treatments have been used on the fit surface of the retainer. These include sandblasting with 50 μm alumina, heat treatment and oxide formation, silicate coating, tin plating or application of a metal primer. It is generally accepted that roughening the fit surface by sandblasting is the most convenient and reliable surface treatment, providing bond strengths comparable to the other methods when appropriate adhesive resin luting cements are used (Figure 18.6).

PRINCIPLES OF TOOTH PREPARATION AND BRIDGE DESIGN – ANTERIOR TEETH

The retention achieved for resin retained bridges will be dependent on the quantity and quality of the enamel to which the retainer(s) can be bonded. It is important to maximize the surface area of tooth tissue covered whilst not compromising the aesthetics. Although it would seem logical to use more than one wing as a retainer to increase the total surface area, it soon became apparent that when fixed–fixed resin-bonded bridge designs were used, one retainer commonly debonded.

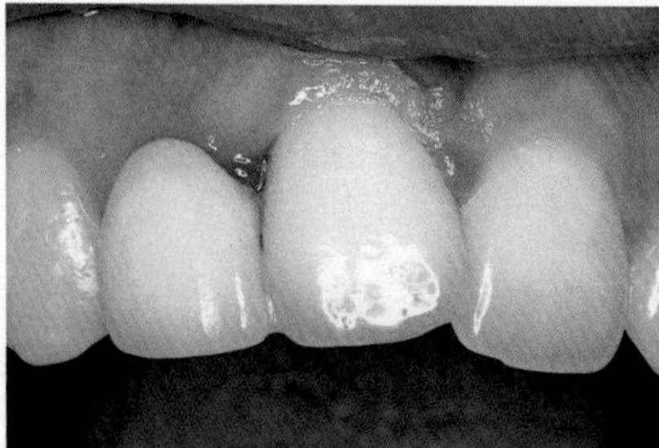
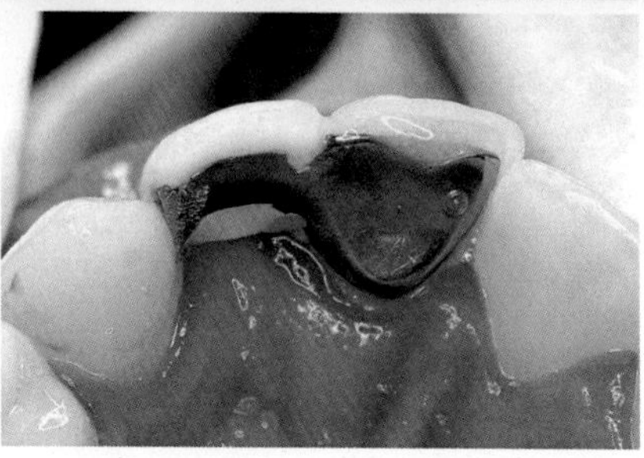

Figure 18.7 A three unit fixed–fixed resin retained bridge was made to replace the upper right lateral incisor. The wing had debonded off the canine and has now been cut off. The bridge has now been successful as a cantilever bridge.

For example, the patient in Figure 18.7 has a missing upper right lateral incisor. This was originally replaced with a fixed–fixed minimal preparation (resin-bonded) bridge using both the upper right canine and central incisor as abutment teeth. It can be seen that the surface area available for bonding to on the palatal surface of the canine tooth is less than that of the central incisor tooth. Thus the retention is also less. This, together with differences in the direction of the occlusal forces on each abutment tooth, led to the canine retainer debonding. The wing on the canine tooth has been removed and the bridge now functions as a cantilever bridge off the upper right central incisor tooth. A recent literature review comparing fixed–fixed three unit resin retained bridges with two unit cantilever designs has shown that the longevity of the latter is better when used in similar clinical situations (van Dalen et al., 2004).

There is some debate as to how much tooth preparation is required for minimal preparation (resin-bonded) bridges. A cingulum rest is important to resist potential shear stresses within the cement lute which would result from occlusal forces (Figure 18.8). The cingulum rest also helps as a locating device for cementation as it can be difficult to determine the correct seating of the wing onto a smooth lingual/palatal tooth surface. Even with such a rest seat it is often difficult to position the bridge during try-in and cementation. To facilitate this, some clinicians prescribe a small incisal extension or rest from the wing which can be cut off once cemented

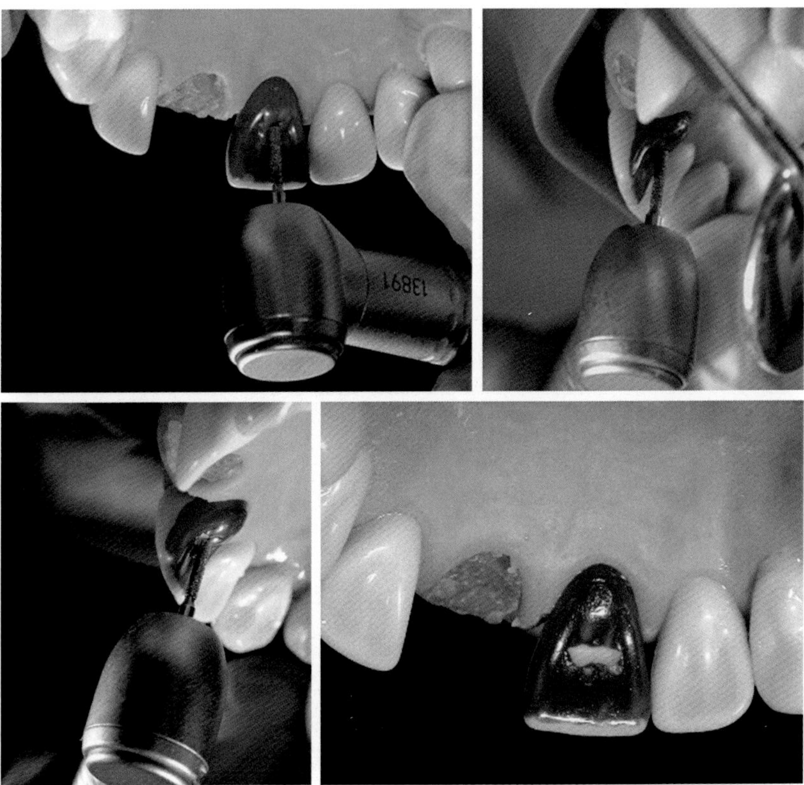

Figure 18.8 Cingulum rest preparation for a cantilever resin retained bridge.

(Figure 18.9). This is done by sectioning the rest along the red dotted line as seen in Figure 18.9 and using an excavator to lever it off whilst protecting the airway with a gauze square or Spontex sponge and high volume suction. The rest is easy to remove as the incisal and labial aspect of the tooth is not etched, the incisal rest fit surface is not sandblasted and no luting cement need be applied to it. Whilst such rests help the operator in positioning the bridge for cementation, they hinder patients when trying to assess the appearance. Once the rest has been removed the metal wing can be polished (Figure 18.10).

Some clinicians also like to cut a cervical chamfer whilst others do not. Those that support this view argue that it aids in checking the seating of the casting onto the tooth and avoids an overhanging cervical margin (Figure 18.11). However, in the area that the chamfer is cut, the enamel cap is very thin and dentine can be exposed. This might lead to sensitivity until the bridge is cemented and the bond of the luting cement to dentine is not as strong as it is to etched enamel. With the seating rests described and a cleansable rounded cervical margin to the wing, the claimed advantages of preparing the tooth cervically are relatively minor.

Occlusal clearance

For patients with a complete tooth-to-tooth overbite, placement of a resin retained bridge in the upper anterior region will lead to premature occlusal contact of the lower incisors with the wing retainer. There are three solutions to this:

- Adjust the opposing tooth when the minimal preparation (resin-bonded) bridge is fitted. This compromises the opposing tooth and may affect the appearance.
- Create occlusal clearance at the time of tooth preparation. However, overeruption of the opposing teeth might take place whilst the bridge is being made in the laboratory, losing the valuable space created. Temporization of the palatal surface of the upper anterior teeth is not possible unless an adhesive material is used. This poses difficulty when trying to remove it accurately at the subsequent fit appointment as it is important not to leave any material behind or inadvertently remove some of the tooth surface which would result in a poor fit of the bridge. If composite is placed, impregnation of the etched enamel with resin also compromises the

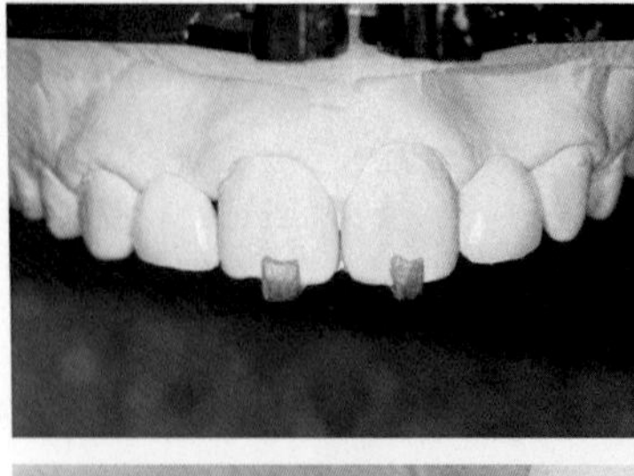
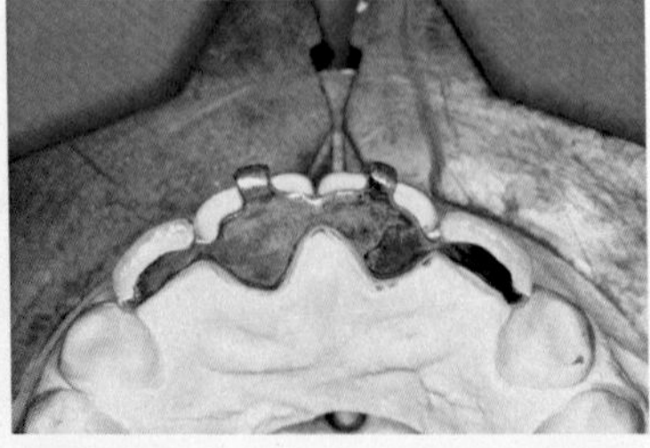
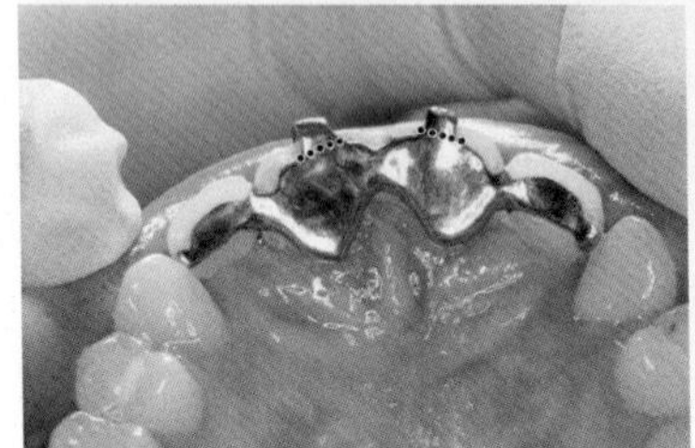
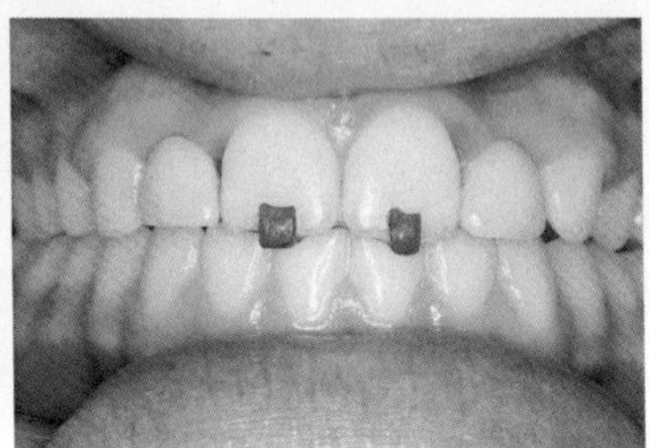
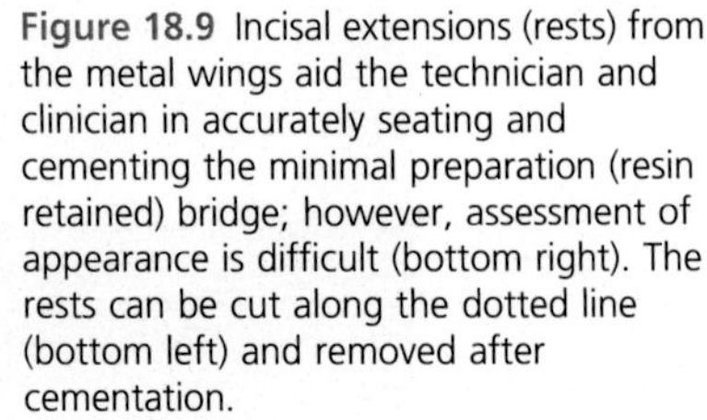

Figure 18.9 Incisal extensions (rests) from the metal wings aid the technician and clinician in accurately seating and cementing the minimal preparation (resin retained) bridge; however, assessment of appearance is difficult (bottom right). The rests can be cut along the dotted line (bottom left) and removed after cementation.

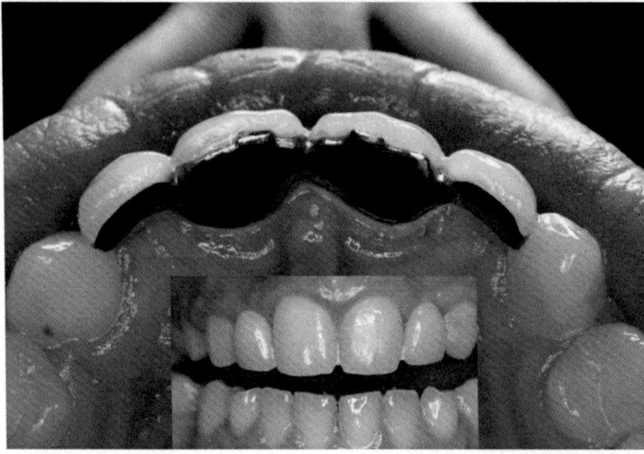

Figure 18.10 A similarly designed bridge to that in Figure 18.9 with the incisal rests removed and polished.

subsequent bond of the bridge. Placement of composite onto the incisal edge of the opposing tooth overcomes these problems and will maintain the occlusal clearance. This can then simply be removed once the bridge is cemented.

- The bridge can be made and cemented without occlusal clearance, provided the patient knows at the treatment planning stage that the bridge will feel 'high on the bite' at the fit appointment. This will then not appear to the patient as a lack of skill or judgement. The bridge will then act as a Dahl appliance (Ricketts & Smith, 1993a,b), causing intrusion of the opposing teeth and allowing the remaining separated teeth to overerupt (see Chapter 16). Patients adapt quickly to this change and a normal occlusion should be achieved within 2–3 months.

Special considerations – missing lateral incisors

Hypodontia (up to six congenitally missing teeth) is common, third molar teeth are most often affected and up to 2% of individuals suffer from one or both missing lateral incisor teeth. In this situation a decision has to be made whether to create space for the upper lateral incisors with orthodontic treatment followed by prosthodontic replacement, which usually results in optimum aesthetics, or to close the space and modify the shape of the canine teeth. The latter often results in a compromised appearance, but the patient has no prosthodontic replacement to be maintained throughout life (see Figure 17.18, Chapter 17).

If space is created for a prosthodontic lateral incisor tooth and a cantilever minimal preparation (resin retained) bridge is planned, either the central incisor or the canine tooth can be used as an abutment. The central incisor benefits from having a larger surface area to bond to than the canine, but often the central incisors are too translucent and unsightly grey shine through from the metal wing can occur (Figure 18.12). In these situations the canine teeth have to be used, even though this might affect guidance in lateral excursion.

The mesial surface of the canine tooth is often markedly convex, with its bulbosity close to the gingival margin. This poses two problems: (1) the connector between the wing and the pontic is too narrow for adequate strength and rigidity (Figures 18.13 and 18.14); and (2) it is too close to the gingival papilla to allow for oral hygiene procedures and best appearance. Preparation of a guide plane on the mesial surface of the canine significantly increases the dimensions of the connector (Figure 18.13) and allows it to be moved further away from the gingiva,

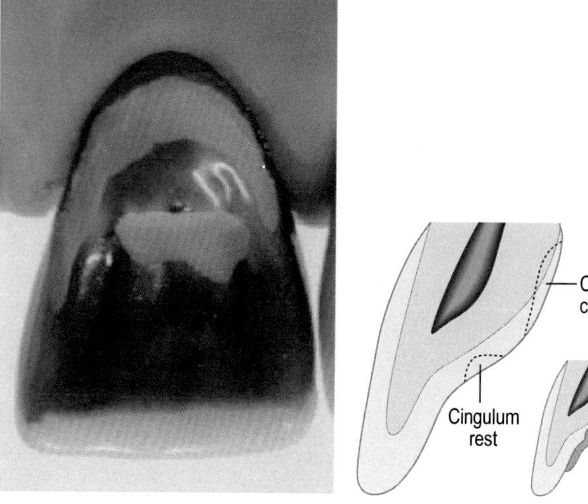

Figure 18.11 Cervical chamfer preparation for resin retained bridge (left). The diagrammatic cross-section through the tooth shows that this can often expose dentine due to the tapered enamel cap (top right). If no cervical preparation is carried out, finishing the wing with a polished and rounded margin should facilitate oral hygiene procedures (right).

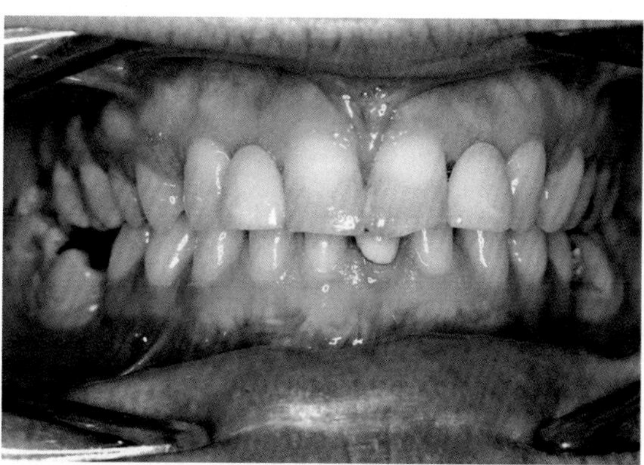

Figure 18.12 Resin retained bridges using the central incisors as abutment teeth has led to shadowing as the incisors are very translucent.

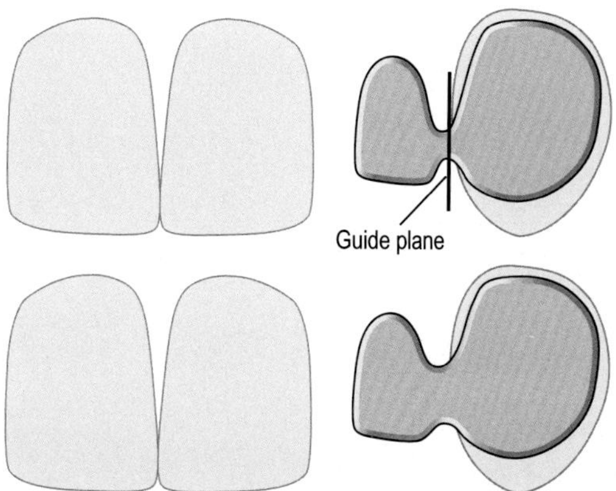

Figure 18.13 Diagrammatic representation of a cantilever resin retained bridge to replace a missing lateral incisor using the canine as an abutment. If no preparation is carried out, the connector is often too thin (top); cutting a small mesial guide plane significantly increases its dimension (bottom).

overcoming these problems. This principle can be applied in a number of clinical situations and allows a definite path of insertion.

Preventing orthodontic relapse

When patients have undergone orthodontic treatment to create space for a prosthodontic replacement tooth (or teeth) there is still the potential for the orthodontic treatment to relapse (Figure 18.15). It is important that at the fit appointment once the bridge has been cemented an impression is taken for a vacuum-formed orthodontic retainer to be made which can be worn over the teeth and bridge at night. Orthodontic retention should be regarded as long term and continued throughout life. Some orthodontic movements are more susceptible to relapse than others and closure of a midline diastema is an example of a particularly unstable procedure. It is possible to use resin retained bridges as orthodontic retainers in this instance. The patients seen in Figures 18.9 and 18.10 have had the wing retainers linked together to prevent the corrected midline diastema from relapsing. Care needs to be taken to ensure that the patient can use super floss beneath the connector between the wings and good follow-up is required to confirm that one retainer does not debond.

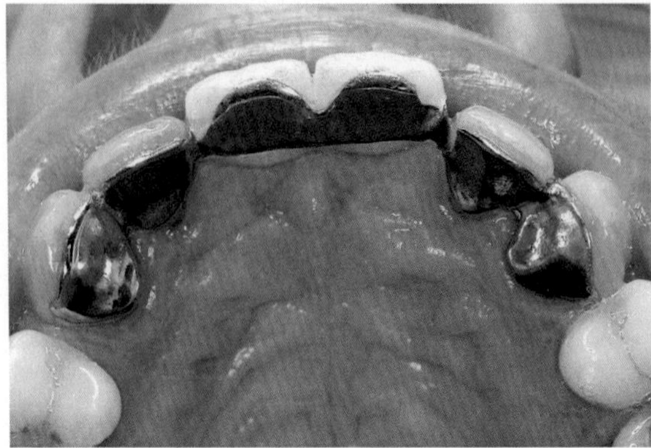

Figure 18.14 The connector between the upper left lateral incisor wing retainer and central pontic is too thin and has fractured. This extensive bridge design was probably chosen as the lateral incisors alone are unlikely to provide adequate retention for two cantilever bridges. Implant retained prostheses would have had a better prognosis.

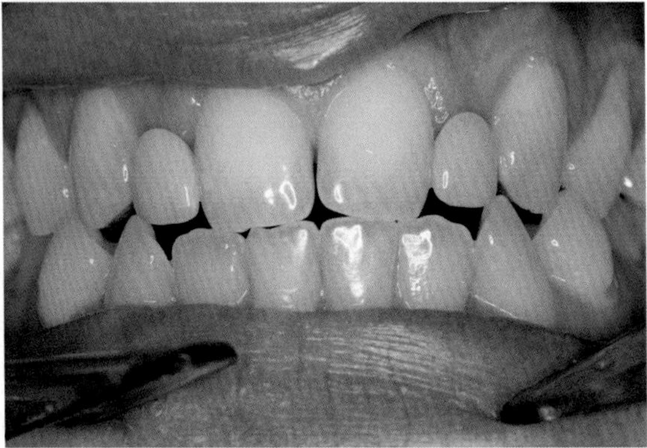

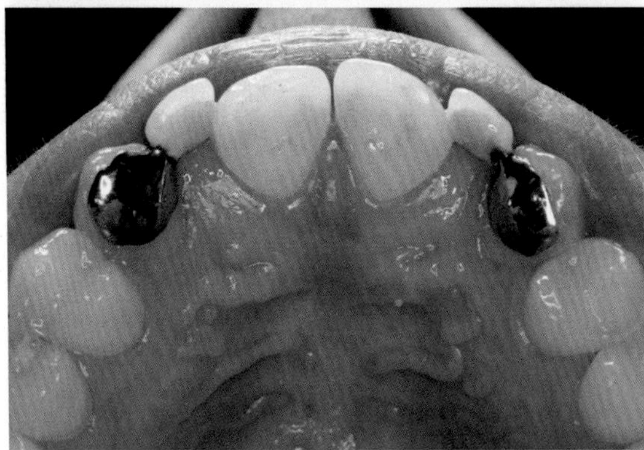

Figure 18.15 This patient has been provided with two cantilever resin retained bridges following orthodontic treatment to create space for the lateral incisors. No orthodontic retainer was provided and as such there has been orthodontic relapse leading to opening of a midline diastema and slippage of the contact point with the pontic moving labially.

PRINCIPLES OF TOOTH PREPARATION AND BRIDGE DESIGN – POSTERIOR TEETH

The same principles of tooth preparation apply to posterior minimal preparation (resin retained) bridges. Like anterior bridges there may be little benefit in preparing a cervical chamfer, but occlusal rest seats are important to resist displacement from occlusal loads and stresses placed on the pontic that would lead to cohesive and adhesive failure at the cement lute interfaces. As occlusal loads are likely to be greater posteriorly, it is important to try to achieve a 180° wrap-around to the wing retainer. Posterior teeth are also bulbous and preparation of a proximal and lingual guide plane increases the tooth surface area above the survey line to which the bridge can be bonded (Figure 18.16).

It is possible to improve the surface area of the tooth to which the minimal preparation (resin retained) bridges can be cemented by covering as much of the occlusal surface as the occlusion will allow. To assist in the preparation and treatment planning, articulated study casts are invaluable (Figure 18.17). It is clear from the articulated

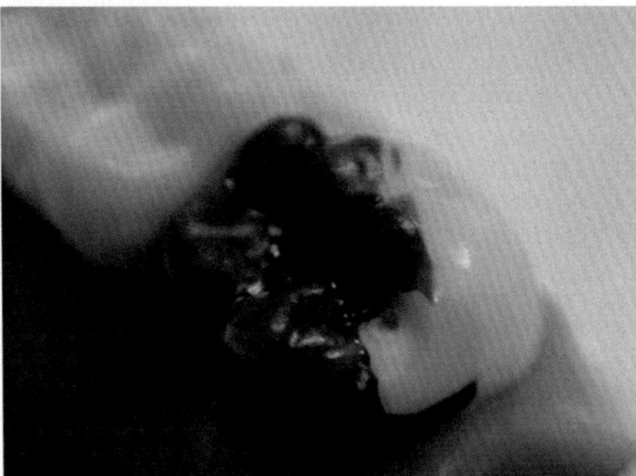

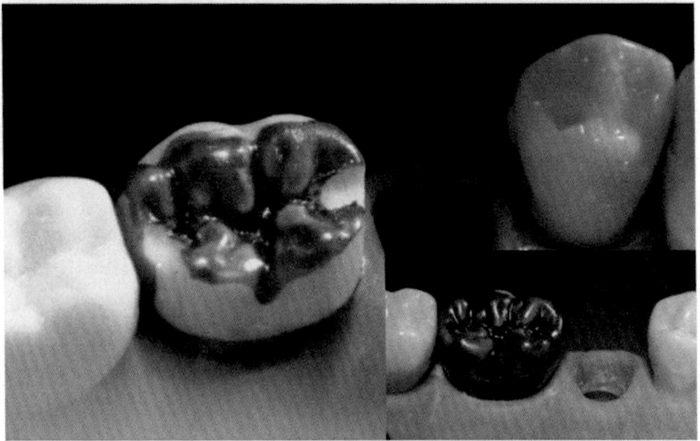

Figure 18.16 Posterior resin retained bridge preparation, showing rest seats mesially and distally and a mesial and lingual guide plane to increase the surface area for bonding.

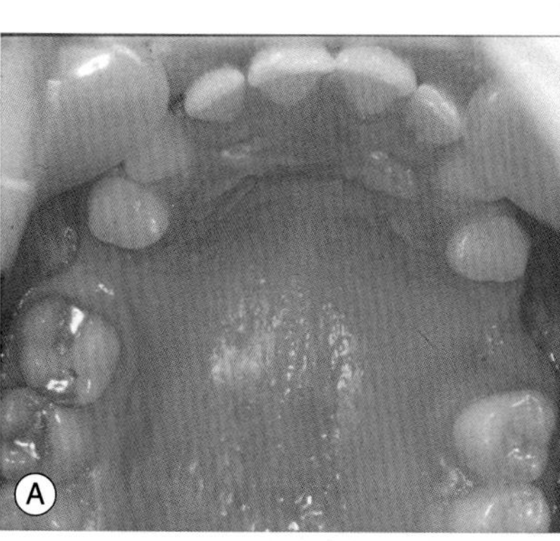

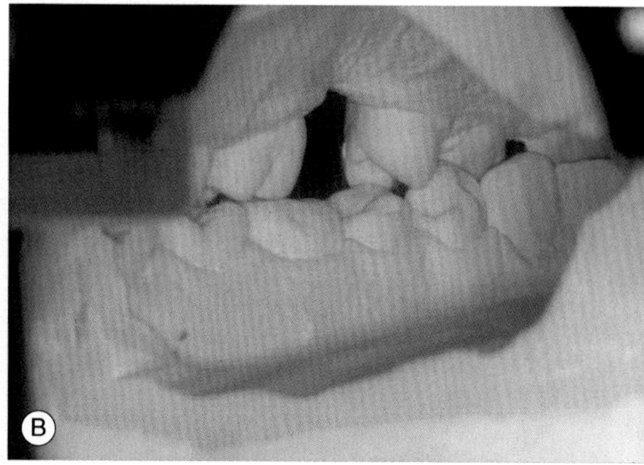

Figure 18.17 Patient with hypodontia requiring prosthetic tooth replacement (A). Articulated study casts show that there is sufficient occlusal clearance over the palatal cusps when in intercuspal position for metal coverage which can be incorporated into the resin retained bridge design (B).

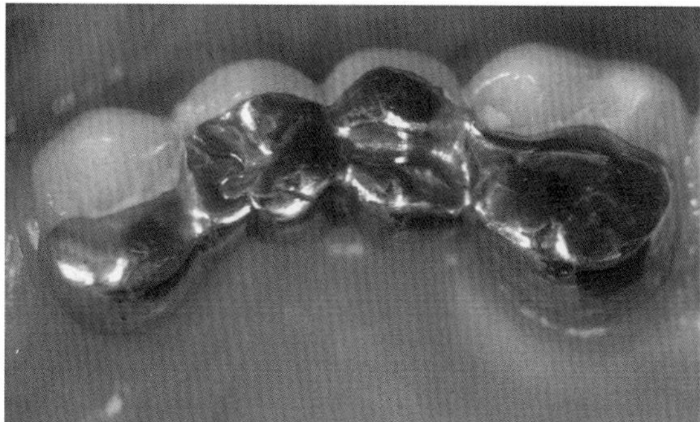

Figure 18.18 Fixed-movable resin retained bridge for the patient seen in Figure 17. Covering the palatal cusps has provided excellent retention and has brought the teeth into function.

casts that there is no occlusal contact between the palatal cusps of the potential abutment teeth in the upper arch and the opposing teeth in the intercuspal position. Extending the wing retainer over the cusp tips would significantly improve retention and support against occlusal forces. An additional advantage is that it also brings the abutment teeth into functional occlusion (Figure 18.18). In situations where appearance is not an issue, buccal wing retainers can also be considered.

Abutment teeth can have existing small to moderate sized intracoronal restorations present which can be incorporated into the design of the minimal preparation (resin retained) bridge (Figure 18.19). This will give a degree of conventional mechanical retention to the retainer. Most intracoronal cavities for direct restorations may contain undercuts due to the natural spread of caries and cavity preparation, but indirect preparations need to be divergent occlusally to allow insertion and removal of the restoration. Thus, when the existing restoration is removed, these undercuts have to be eliminated, either by removing more tooth tissue with a tapered bur or by blocking out the undercut with (ideally) an adhesive restorative material. The former is usually overly destructive of tooth tissue, so the latter is preferred, but can be difficult to perform accurately (Figure 18.20). An alternative approach is to restore the entire cavity with the adhesive material and then cut an inlay preparation within it, ensuring all preparation margins are onto tooth tissue (Figure 18.21). For deeper cavities it is wise to ensure that the occlusal aspect of the inlay is only about 3 mm or so deep. This will give adequate retention, but should allow easy access to the pulp chamber through the metal framework if root canal treatment was ever required.

For longer span resin-bonded bridges which have abutment teeth of different root surface areas there is a problem if one tooth potentially has more physiological movement than the other, with the result that debonding occurs at the retainer with least retention (usually at the smaller tooth with the greater potential for movement). To overcome this problem, consider the patient in Figures 18.17 and 18.18. On the left-hand side the edentulous space can be restored with either two separate cantilever bridges, one pontic retained off the premolar tooth and one off the molar tooth, or by using a fixed–movable bridge design which allows some differential tooth movement of the two abutment teeth by virtue of the movable joint.

The movable joints incorporated into the castings usually have a factory-made precision fit and little movement other than along the long axis of the joint occurs. If the abutment tooth is restored it is possible to simply cut a rest seat within the restoration. This will give support to the pontic at its furthest point from the retainer but little bracing in excursive movements. For this type of bridge design careful attention needs to be paid to the occlusion to avoid heavy lateral loads on the pontic.

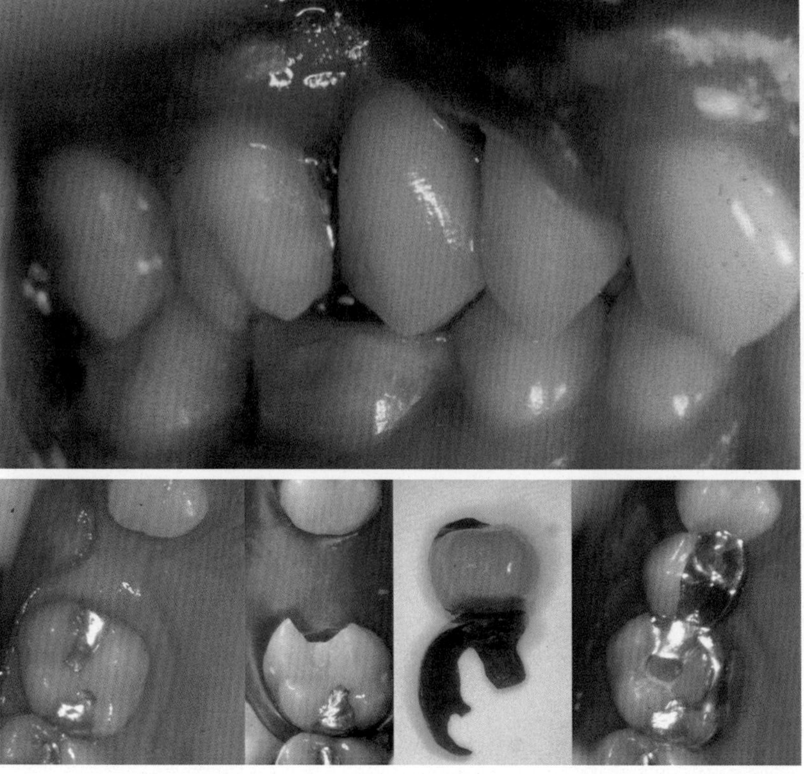

Figure 18.19 The mesio-occlusal restoration has been removed from the upper first molar tooth and the cavity has been incorporated into the resin retained bridge design giving superior retention.

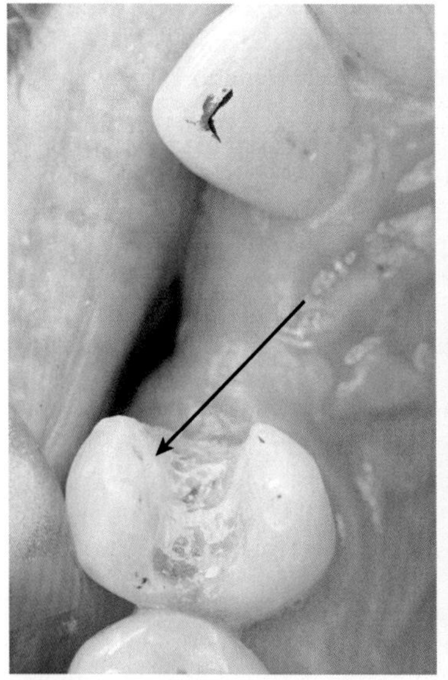

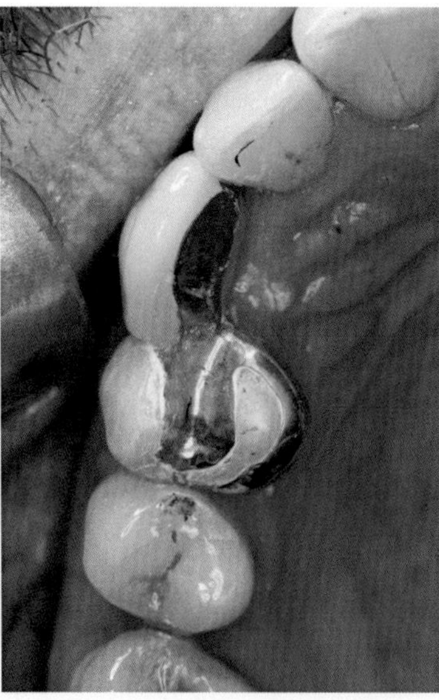

Figure 18.20 Undercut on the buccal aspect of the cavity has been blocked out with composite (arrowed), producing a divergent inlay preparation. Care has been taken in this situation to avoid occlusal contacts on the canine pontic in lateral excursion.

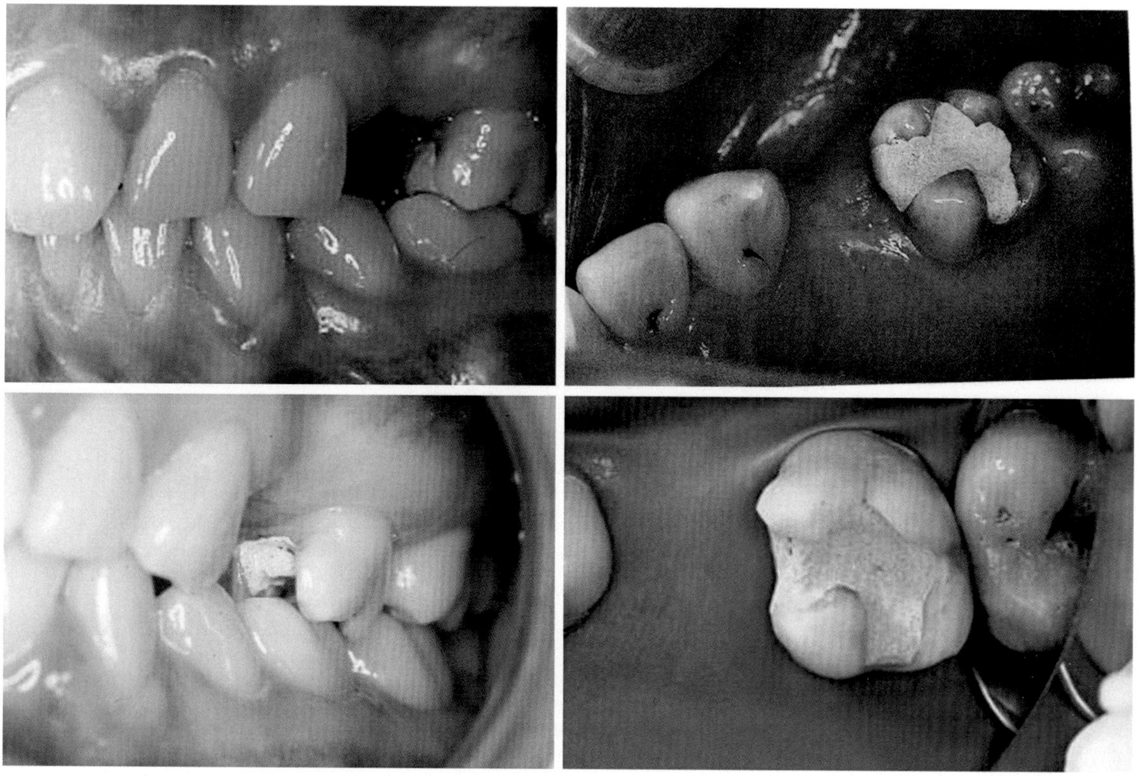

Figure 18.21A The first molar tooth has been restored with a silver re-enforced glass ionomer cement and a classic inlay preparation has been cut leaving the cement to block out the undercuts. The cement at the floor of the box still needs to be removed to finish all margins onto tooth tissue. (bottom left).

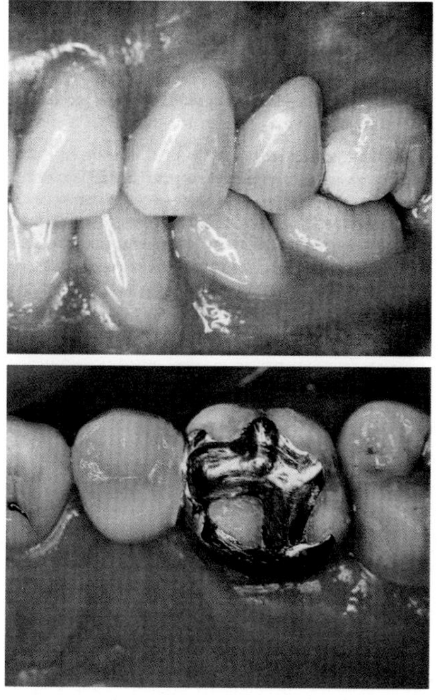

Figure 18.21B The minimal preparation (resin retained) bridge cemented.

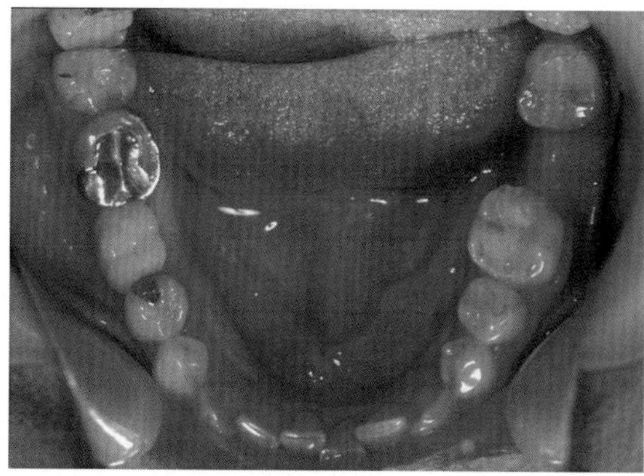

Figure 18.22 The resin retained bridge in the lower right quadrant has an inlay retainer on the second molar tooth and a rest seat has been cut in a disto-occlusal composite in the second premolar tooth to gain support at the mesial end of the pontic.

Such bridge designs are useful posteriorly where there is canine guidance in lateral excursion which results in posterior disclusion and a posterior protected occlusion (Figure 18.22).

It is important that rest seats are only used within restorations and not natural tooth tissue, as – unlike removable cobalt chromium prostheses – the restoration cannot be removed to clean beneath the rest and there is a risk that caries will occur beneath it. The rest seat is not cemented to the restoration, but sits passively on it. As there should be no obvious movement of the rest seat, wear of the restorative material should not be an issue.

SUMMARY

The introduction of adhesive resin luting cements has completely changed the way in which dentists manage the replacement of missing teeth in a dentition which is minimally restored. If care is taken in optimizing the retention of resin retained bridges through the principles outlined in this chapter and the use of a meticulous cementation technique, long-term success can be guaranteed.

FURTHER READING

Brosh, T., Pilo, R., Bichacho, N., Blutstein, R., 1997. Effect of combinations of surface treatments and bonding agents on the bond strength of repaired composites. Prosthet. Dent. 77, 122–126.

Cobourne, M.T., 2007. Familial human hypodontia – is it all in the genes? Br. Dent. J. 203, 203–208.

Ricketts, D.N., Smith, B.G., 1993a. Clinical techniques for producing and monitoring minor axial tooth movement. Eur. J. Prosthodont. Restor. Dent. 2, 5–9.

Ricketts, D.N., Smith, B.G., 1993b. Minor axial tooth movement in preparation for fixed prostheses. Eur. J. Prosthodont. Restor. Dent. 1, 145–149.

Thompson, V.P., Livaditis, G.J., 1982. Etched casting acid etch composite bonded posterior bridges. Pediatr. Dent. 4, 38–43.

van Dalen, A., Feilzer, A.J., Kleverlaan, C.J., 2004. A literature review of two-unit cantilevered FPDs. Int. J. Prosthodont. 17, 281–284.

Chapter | 19 |

Conventional bridges

David Bartlett, David Ricketts

CHAPTER CONTENTS

CONVENTIONAL BRIDGES OR IMPLANTS?

The advent of implant supported restorations has, to some extent, reduced the need for conventionally prepared bridges. However, the financial cost of implant retained restorations is higher than conventional bridges, due to the additional cost of the implant components. Others claim that there is little long-term difference due to the biological impact conventional bridge preparation has to abutment teeth and the potential need for further treatment. Despite the cost, implants require surgical procedures demanding sufficient quantity and quality of bone (see Chapter 17). These issues, together with the status of the remaining dentition, may influence the choice as to how to replace teeth and, as such, conventional bridges remain useful options in prosthodontics.

TERMINOLOGY

The terminology used for bridges or fixed partial prostheses/dentures includes the following (Figure 19.1):

- *Abutment*. The tooth or teeth that support the bridge.
- *Retainer*. The restoration that attaches the bridge to the abutment tooth or teeth.
- *Pontic*. The false tooth.
- *Connector*. The part of the bridge that connects the pontic to the retainer and is frequently overlooked.
- *Span*. The mesio-distal length of the edentulous space.

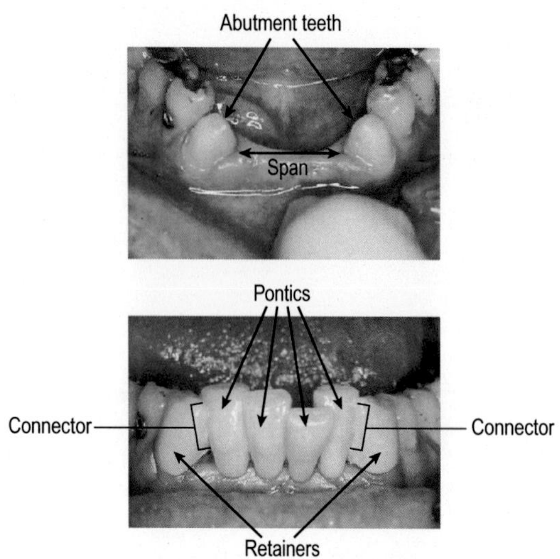

Figure 19.1 Terminology used in relation to bridges.

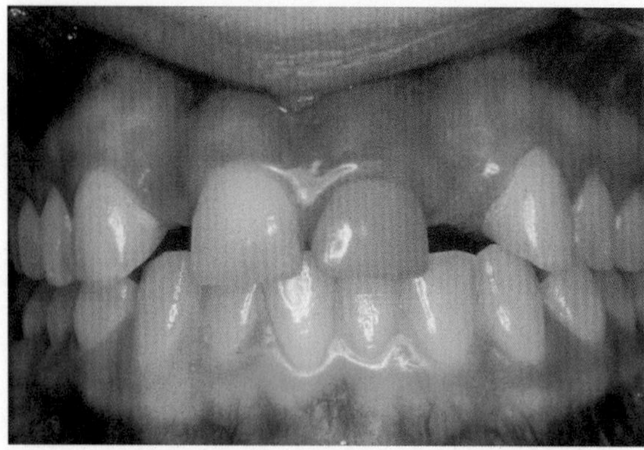

Figure 19.2 Patient with congenitally missing lateral incisor teeth and discoloured upper left central. Preparation of this tooth for a full coverage bridge retainer will also mask the discolouration.

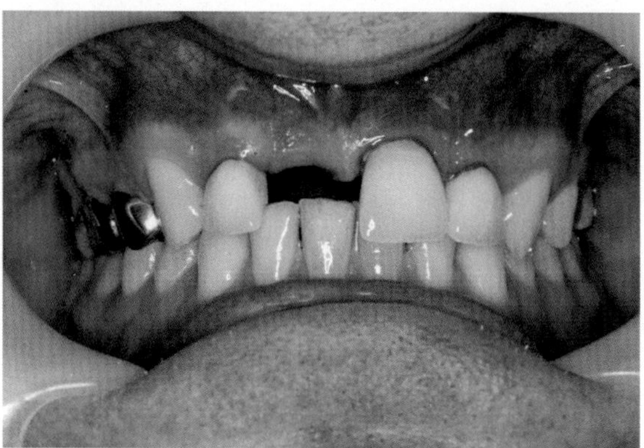

Figure 19.3 The upper right central incisor space is larger than the upper left central incisor crown. Removal of crowns on the adjacent teeth will allow construction of a fixed–fixed bridge distributing the tooth sizes evenly and proportionally.

CONVENTIONAL VERSUS RESIN RETAINED BRIDGES

Conventional bridges are indicated when the abutment teeth are extensively restored and preparation of the tooth for an indirect restoration (usually a full coverage retainer or crown) is justified. As with a full coverage crown, the retainer has the additional benefit of protecting the remaining tooth tissue and core. Extensively restored teeth are usually unsuitable for minimal preparation (resin retained) bridges because of the presence and extent of the material–tooth interfaces.

Occasionally the shape and/or appearance of the abutment teeth may require alteration and this can be incorporated into the bridge design. The patient seen in Figure 19.2 has congenitally missing upper lateral incisor teeth. The image shows that the left central incisor is discoloured and the composite veneer used to mask this has not been successful. Preparation of the central incisor for a metal–ceramic retainer on a cantilever designed bridge will improve the appearance of the tooth and provide support for the pontic.

Preparation of teeth for full coverage crowns also allows some control over distribution of space and size of teeth. For example, Figure 19.3 shows the upper right central incisor tooth is missing, but the span (mesio-distal space) is greater than the mesio-distal width of the contralateral incisor crown. Removal of the crowns on the adjacent teeth will allow the retainers to be made with a slightly larger mesio-distal width and hide the space and tooth size discrepancy. In a similar way, tilted or angled abutment teeth can be aligned to some degree to improve the appearance in the anterior region.

Bridges with more than one pontic require a fixed–fixed or fixed–movable design rather than a cantilever design. This allows support and retention to be gained from the abutment teeth either side of the pontic. When the abutment teeth are minimally restored, minimal preparation (resin retained) bridges can be considered, but longer span bridges demand greater retention from the abutment teeth and this can only be achieved from conventional preparations. The risk of decementation of minimally prepared (resin retained) bridges becomes too great once the span increases by more than one pontic. For example, the edentulous span for the elderly patient seen in Figure 19.1 is too long for a minimally prepared (resin retained) bridge and the abutment teeth have been prepared for metal–ceramic retainers to optimize retention. The age of the patient, the mild wear on the teeth and the exposed root surface will ensure sufficient secondary and tertiary dentine formation to reduce potential pulpal trauma during tooth preparation.

OPTIMIZING AESTHETICS

All bridges made in the smile line need to ensure an aesthetic symmetrical result. The space needed for the pontic has to mirror the ideal size of the tooth which it is to replace. The contralateral tooth should give a guide to the dimensions. If the space is too small, a number of solutions can be considered:

- The teeth either side can be increased in size by the addition of composites, veneers or crowns, depending on the restorative status of the teeth.
- The space can be closed orthodontically.
- The space can be increased orthodontically for the ideal sized tooth; however, there has to be a space for the adjacent tooth/teeth to be moved into and this often requires extraction of a tooth.
- Bridge designs showing some degree of tooth crowding can be used (Figures 19.1 and 19.4).

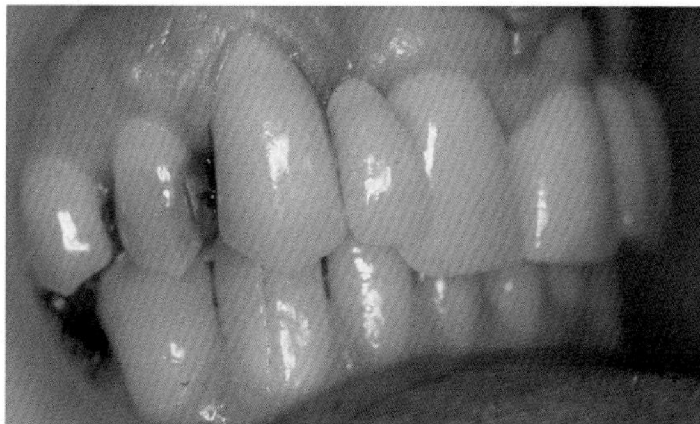

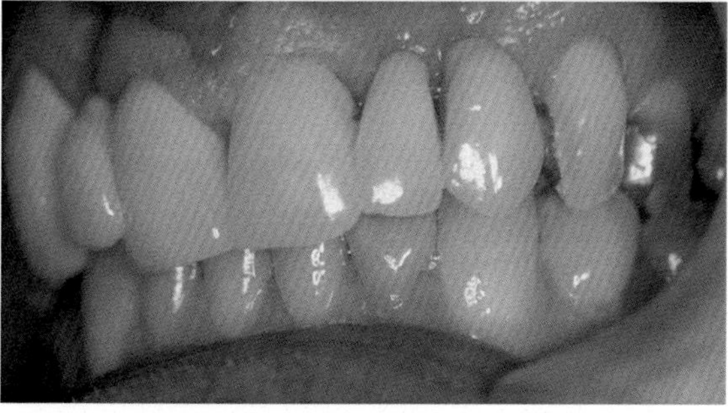

Figure 19.4 This patient has a crown on the upper right canine, and two separate cantilever conventional bridges with metal–ceramic retainers on the central incisors and lateral incisor pontics. There is a third minimum preparation (resin retained) cantilever bridge replacing the upper left canine using the first premolar tooth as an abutment.

When the space is too large compared to the contralateral tooth (Figure 19.3):

- The adjacent tooth/teeth can be crowned or recrowned to redistribute the size of the teeth and avoid any spacing or, if sound, composite can be added to the teeth.
- A cantilever bridge design can be considered, leaving residual spacing to one side of the pontic only.
- Orthodontic space closure to ideal size
- If the prosthetic tooth is to be placed in the centre of the space and residual spacing accepted, two options are available: a removable prosthesis or an implant.

BRIDGE DESIGN

The principles involved in the design of conventional and minimal preparation (resin retained) bridges are similar. The generic designs are cantilever, fixed–fixed and fixed–movable; the terminology is based on how the pontic is attached to the retainer(s).

Cantilever bridges

Cantilever bridges are designed so that the pontic is attached to a retainer on one side only, and are therefore usually more conservative of tooth tissue, especially if the other potential abutment tooth is minimally restored or sound. Retrievability is also easier if cantilever bridge designs are used. Consider the patient in Figure 19.4: three separate cantilever bridges have been placed instead of a fixed–fixed bridge design (see next section). Thus, if one abutment tooth fails due to secondary caries for example, only one tooth and bridge need replacing, so reducing the complexity of treatment and cost to the patient. Longer span bridges, particularly those where the pontic or retainers are involved in lateral guidance, increase the occlusal forces on the bridge and potentially reduce their survival. Historically, attempts were made to overcome this problem by using two abutment teeth. A typical example was a bridge to replace an upper canine; two premolar teeth were prepared for three-quarter crown retainers and linked to form a three unit cantilever bridge with a mesial pontic to replace the canine. This should be avoided as maintaining good oral hygiene beneath linked retainers is difficult, increasing the risk of caries and periodontal disease.

Occasionally cantilevered pontics can be used in conjunction with more extensive bridge designs. The patient seen in Figure 19.5 has a four unit fixed–fixed conventional bridge with the upper second premolar and second molar teeth used as abutments and the upper first premolar and molar teeth as pontics. The second premolar abutment has a pontic on either side and is referred to as a

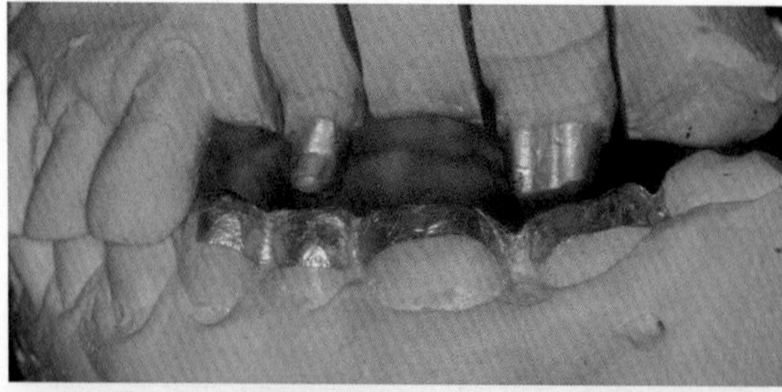

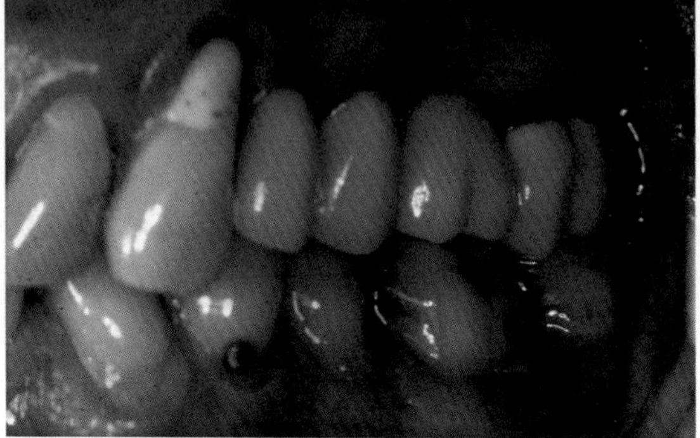

Figure 19.5 Patient with a four unit fixed–fixed bridge design with the upper second premolar tooth as pier abutment and the first premolar cantilevered pontic.

pier abutment, the first premolar pontic being cantilevered off the bridge.

Spring cantilever bridges

Spring cantilever bridges are mainly of historic interest and were used when an anterior tooth was missing and the adjacent teeth were unrestored or where there was anterior spacing. Usually, molar teeth, which were extensively restored, were crowned and used to support a long palatal connector for the pontic in the anterior region. The introduction of dental implants has made these bridge designs obsolete; on rare occasions, however, clinicians may still see these bridges in service.

Fixed–fixed bridges

A fixed–fixed bridge has a pontic rigidly connected to retainers on both sides and has one path of insertion. The vertical orientation of both abutment teeth needs to be reasonably well aligned and parallel to each other (Figures 19.1, 19.5 and 19.6) to avoid undercuts. Most fixed–fixed bridges have full coverage crown retainers: if one abutment tooth had a relatively small restoration and an inlay was use as a retainer, occlusal contact on the tooth would lead to shear stresses being generated in the cement lute, with eventual debonding and risk of secondary caries (Figure 19.7). In theory, the use of a movable joint within the inlay would allow independent micromovement of that abutment tooth in an axial direction in line with the moveable joint (Figure 19.8).

The most important principle in planning tooth preparations on abutment teeth is retention. Preparations

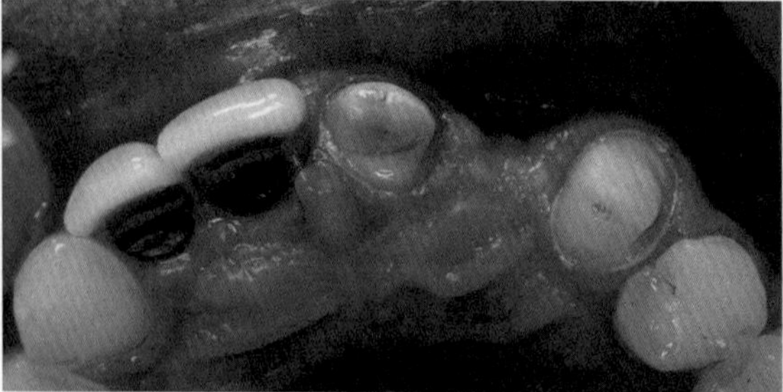

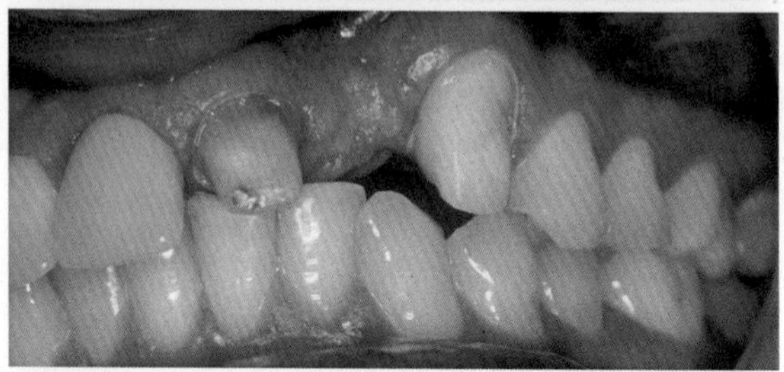

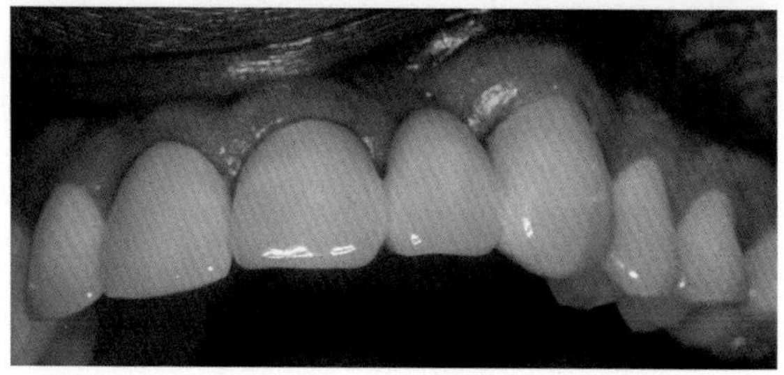

Figure 19.6 Fixed–fixed anterior bridge preparation and cemented bridge. Note the abutment teeth are well aligned.

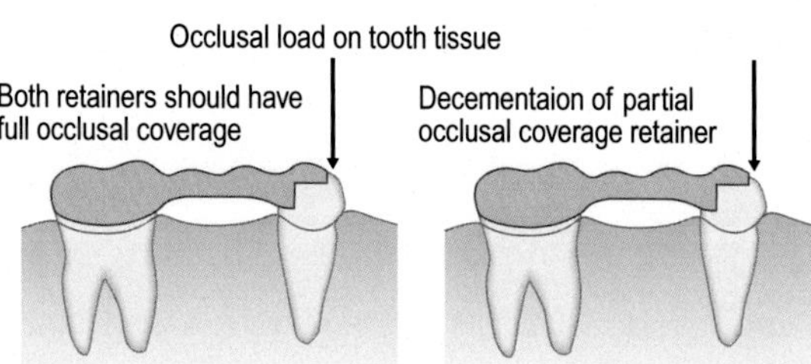

Figure 19.7 Diagram depicting an incorrect fixed–fixed bridge design linking a full occlusal coverage retainer on the molar tooth with a partial occlusal coverage retainer (inlay) on the premolar tooth. Occlusal loading on the premolar tooth generates shear stresses in the cement lute with eventual debonding of the inlay retainer. The retainers for fixed–fixed bridge designs should always have full occlusal coverage.

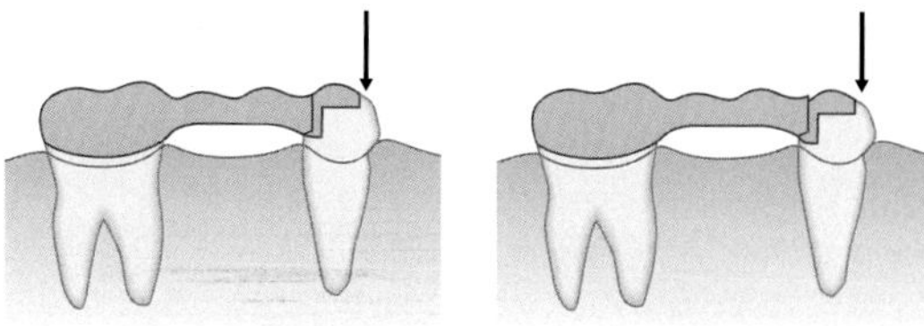

Figure 19.8 Incorporation of a moveable joint in the inlay retainer will allow some differential axial movement between the abutment teeth, providing the joint is in line with the long axis of the premolar tooth.

should follow the general principle of long and near parallel (at least 10–15° taper) sides. Fixed–fixed conventionally designed bridges present challenges to ensure that undercuts are not introduced between abutment teeth, and whilst anterior preparations are often easier because of direct vision, posterior ones are more challenging. Take the patient in Figure 19.9 for example: the first premolar tooth has been prepared with a labial shoulder and palatal chamfer to accept a full coverage metal–ceramic retainer. The first molar tooth is not in the smile line and a preparation for a full gold crown with a buccal and palatal chamfer finish to preserve as much of the tooth tissue as possible has been carried out. Note that no undercuts are evident between the two abutment preparations.

Fixed–movable bridges

A fixed–movable bridge has a pontic which is rigidly connected to a retainer at one end and to a moveable joint at the other. The retainer to which the pontic is rigidly attached is called the major retainer and the one that houses the movable joint is called the minor retainer (Figure 19.10). The size of the retainer has no bearing on

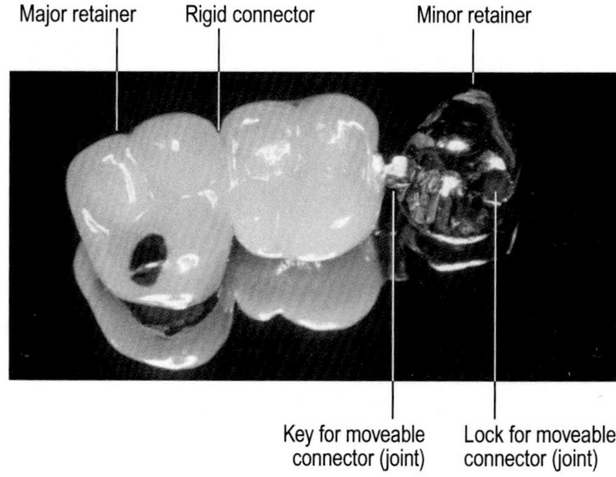

Figure 19.10 Components of a conventional fixed–movable designed bridge.

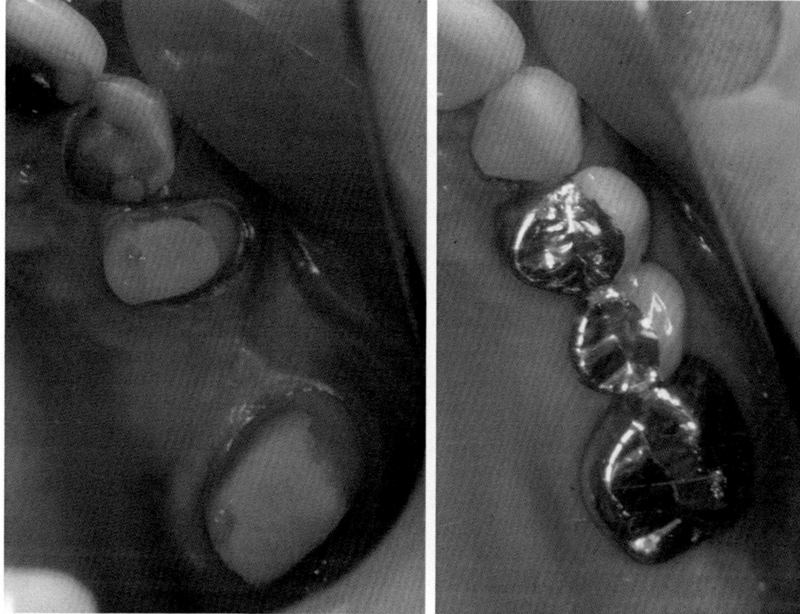

Figure 19.9 Fixed–fixed bridge with full coverage metal retainer on the upper left molar tooth and metal–ceramic retainer on the premolar tooth. Note metal occlusal coverage on both abutment teeth preserving the clinical crown height and improving retention.

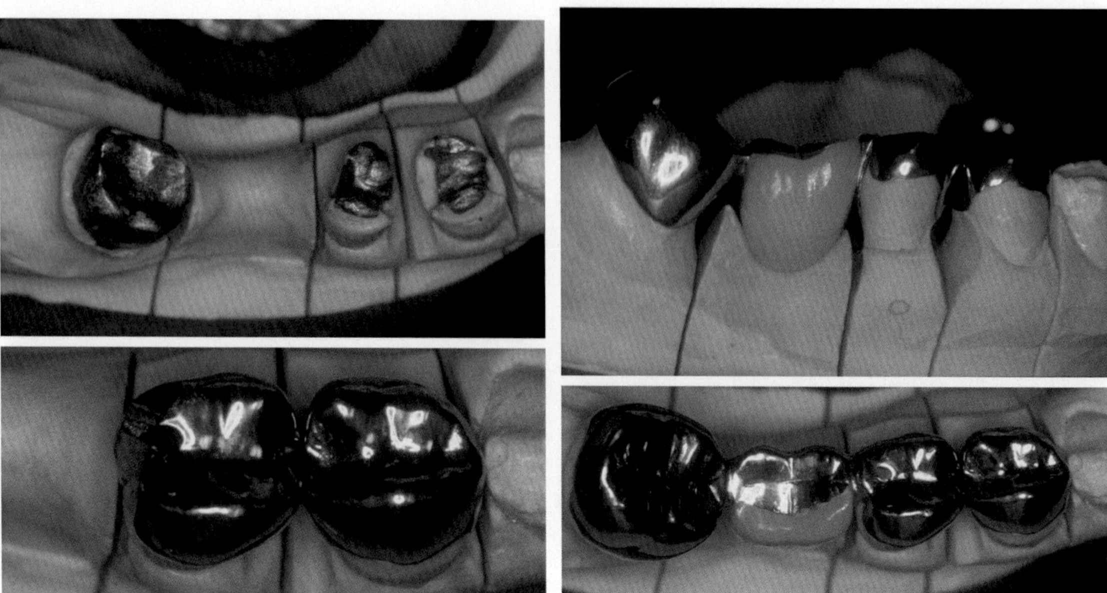

Figure 19.11 The lower right second premolar tooth has been prepared for a three-quarter gold minor retainer. The lock can be seen in the distal aspect of the minor retainer. The key on the mesial aspect of the pontic seats into the lock of the minor retainer. The base of the lock resists mesial tilting of the molar abutment which has a full metal coverage major retainer.

the terminology. Normally, the movable joint is attached to the mesial retainer and is the smaller abutment tooth (Figure 19.11). The joint is usually placed in the mesial retainer as teeth tend to drift and tilt in a mesial direction. The potential for this to occur in a distal abutment tooth is resisted by the key pressing against the base of the movable joint (Figure 19.11 bottom two images). If care is taken with the occlusion and there is good interdigitation of teeth, tooth movement is unlikely to occur and the movable joint could be placed in the distal (larger) retainer.

The movable joint must have a base to achieve support for the pontic and must be within the retainer. Consider the bridge design for the patient in Figure 19.12. This design is wrong as the key is cantilevered off the retainer and whilst it sits in the lock in the mesial of the pontic, no support is given to the pontic. As a result, the molar pontic is essentially cantilevered off the distal abutment tooth and mesial tilt of this tooth has occurred with the key emerging from the lock.

Generally, fixed–movable bridges are indicated for posterior bridges where the space needed for the movable joint can be incorporated into the retainer without interfering with the appearance of the bridge. The major advantage of the fixed–movable bridge design is that the movable joint can overcome differences in angulation of abutment teeth; retainers on each abutment tooth can have optimum retention and path of insertion irrespective of the alignment of the abutment teeth (Figures 19.13 and 19.14).

The movable joint of a fixed–movable bridge is usually achieved by using factory-made plastic precision fitting components (Figure 19.15) which are incorporated into the laboratory wax-up of the bridge. Figure 19.16 shows the laboratory construction of a hybrid fixed–movable bridge. The minor retainer is a conventional full coverage metal–ceramic retainer, whilst the major retainer is a

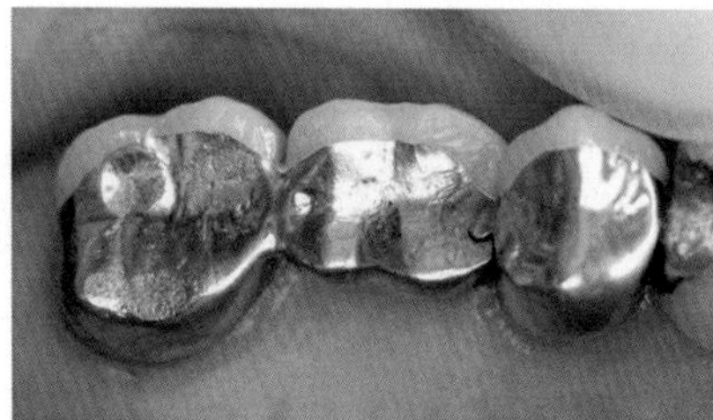

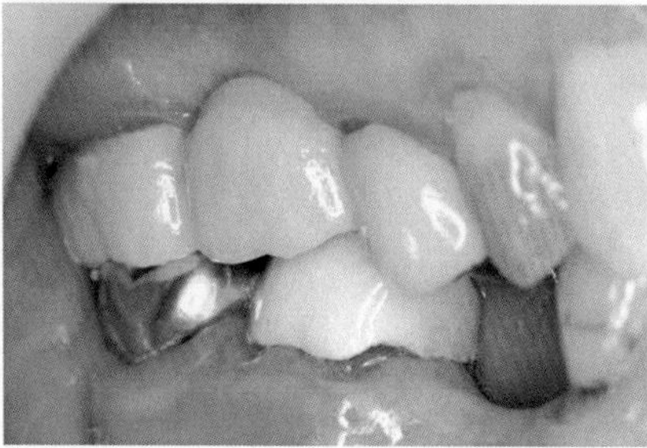

Figure 19.12 Incorrect fixed–movable bridge design. The lock is incorrectly placed in the pontic and even if it has a base to it, it has not resisted mesial tilting of the major retainer and the key appears to be coming out of the lock.

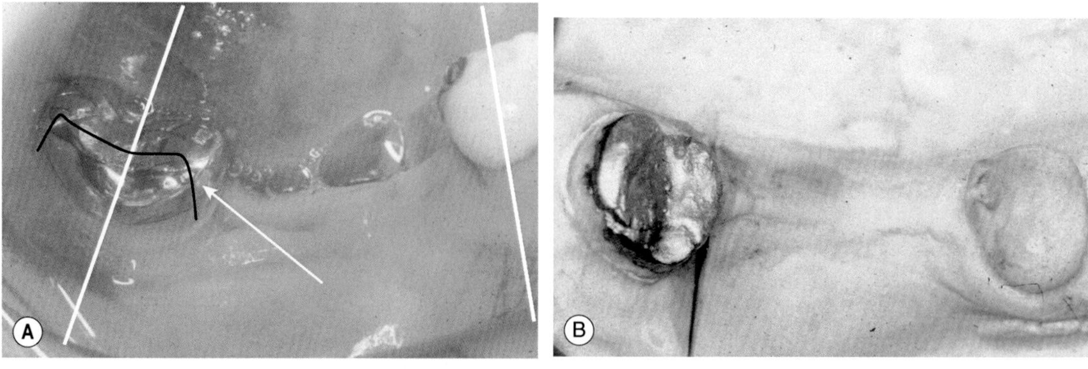

Figure 19.13 **A** Two potential abutment teeth which are poorly aligned. Any attempt at preparing the distal abutment tooth in alignment with the long axis of the mesial tooth for a fixed–fixed bridge design will lead to overpreparation of the mesial aspect of the tooth (arrowed). This may cause greater pulpal damage and an overtapered preparation, and hence poorer retention. **B** The working model of the patient seen in **A**. Note that the minor retainer has already been cemented and the lock is angled in line with the long axis of the distal abutment. The preparation on this tooth can therefore have the optimum taper and a different path of insertion to the minor retainer. Usually the entire bridge is made and cemented in the same appointment, obviously seating the minor retainer first and then the major retainer and pontic.

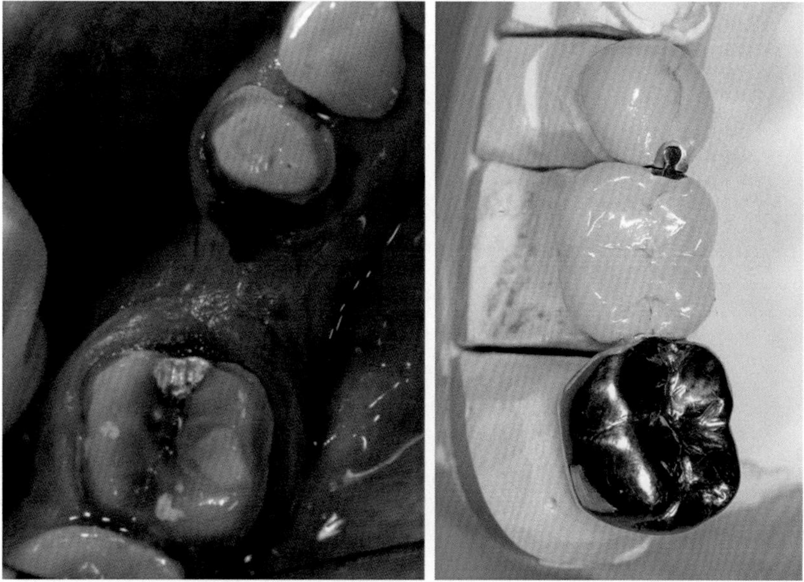

Figure 19.14 Another example of a fixed–movable bridge design allowing both abutment teeth to have optimal retention without the need for ensuring that they are parallel.

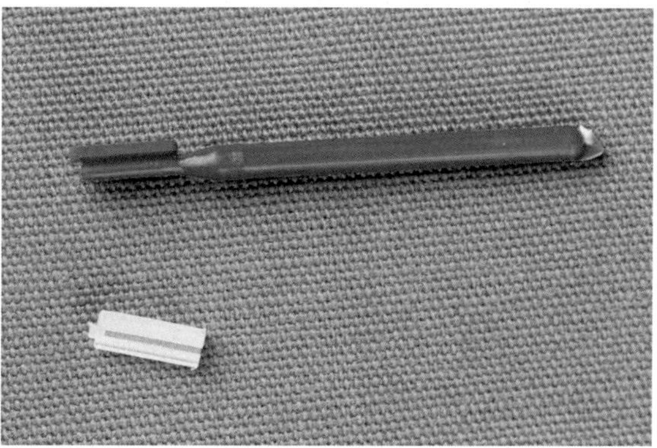

Figure 19.15 Factory-made Tube Lock joint (Sterngold Attachments, MA, USA).

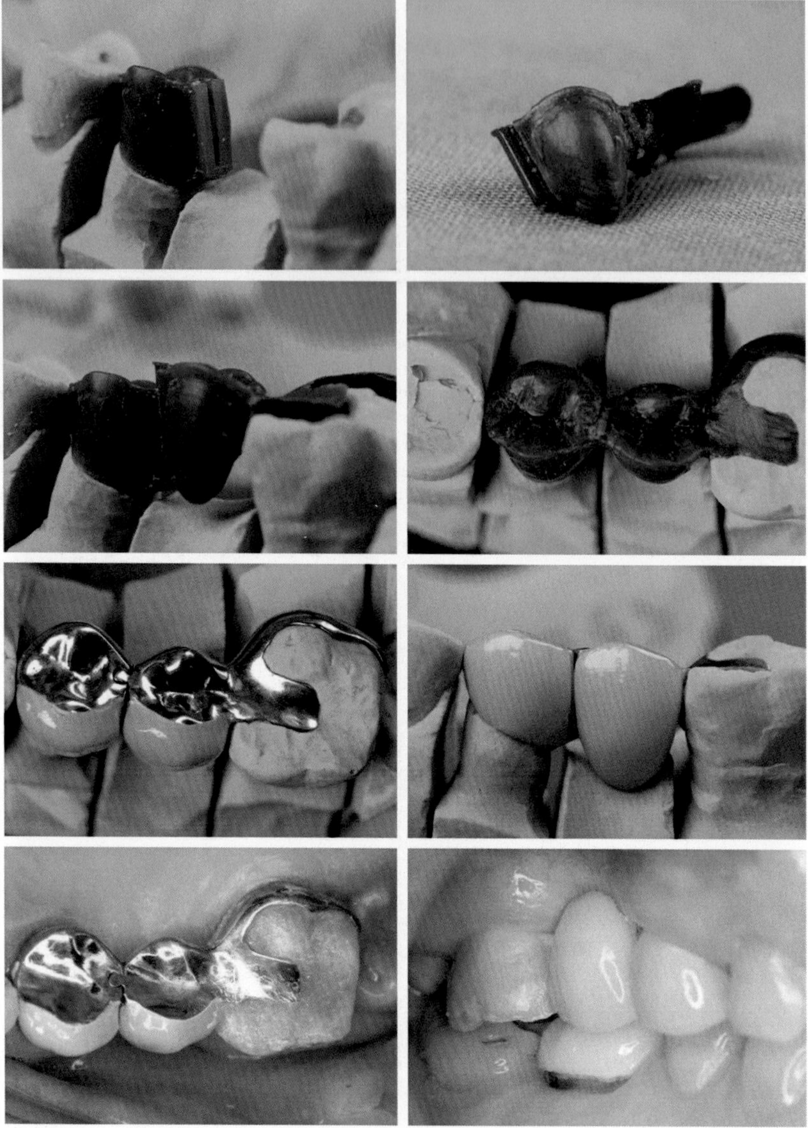

Figure 19.16 Laboratory stages of making a fixed–movable hybrid bridge incorporating the Tube Lock joint (top six images) and when cemented intraorally.

minimal preparation (resin retained) inlay and wing (see Chapter 18).

There is a theoretical advantage that the presence of a movable joint between the retainers may allow some movement (called stress breaking) and reduce the effect of lateral forces applied to the abutments. However, since most joints are precision made (Figure 19.15), any movement between the major and minor connectors is unlikely to have any significant clinical effect and can only take place along the long axis of the joint.

PREPARATION FOR CONVENTIONAL BRIDGES

Most preparations for conventional bridges will involve full coverage retainers. When preparing teeth for fixed–fixed bridge designs, it is often better to prepare the teeth together to avoid introducing undercuts between abutments. For example, when preparing the axial walls it is advisable to visualize the long axis of each abutment tooth and check that the preparations are aligned without overpreparing either tooth. Preparing corresponding surfaces a little at a time and frequently moving from one preparation to another without altering the angle of the tapered bur ensures that the preparations are better aligned with no undercuts; the longer the span, the greater the difficulty in keeping preparations aligned. It is equally important not to alter the angle of the dental mirror when moving it to visualize one preparation and then another.

PONTIC DESIGN

The design concepts for pontics are the same for minimum preparation (resin retained) bridges and conventional bridges and should always be prescribed to the technician. The different pontic designs are:

- Wash through or sanitary (Figure 19.17)
- Saddle (Figure 19.17)
- Dome (Figure 19.17)
- Ridge lap (Figure 19.17)
- Modified ridge lap (Figure 19.17)
- Ovate.

When a bridge is removed, the underlying edentulous ridge often appears red and inflamed, and this has been attributed to poor oral hygiene and the presence of a bacterial biofilm in contact with the surface of the alveolar ridge. When bridge hygiene is poor the inflamed tissue can often become hyperplastic in nature (Figures 19.18 and 19.19). The regular use of super floss beneath the pontic is necessary and should remove the plaque, preventing this from occurring. Some argue that the ridge appears red because it has become less keratinized as the tissue is protected from the frictional contacts made during mastication. In most situations it would be preferable to use a more cleansable pontic design.

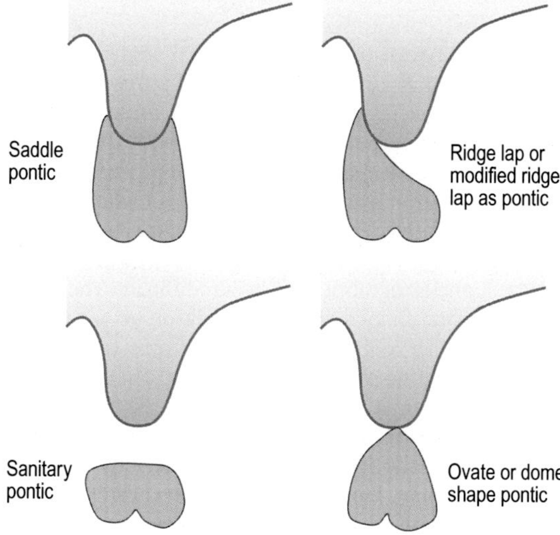

Figure 19.17 Diagrammatic representation of a section through pontics of different designs and their relationship to the edentulous ridge.

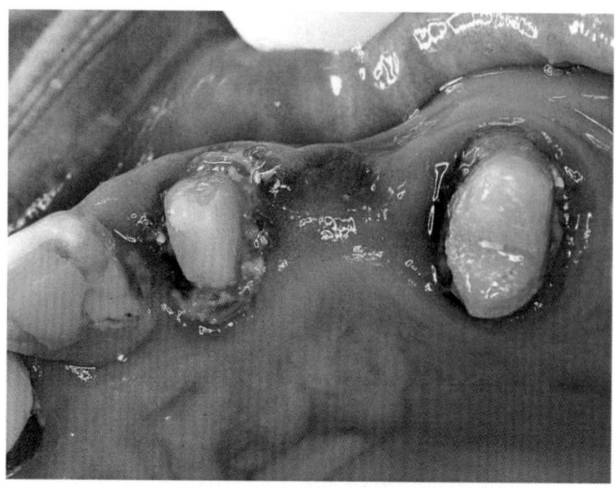

Figure 19.18 This patient's bridge has decemented. Oral hygiene is poor generally, but where the pontic sat the tissues are inflamed and becoming hyperplastic.

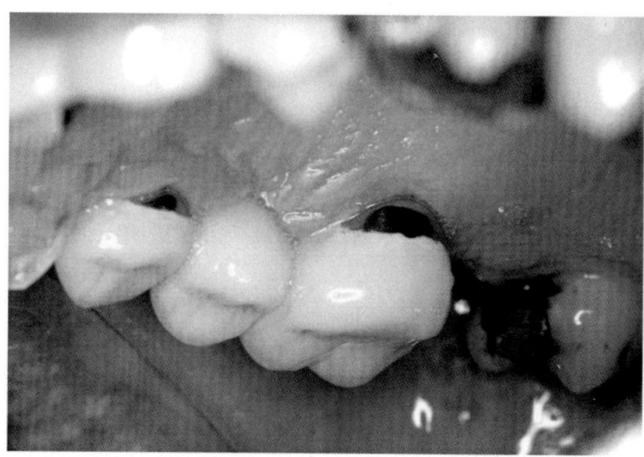

Figure 19.19 A saddle pontic in situ. Super flossing beneath this pontic has been difficult and the gingival tissues are inflamed and swollen.

The wash through or sanitary pontic (Figure 19.20) is only appropriate to replace posterior teeth which are not seen in the smile line. This historical bridge design ensures that there is no contact beneath the pontic and the edentulous ridge, and that there is sufficient space beneath the pontic not to trap food, which is easily 'washed away'. Whilst not often used, this design is useful when needed to provide a functional and stable occlusion and where oral hygiene procedures need to be kept simple. Adequate oral hygiene can be achieved with the use of an interdental bottle brush, such as a TePe brush.

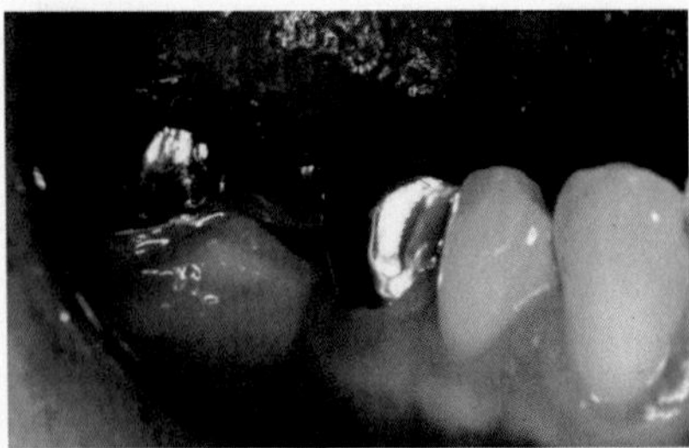

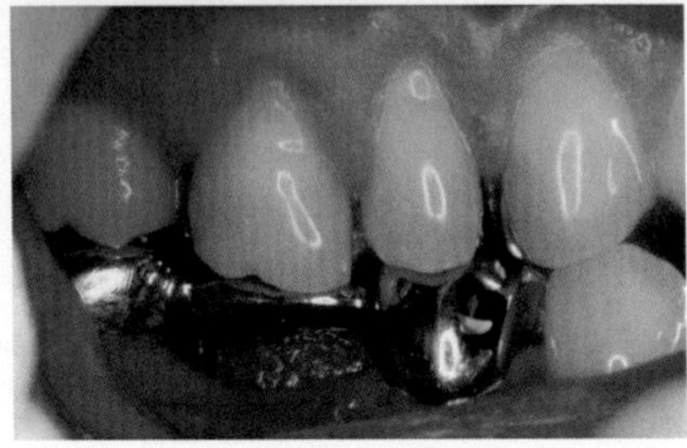

Figure 19.20 Wash through or sanitary pontic used to achieve a stable occlusion and improve function.

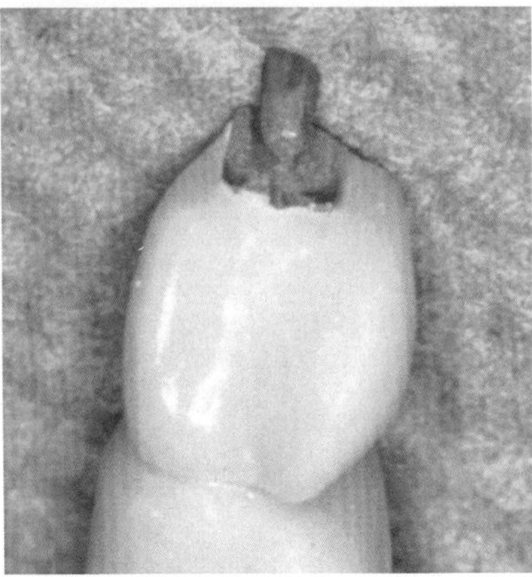

Figure 19.21 Saddle pontic.

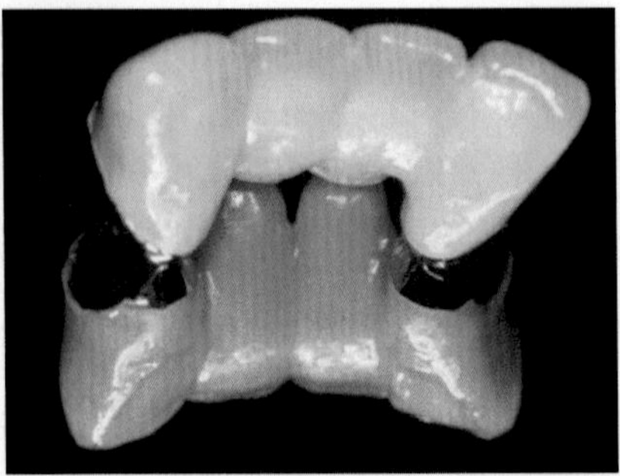

Figure 19.22 Ridge lap pontic on a conventional fixed–fixed designed bridge.

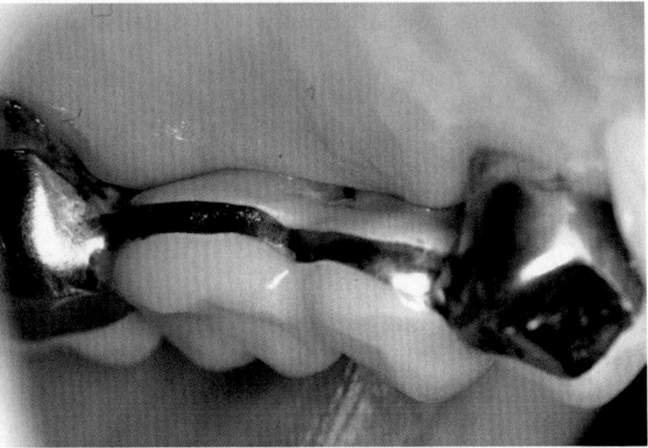

Figure 19.23 Palatal view of a modified ridge lap pontic having minimal contact with the edentulous ridge buccally.

The most popular choice from a patient's perspective is the saddle pontic which has a similar profile to natural teeth (Figure 19.21). The inevitable scalloped shape of the surface along the edentulous ridge buccally and lingually provides a more realistic 'feel' to the bridge but its concaved ridge surface makes it more difficult to clean than the ridge lap designs.

The ridge lap and modified ridge lap designs, like the saddle-shaped pontic, provide a conventional buccal contour to create a tooth pontic that has a realistic appearance visible on the buccal surface but is cut back on the palatal or lingual surface to allow better access for cleaning (Figures 19.22 and 19.23). The modified ridge lap has an even more extensive removal of the palatal surface to allow greater access for cleaning with super floss and other oral hygiene products.

The dome-shaped pontic is used when aesthetics at the gingival margin is not important. It has a convex ridge surface which makes point contact with the crest of the edentulous ridge, again keeping contact with the ridge to a minimum and facilitating oral hygiene procedures.

The ovate pontic is an uncommon design which is used in implant restored dentitions where extensive edentulous ridges make the creation of an interdental papilla between adjacent pontics or abutment teeth difficult. The ovate pontic is tooth shaped with the addition of a bulbous end, shaped like a short root, which forms by pressure an indentation into the edentulous ridge. The shaping of the ridge is normally produced during the provisional bridge construction and when the definitive bridge has been produced the indentation gives the illusion of an interdental papilla. Electrosurgery has also been suggested to remove soft tissue from the edentulous ridge, recontouring it to receive an ovate pontic. This gives an emergence profile to the pontic comparable to that of a natural tooth (Elder & Djemal, 2008).

THE CONNECTOR

Little attention is often paid to the connector between the pontic and the retainer but this is an important aspect to the bridge. The connector has to be of an adequate dimension for strength and rigidity, but it is important that it is not too large so as to encroach upon the gingival margin of the abutment tooth. This can be a common mistake because the laboratory technician sections the model to remove the individual dies. In order to contour the cervical aspect of the retainer correctly and to produce an acceptable emergence profile without ledges, the technician trims away the gingival area from the die (see Figure 19.5). Reference to the gingival area is therefore lost and the connector can become too large (Figure 19.24). At try-in it is important to check this aspect of the bridge and ensure that oral hygiene procedures are possible.

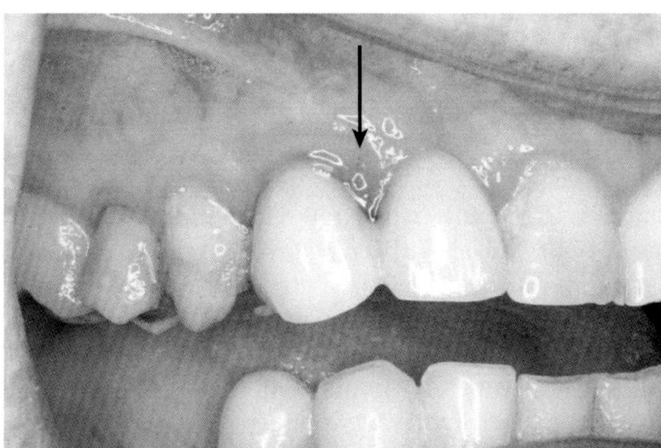

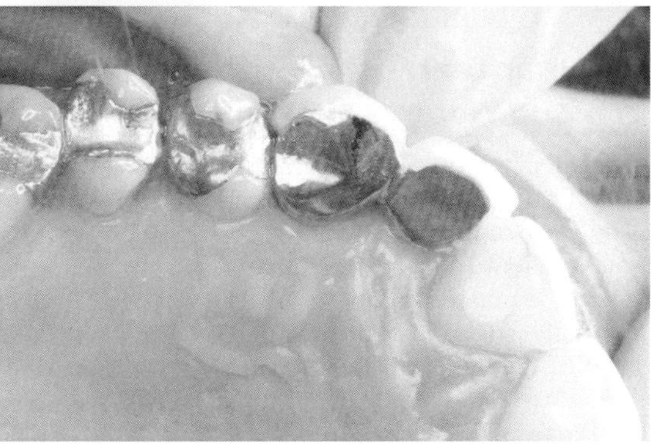

Figure 19.24 The connector between the pontic and retainer for the cantilever bridge on the upper right canine is too large, making oral hygiene difficult and resulting in periodontal problems (arrowed).

THE OCCLUSION

The aim of a bridge is to replace teeth and provide function. However, loading abutment teeth with pontics will increase the forces transmitted to the periodontium. Therefore, occlusal contacts on bridges need to be carefully controlled. The abutment teeth and pontics should have contacts in the intercuspal position but excursive contacts should only be directed onto the abutment teeth when necessary. If guidance is also established on the pontics, damaging lateral forces may occur, especially with cantilever bridge designs, increasing the risk of failure.

In a Class I incisor relationship canine guidance causes posterior disclusion. This immediate disclusion of the posterior teeth simplifies the construction of posterior bridges as it removes any need to ensure that the palatal cusps on the upper teeth and the buccal cusps on the lower teeth meet during lateral excursions. The immediate disclusion of the teeth in canine guidance in a Class I incisor relationship means that the cusps can be made to their optimum height. During group function the need to have multiple tooth contacts during lateral excursion complicates the construction of the occlusal shape of bridges and increases the load transferred to the abutment teeth.

How many teeth can we replace with a bridge?

This is a frequently asked question and historically dentists referred to 'Ante's Law' (1926) which states that 'the total periodontal membrane area of the abutment teeth must equal or exceed that of the teeth to be replaced' (Lulic et al., 2007). This law gives an oversimplified guide to the clinician; however, it is based on engineering and not biological principles and is far too dogmatic. Teeth differ in root length, coronal size and restorative status, and occlusal forces differ between individuals and occlusal schemes. All of these factors have a potential impact on the number of teeth that can be replaced and should be taken into consideration when planning a bridge. By virtue of periodontal mechanoreceptors, proprioceptors and pain receptors, patients are able to adapt to changes in the occlusal load placed on abutment teeth, and in certain circumstances more extensive bridges can be made, providing care is taken with the occlusion (Figure 19.25).

LONGEVITY OF CONVENTIONAL BRIDGES

The data to support the lifespan of conventional bridges are not extensive but suggest that the survival is longer than minimal preparation (resin retained) bridges.

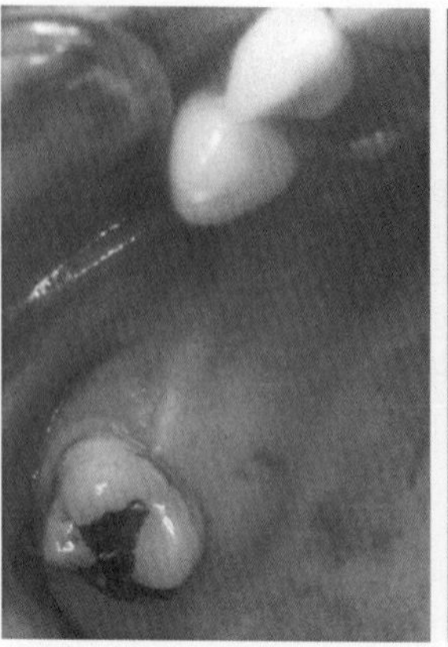
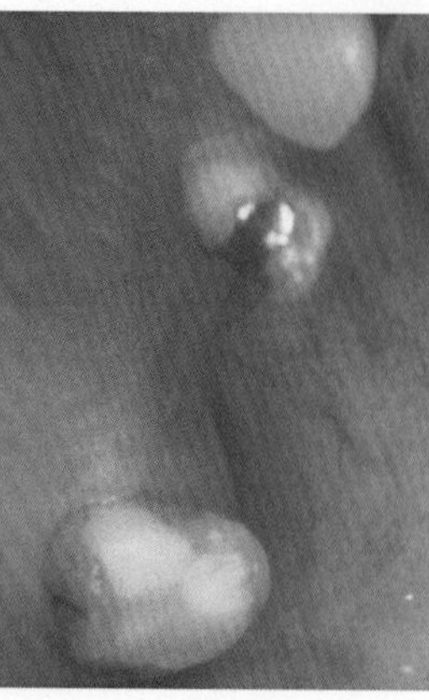

Figure 19.25 Longer edentulous spans where good periodontal bone support means that more extensive bridges could be considered, taking care with the occlusion.

A number of systematic reviews indicate that the long-term expectation of conventional fixed–fixed bridges is over 10 years and at around 15 years the increase in annual failure rate suggests that they become less viable (Pjetursson et al., 2004). These figures compare well with current data for implant supported restorations. The data from these studies also suggest that bridges fail within two main categories: decementation in the early stages and later mechanical failure of the retainer or pontic. Failure due to caries or periodontal disease is less common. The other major finding from systematic reviews is that fixed–fixed designs have a better prognosis than cantilevers. Fixed–movable designs are not as commonly used outside the UK as other forms and so comparison is not possible. For comparison, the longevity of minimal preparation (resin retained) bridges is around 5–7 years.

EXAMPLES OF BRIDGE DESIGN AND REPLACING TEETH

Canines

The most challenging tooth to replace in the arch is the canine, particularly in the maxilla when the palatal surface is involved with lateral guidance. The adjacent teeth are normally the lateral incisor and the first premolar, neither of which is particularly large for retention of a bridge (Figure 19.26). In these situations alternative restorative options such as an implant or more extensive bridgework may need to be considered. The possibility of using double abutments (two or more retainers positioned on the same side as the edentulous space) for a cantilever design bridge has already been addressed and should be avoided wherever possible. Generally, double-abuting teeth increase the risk of failure as a pivot is established between the pontic and the closest retainer. Potential differential movement of the retainers on the abutment teeth creates the possibility of movement at the distal margin and theoretically increases the risk of partial decementation and consequently caries.

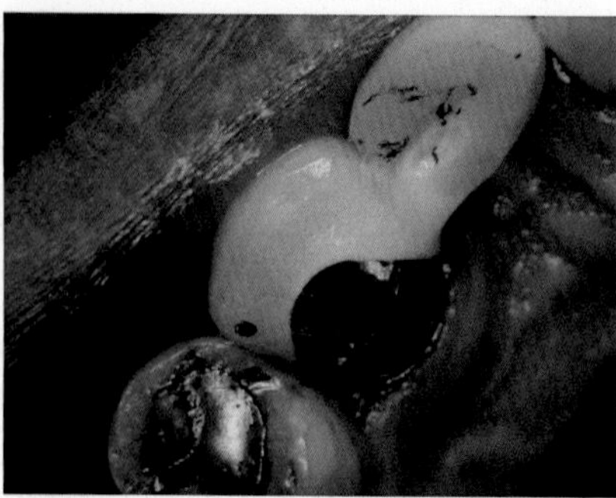

Figure 19.26 The canine pontic is cantilevered off the premolar tooth. The occlusion is being checked in lateral excursion to ensure the guidance is not on the canine pontic.

The other major consideration is the occlusion, particularly if the canine guides the mandible in lateral excursion. If the palatal surface of an upper canine pontic guides the mandible in lateral excursion, the stress placed upon either one (cantilever design) or two abutment (fixed-fixed or fixed-movable designs) teeth may exceed their retentive capacity. Even if small degrees of movement occur on the retainers, the risk of partial decementation and caries developing or complete decementation of the bridge increases. Generally, when planning bridges to replace canine teeth which have been involved in guidance, consideration should be given to changing the guidance to group function. This protects the retainers and the bridge but increases the complexity of the bridge, particularly when fitting the bridge in the mouth. Often adjustment of the opposing canine is necessary in order to produce an upper canine of adequate aesthetic length.

Premolar teeth, the shortened dental arch and removable prostheses

Distal cantilever designed bridges are normally considered to be a risk due to adverse occlusal forces and are consequently not commonly used. The one situation where a distal cantilever design is useful is when the opposing dentition is restored with a removable prosthesis. This is particularly relevant to the mandible when there is a shortened clinical arch. Research has shown that using bilateral free-end partial dentures to replace all the molar teeth is often unsuccessful. Provided at least one premolar tooth is present bilaterally, together with the canines and incisors, there is little functional benefit from replacing the molar teeth. Using the first premolars to support a distal cantilever designed conventional or resin retained

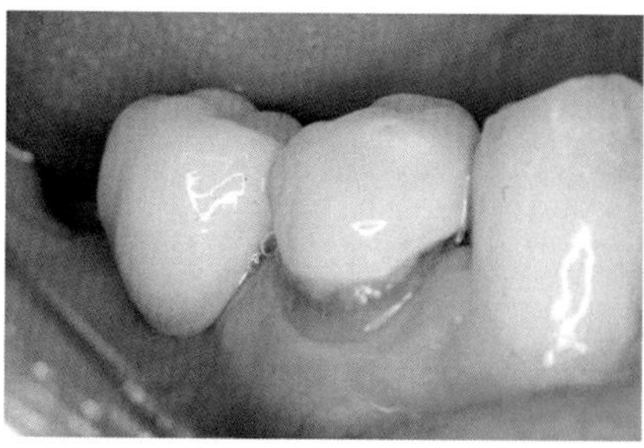

Figure 19.27 Distal cantilever bridge design. In the opposing arch is a complete removable prosthesis. The bridge design provides the patient with a shortened dental arch without the need for a lower removable prosthesis.

bridge will improve the function of the dentition without necessarily increasing risk of failure (Figure 19.27).

LABORATORY CONSTRUCTION OF BRIDGES

Most bridges are made from metal and ceramic. The metal provides the substructure and strength whilst the ceramic gives the shape and colour of the bridge. The metal needs to be of sufficient thickness to provide support and strength to the bridge; if it is too flexible the ceramic will undergo tension and crack. Therefore, a balance is needed between the thickness of the metal and sufficient space needed for the ceramic to hide the appearance of the metal. The ceramic is built up in a layering technique with opaque ceramic added first and then increasingly more translucent shades are added to provide the final appearance of the restoration (see Chapter 10 on metal–ceramic crowns).

With the advent of computer-aided design and computer-aided manufacture (CAD-CAM) technology and improvements in ceramics such as zirconia, all-ceramic bridges are now possible. The increased strength of the zirconia coping enables it to be used in bridge construction where the aesthetic demands are high and lifelike translucent restorations are required (Figure 19.28). To

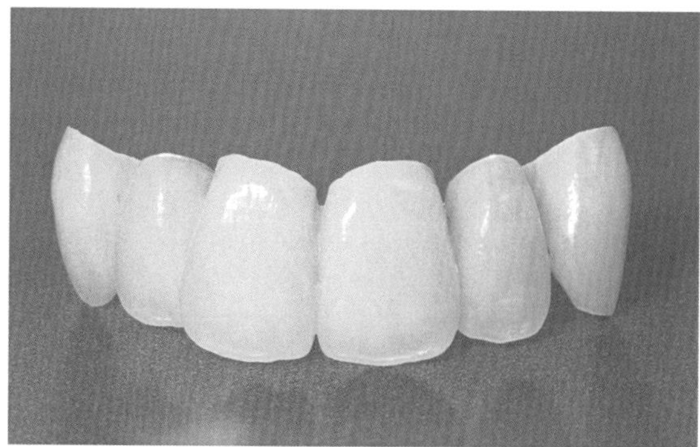

Figure 19.28 All-ceramic six unit fixed–fixed Lava bridge. *(Courtesy of 3M ESPE)*

achieve an adequate strength between the pontic and the retainer, the connector for all ceramic bridges must be of sufficient size; as such, care needs to be taken to ensure adequate oral hygiene procedures. There is growing evidence that posterior all-ceramic bridges are more liable to mechanical failure whereas anterior bridges have a better prognosis.

SUMMARY

Conventional bridges still remain an important part of the dentist's armamentarium for replacing missing teeth. Their use is mainly confined to situations where the abutment teeth are heavily restored. Preparation of teeth for full coverage retainers gives greater control over aesthetics in the anterior region and greater retention generally compared to resin retained bridges. Careful selection of bridge design is important and consideration needs to be given to the retainer, pontic and connector in addition to aspects of appearance (see Chapter 15). Tooth preparation (especially for fixed–fixed bridge designs) is demanding, not only from a mechanistic point of view but also from a biological and preservation of healthy tissues perspective.

FURTHER READING

Elder, A.R., Djemal, S., 2008. Electrosurgery: a technique for achieving aesthetic and retentive resin-bonded bridges. Dent. Update 35, 371–374, 376.

Lulic, M., Bragger, U., Lang, N.P., Zwahlen, M., Salvi, G.E., 2007. Ante's (1926) law revisited: a systematic review on survival rates and complications of fixed dental prostheses (FDPs) on severely reduced periodontal tissue support. Clin. Oral Implants Res. 18 (Suppl. 3), 63–72.

Pjetursson, B.E., Tan, K., Lang, N.P., Bragger, U., Egger, M., Zwahlen, M., 2004. A systematic review of the survival and complication rates of fixed partial dentures (FPDs) after an observation period of at least 5 years. Clin. Oral Implants Res. 15, 625–642.

Index

Note: Page numbers followed *f* indicate figures and *t* indicate tables.

ADVANCED OPERATIVE DENTISTRY: RICKETTS AND BARTLETT

A

B

C

E

F

G

L

M

N

O

P

Q

R

S

T

Printed in the United States
By Bookmasters